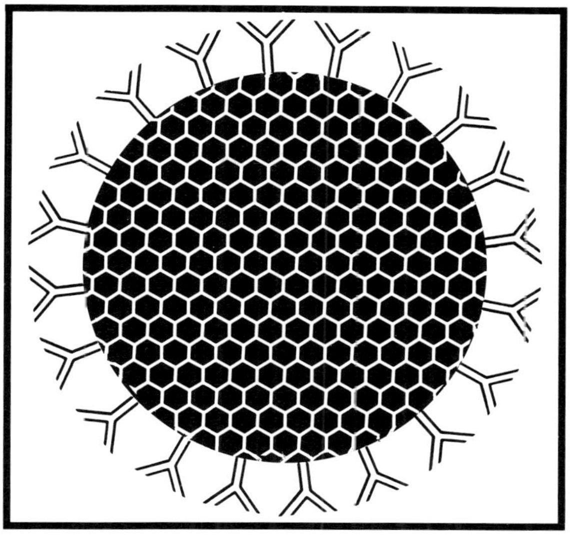

Otolaryngic Allergy and Immunology

Helen F. Krause, M.D., F.A.C.S.

Clinical Assistant Professor
Department of Otorhinolaryngology
University of Pittsburgh School of Medicine
Private Practice
Pittsburgh, Pennsylvania

1989
W.B. SAUNDERS COMPANY
Harcourt Brace Jovanovich, Inc.
Philadelphia • London • Toronto • Montreal • Sydney • Tokyo

W. B. SAUNDERS COMPANY
Harcourt Brace Jovanovich, Inc.

The Curtis Center
Independence Square West
Philadelphia, PA 19106

Library of Congress Cataloging-in-Publication Data

Otolaryngic allergy and immunology/[edited by] Helen F. Krause.
p. cm.

1. Otolaryngology—Immunological aspects. 2. Allergy.
I. Krause, Helen F. [DNLM: 1. Immunologic Diseases.
2. Otorhinolaryngologic Diseases—immunology.
WV 100 0864]

RF46.5.085 1989 616.97—dc19

ISBN 0–7216–2867–2

DNLM/DLC 88–39227

Editor: W. B. Saunders Staff
Designer: Dorothy Chattin
Production Manager: Carolyn Naylor
Manuscript Editor: RoseMarie Klimowicz
Illustration Coordinator: Walt Verbitski
Indexer: Diana Fitt
Cover Designer: Michelle Malony

Otolaryngic Allergy and Immunology ISBN 0–7216–2867–2

Last digit is the print number: 9 8 7 6 5 4 3 2 1

CONTRIBUTORS

JOHN H. BOYLES, JR., M.D.
Clinical Instructor, University of Cincinnati; Assistant Clinical Professor, Wright State University; Active Staff, Kettering Medical Center, Miami Valley Hospital, Children's Medical Center, Cincinnati, Ohio
Introduction to Food Allergy: History and Characteristics
Introduction to Chemical-Environmental Allergy
Therapy of Chemical and Environmental Factors in Allergic Disease

JOAN E. CUNNICK, PH.D.
Research Associate, University of Pittsburgh School of Medicine, Pittsburgh, Pennsylvania
Stress and the Immune System

JOSEPH P. KEENAN, M.D., F.A.C.S.
Assistant Clinical Professor of Surgery, Division of Otorhinolaryngology, University of Connecticut Health Center, Farmington; Staff, Noble Hospital, Westfield, Massachusetts
Office Evaluation of the Allergic Patient
General Management of the Allergic Patient
Management of Problems and Immunotherapy Failures
Therapy of Chemical and Environmental Factors in Allergic Disease

HUESTON C. KING, M.D., F.A.C.S., F.A.C.A.
Clinical Associate Professor, Department of Otolaryngology, University of Texas, Southwestern Medical School, Dallas; Active Staff, Venice Hospital, Venice, Florida
Inhalant Allergy
Stinging Insect Allergy
Antigen Selection for Testing and Therapy
Stinging Insect Therapy
Antigen Selection for Food Allergy Testing
In Vitro Evaluation of Food Allergy: Current Status

WILLIAM P. KING, M.D.
Clinical Assistant Professor, Department of Otorhinolaryngology and Communicative Sciences, Baylor College of Medicine, Houston; Chief of Otolaryngology Department, Spohn Hospital; Staff Member, Alice Physicians and Surgeons Hospital, Memorial Medical Center, Southside Community Hospital, Driscoll Foundation Children's Hospital, Humana Hospital, Corpus Christi, Texas
Skin Endpoint Titration and the Modified RAST: Current Status
Diagnostic Provocation Testing and Neutralization Therapy for Food Allergy
Diagnostic and Therapeutic Techniques for Chemical-Environmental Allergy and Hypersensitivity

HELEN F. KRAUSE, M.D., F.A.C.S.
Assistant Clinical Professor, Department of Otolaryngology, University of Pittsburgh School of Medicine, Pittsburgh, Pennsylvania
Interface: Immunology-Allergy-Otorhinolaryngology

Diagnostic Patterns of Otolaryngic Allergy: Symptoms
Nasal Cytology in Clinical Allergy
Pharmacotherapy in the Management of Allergic Diseases
Surgery and the Allergic Patient
Aspirin, Rhinosinusitis, and Asthma

DONALD T. LYSLE, PH.D.
Research Associate, University of Pittsburgh School of Medicine, Pittsburgh, Pennsylvania
Stress and the Immune System

RICHARD L. MABRY, M.D.
Clinical Professor in Otorhinolaryngology, University of Texas Southwestern Medical Center, Dallas; Active Staff, Methodist Hospital; Senior Active Staff, Parkland Memorial Hospital; Attending Staff, Veterans Administration Hospital, Dallas, Texas
Intranasal Medications: Sprays and Aerosols, Corticosteroid Injection
Corticosteroids: General Considerations of Systemic Therapy
Management of Allergic Emergencies

SHIRLEY MURPHY, M.D.
Professor of Pediatrics; Director, Division of Pulmonary/Critical Care Medicine, Department of Pediatrics, University of New Mexico School of Medicine, Albuquerque, New Mexico
Asthma Concepts
Management of Asthma

DONALD J. NALEBUFF, M.D.
Associate Clinical Professor, Department of Otolaryngology, New Jersey College of Medicine and Dentistry; Chief, Department of Otolaryngology, Holy Name Hospital, Teaneck, New Jersey; Consultant, Manhattan Eye and Ear Infirmary, New York, New York
In Vitro Tests in the Diagnosis of Allergic Disorders
In Vitro–Based Allergen Immunotherapy

WILLIAM B. PIERCE, M.D.
Private Practice; Chief of Staff and Chief of Otolaryngology, Genesee Memorial Hospital, St. Jerome's Hospital, Batavia, New York
Diets in Food Allergy: Testing and Therapy

BRUCE S. RABIN, M.D., PH.D.
Professor of Pathology and Psychiatry, University of Pittsburgh School of Medicine, Pittsburgh, Pennsylvania
Structure and Physiology of the Immune System
Immunopathology: Immunologic Deficiency Disease and Evaluation of the Patient with Abnormal Immunity
Immunopathology of Autoimmune Disease
Clinical Use of Monoclonal Antibodies
Immunologic Aspects of Aging and Nutrition
Stress and the Immune System

RICHARD J. TREVINO, M.D.
Assistant Professor of Otolaryngology/Head and Neck Surgery, Louisiana State University, Shreveport; Staff, Alexian Brothers Hospital, San Jose Hospital, Good Samaritan Hospital, O'Connor Hospital, Santa Teresa Community Hospital, San Jose, California
Pathophysiology of Food Allergies and Hypersensitivities

WALTER A. WARD, JR., M.D.
Private Practice, Winston-Salem, North Carolina
Molds: Good News—Bad News
Pathogenic Fungi Allergy
Diagnostic Skin Testing: Skin Endpoint Titration
Skin Endpoint Immunotherapy
Pathogenic Fungi Therapy

FOREWORD

Dr. Krause deserves congratulations for originating and coordinating this project, which brings together authors from different specialties to contribute their knowledge and expertise. Gathering the work of these experienced physicians in this book should benefit those members of the profession who treat patients with problems of otolaryngic allergy. If the profession benefits, then so should their patients through improved care.

As the author points out in her introduction, the diagnosis and treatment of allergy constitutes a significant portion of the practice of various specialties, and so the goal of this book is to offer instruction to all those interested, regardless of their chosen medical field. This book should be of special value to the astute head and neck surgeon who realizes that surgery, necessitated by the complications of allergy, has done nothing to elucidate the etiology of the disease. Unless the allergic basis is recognized and effectively treated, the problems are likely to recur, to both the surgeon's and the patient's chagrin.

This book should be of interest and practical value to all students of allergy of the head and neck. Since the capable clinician is a student throughout his or her professional career, medical students, residents, and practitioners alike should find this volume a valuable part of their library.

JEROME C. GOLDSTEIN, M.D., F.A.C.S.
WASHINGTON, DC

INTRODUCTION

The field of diagnosis and treatment of allergy constitutes a significant portion of several medical specialties. It overlaps with the fields of otorhinolaryngology, general and internal medicine, pulmonology, pediatrics, and dermatology, and touches on several others. Otorhinolaryngology in particular has a broad scope in which allergies of the head and neck are significant. Allergies, in fact, affect over 15 per cent of the population of the United States, at considerable cost to both patients and employers.

Otorhinolaryngologists have been actively involved in the study and treatment of allergy for more than 50 years. In the early 1930s, Dr. French Hansel related then-current concepts of allergy to otolaryngology, for which he might well be considered the father of otolaryngic allergy. In later years he helped establish the American College of Allergists to encourage ongoing vitality in the specialty. On a personal note, Dr. Hansel introduced allergy to your editor in 1962, during her otolaryngology residency.

It is the goal of this book to furnish physicians and technical assistants with the fundamentals necessary to recognize allergic symptomatology, including the guidelines to differentiate the diagnosis and a method of accurately determining etiology. The novice will gain the background and specific knowledge needed to approach allergy as the pillar of medicine that it has become. For those already practicing in the field, the book should help answer questions that arise in daily practice as well as update various aspects of allergy and immunology. Development of new immunotechnology, better standardization of materials, and greater understanding of the relevant pathophysiology all progress in research facilities worldwide. In this book, the late 1980s' science of otolaryngic allergy is brought into sharp focus.

It is the intent of the authors to offer educational material for the practice of allergy care and immunology to all those physicians, whatever their specialty, who wish to study these effective, proven techniques of modern allergy treatment. Although it is oriented to the particular needs of the otolaryngologist, it offers much to those in other fields of medicine. The techniques described are not static, antiquated, or experimental. On the contrary, they are eminently practical, having been developed and refined by knowledgeable physicians and other scientists over many years.

Although our major interests lie in diseases of the head and neck, we must be constantly aware of the whole patient. We cannot disregard the rest of the body, for diseases occurring elsewhere may have an impact on our diagnosis and therapy. Total patient care is an ideal that most of us strive to attain in treating any diseases in the head and neck (and, by extension, those in the lungs and gastrointestinal tract). The otolaryngologist, by virtue of four to six years of highly specialized training, concentrating in the head and neck, is uniquely equipped to diagnose, treat, and follow the course of patients with such diseases as rhinitis, sinusitis, nasal polyps, otitis media, and laryngeal edema; and it is the otolaryngologist who should decide if medical management, including allergy care, is sufficient or if surgical intervention is necessary.

Recognition of allergy as a significant factor may change both the concept of disease and its management. We must keep current with advances in immunology, immunotechnology, and therapeutic modalities, incorporating them into our clinical approaches to allergy, tumor management, and autoimmune diseases. The field of clinical immunology and otolaryngic allergy, now so viable and exciting, will then afford an open, stimulating perspective on the practice of medicine.

This book has been written with all these concepts in mind. The first section discusses immunology as it pertains to otolaryngology. The next, on clinical otolaryngic allergy, describes the diagnosis of the multiple expressions of allergy, testing techniques, and therapies for inhalant and epidermal allergies. Section Three updates the current knowledge of food allergy, while Section Four discusses chemical sensitivity as we understand it today. The last section relates surgery and emergency care, important parts of our practices, to the concept of allergy.

Drawing on incredible advances in the understanding of immunology, metabolic processes, and therapeutic potentials and on the development of altered antigenic materials for therapy and potential genetic correction, the book describes basic science as well as state-of-the-art clinical medicine. Both current literature and scientific programs are vital for providing the best, most progressive care to our patients. And, of course, practical hands-on experience under the guidance of expert teachers must be an accompaniment to this and all textbooks.

Guest authors were chosen for their special areas of expertise and their ability to write concise, clear presentations. I am most grateful for their willingness to share their knowledge in the effort to advance the teaching of otolaryngic allergy.

I wish to thank my office personnel for their time and effort in preparation of this book, especially Lee Foley, R.N., and MaryAnn Blake. The Medical Librarian at the North Hills Passavant Hospital, Peggy Trevanion, deserves special recognition for her assistance. Dr. Volker Breitfeld is thanked for his preparation of special slides and his advice in cytology, and Karen Hall Siegel, Ph.D., for her editorial assistance. Several commercial companies—Pharmacia, Fisons, Synbiotics, 3M Diagnostics, and Schering Corporation—have provided funds or materials to enhance the quality of this book. Finally, I wish to thank my husband, M. Marvin Krause, D.M.D., for his constant encouragement.

HELEN F. KRAUSE, M.D., F.A.C.S.

CONTENTS

SECTION TWO OTOLARYNGIC ALLERGY: INHALANT AND EPIDERMAL 49

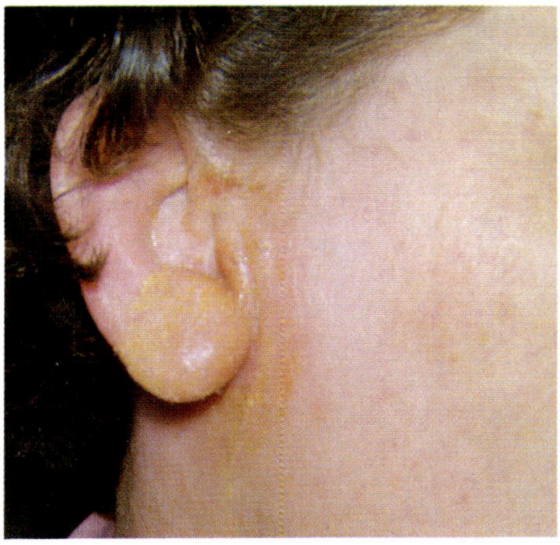

FIGURE 8–1. Eczema of external auditory canal with early perichondritis.

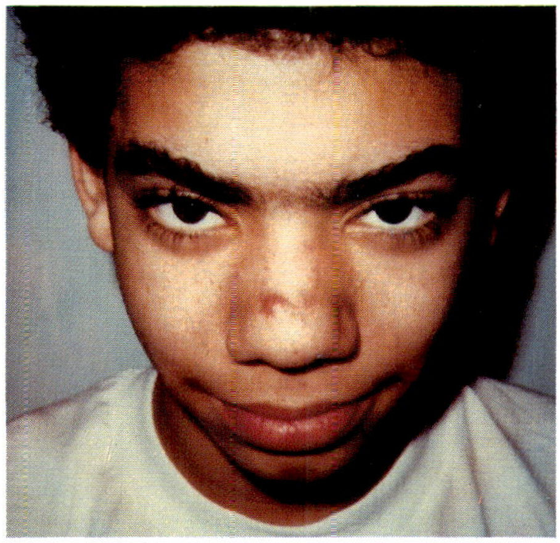

FIGURE 8–5. Nasal crease with acne lesions.

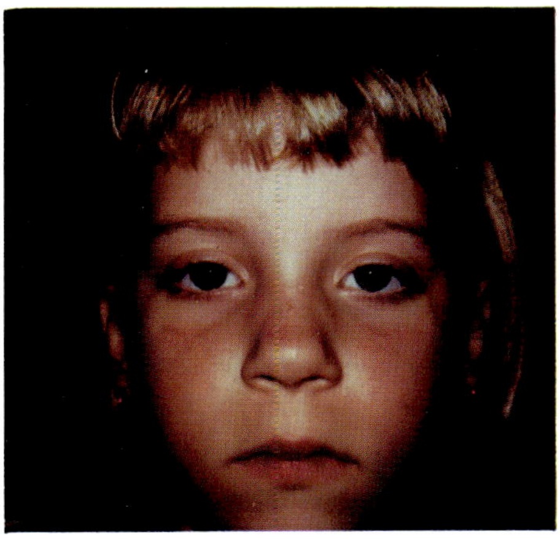

FIGURE 8–6. Allergic "shiners" are the black eyes of allergy in this 7-year-old girl.

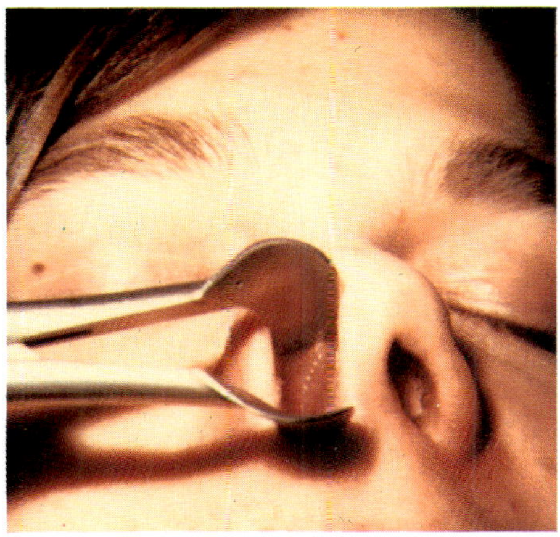

FIGURE 8–8. Nasal polyp.

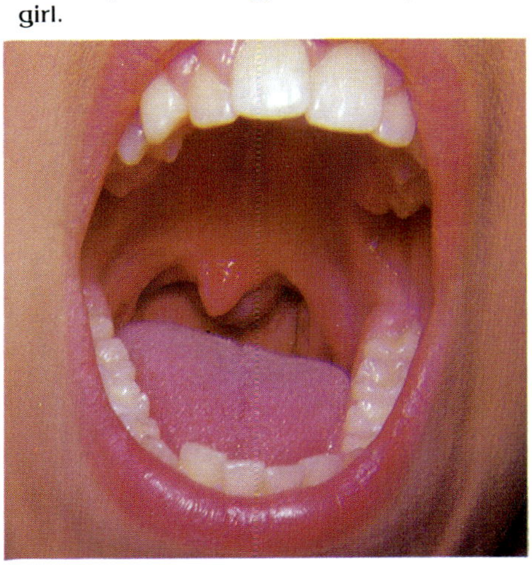

FIGURE 8–9. Choanal polyp in an 11-year-old boy.

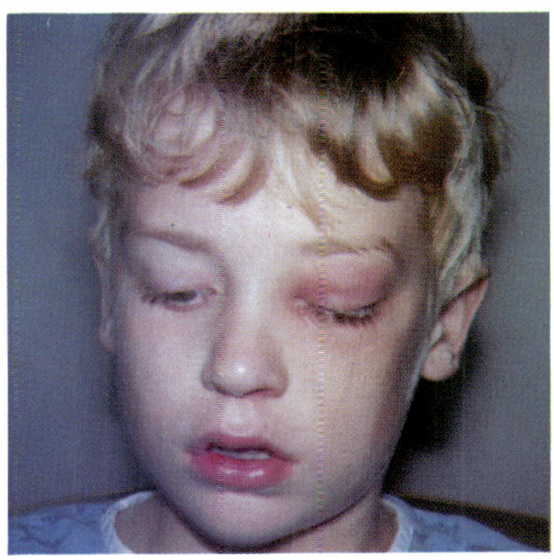

FIGURE 8–11. Left orbital cellulitis of 10-year-old; early resolution stage 14 hours after onset of therapy.

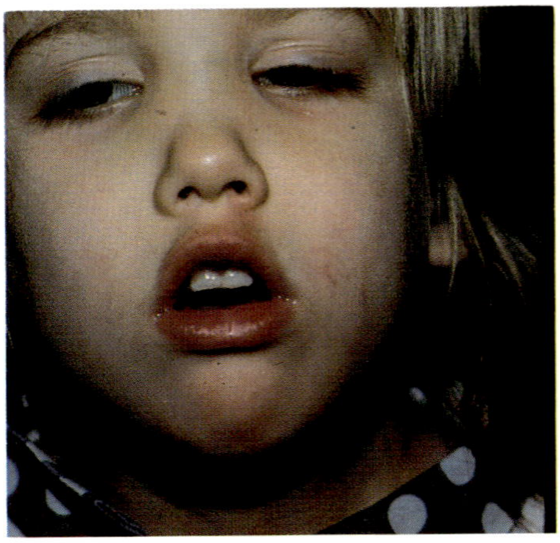

FIGURE 8–14. "Allergic facies" of 5-year-old girl.

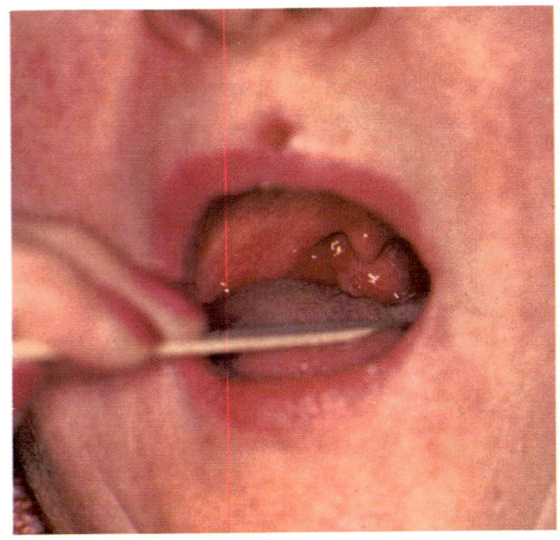

FIGURE 8–17. Inflamed posterior pharyngeal tissue and herpetic lip lesion.

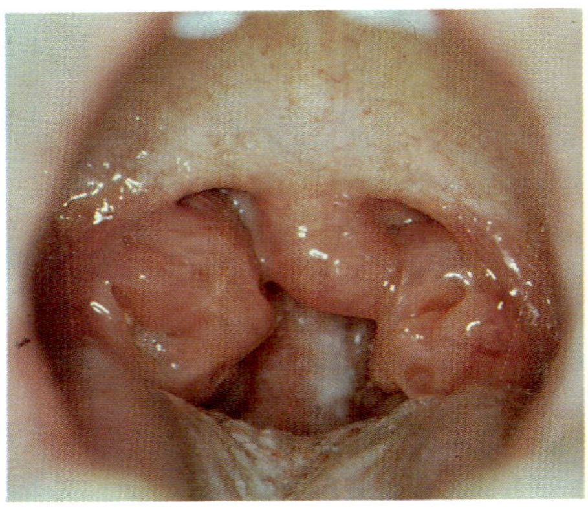

FIGURE 8–18. Hypertrophied tonsils with thick postnasal drainage.

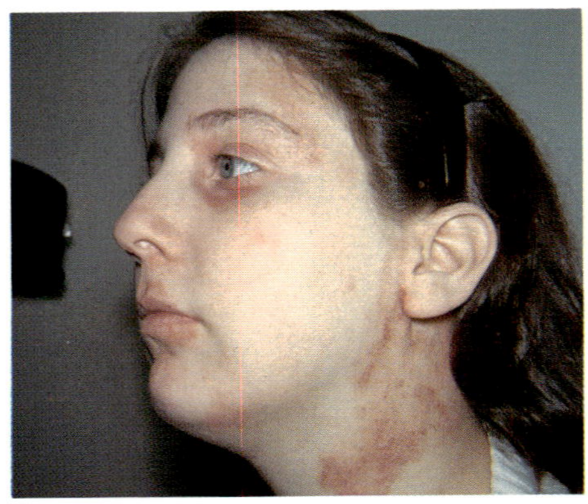

FIGURE 8–22. Recurrent eczema of 18-year-old girl, especially marked on face and neck but also present on arms and legs; resolving with therapy for inhalant and food allergies.

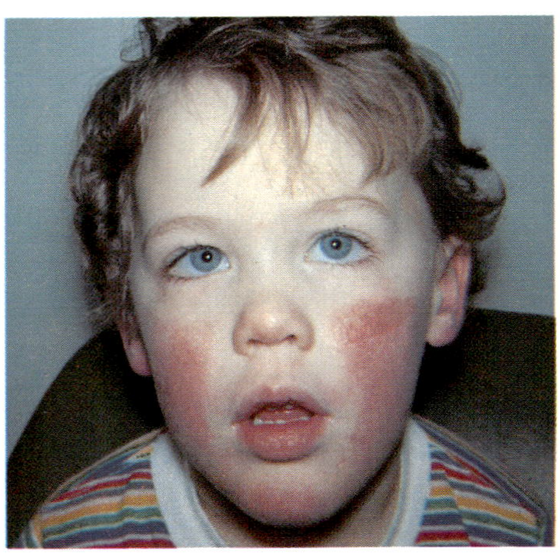

FIGURE 8–23. Facial eczema of 3-year-old boy due to inhalant and milk allergies.

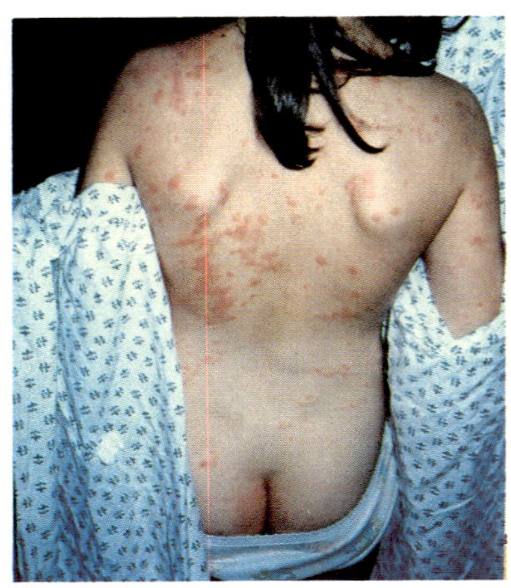

FIGURE 8–24. Generalized hives in 7-year-old girl with inhalant and food allergies.

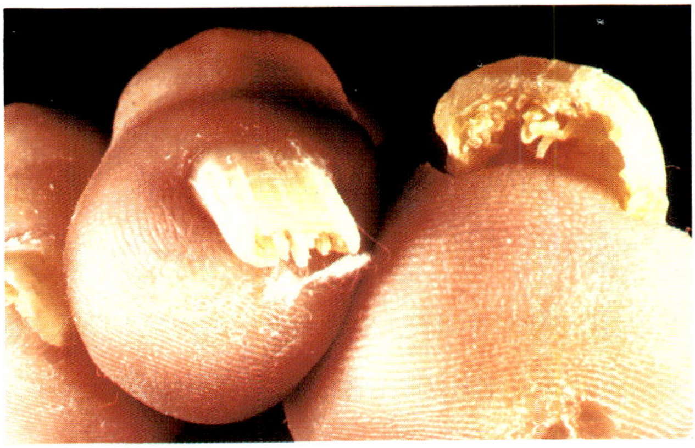

FIGURE 12–2. Onychomycosis, fungal infection of the toenails.

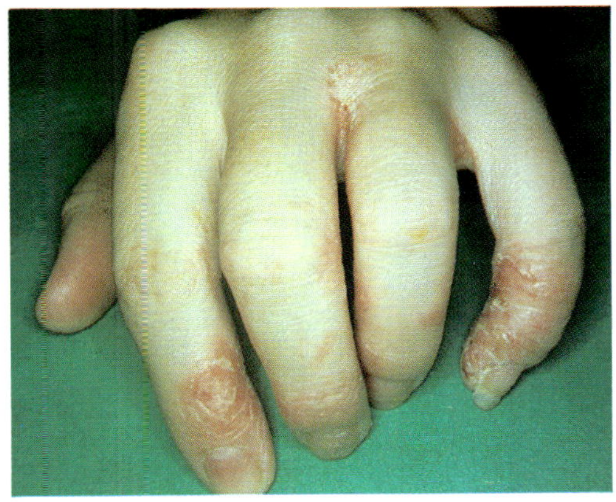

FIGURE 12–3. Id reaction of the hand.

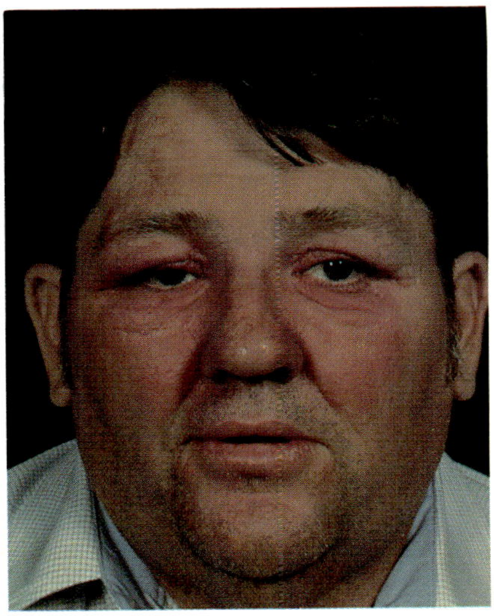

FIGURE 12–5. Facial id reaction.

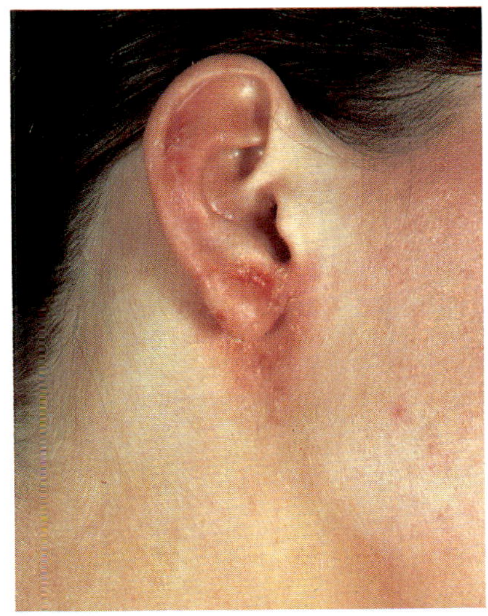

FIGURE 12–6. Id reaction involving an ear—acute and highly inflamed.

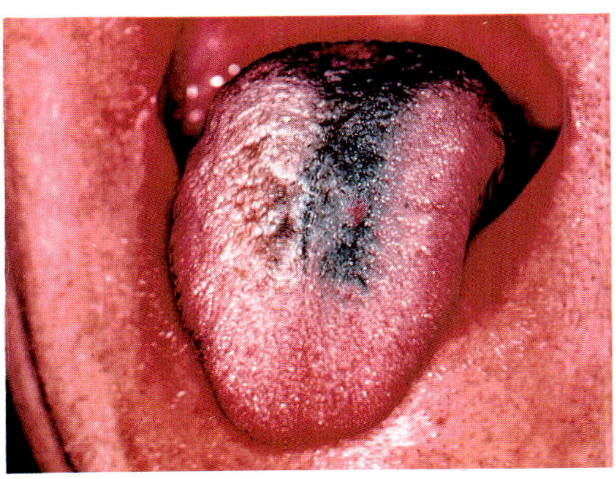

FIGURE 12–7. Black hairy tongue.

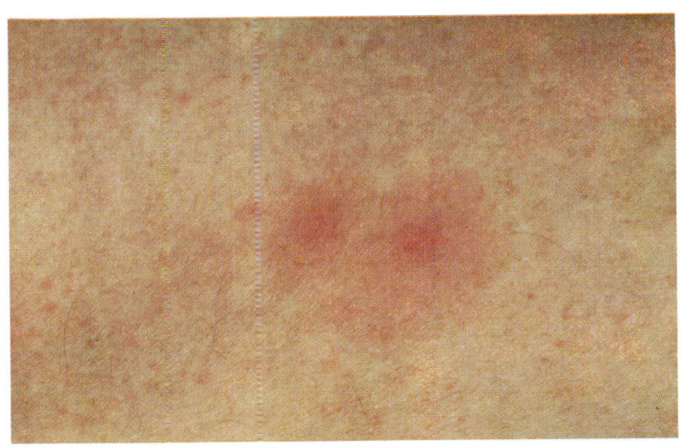

FIGURE 12–8. Delayed tuberculin-like skin reaction.

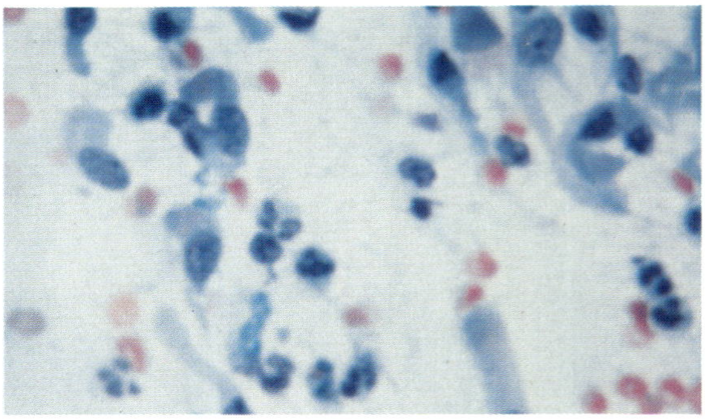

FIGURE 15–5. Epithelial cells, characterized by blue cytoplasm with a large, nearly clear nucleus; some have cilia.

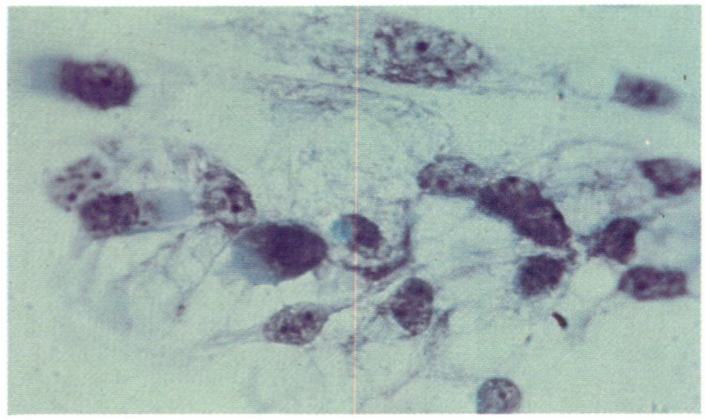

FIGURE 15–6. Goblet cells. Their frothy secretions push nuclei to base of cells.

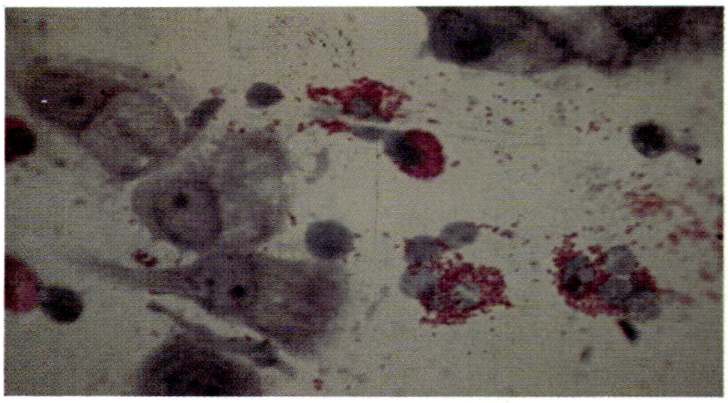

FIGURE 15–7. Eosinophils, including intact cells and disintegrating cells with spilling of pink-red granules. Goblet cells are nearby.

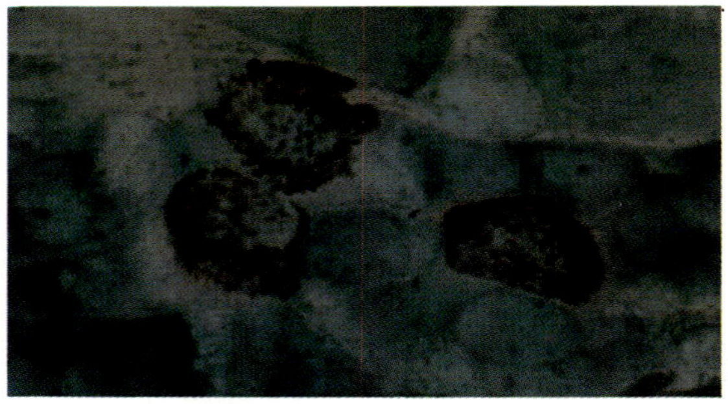

FIGURE 15–8. Mast cell cytoplasm is filled with reddish-purple granules nearly obliterating the oval central nucleus.

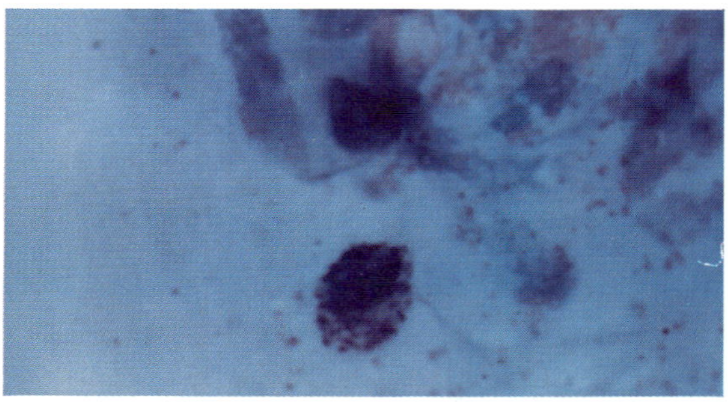

FIGURE 15–9. Basophil, having a distinct cell membrane with sharp purple granules.

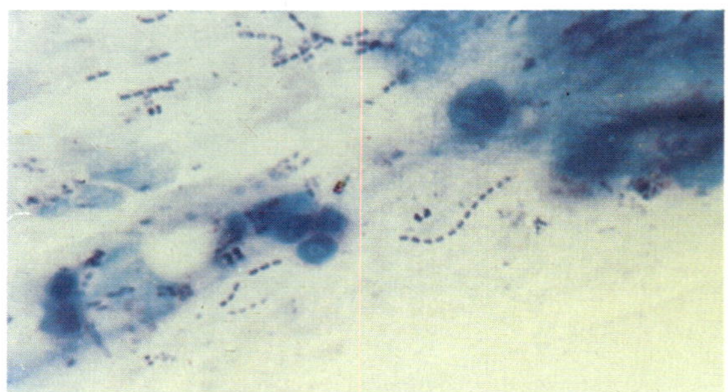

FIGURE 15–10. Polymorphonuclear leukocytes with multilobulated nuclei, occurring with both intracellular and extracellular bacteria.

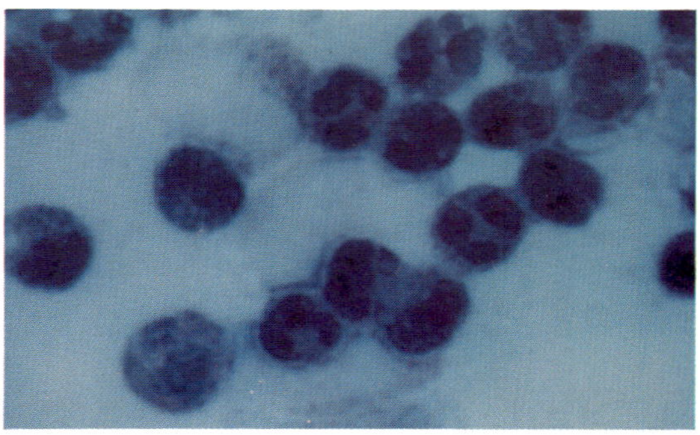

FIGURE 15–12. Lymphocytes with large, dark, central nuclei. The ovid plasma cells are larger and have smaller nuclei.

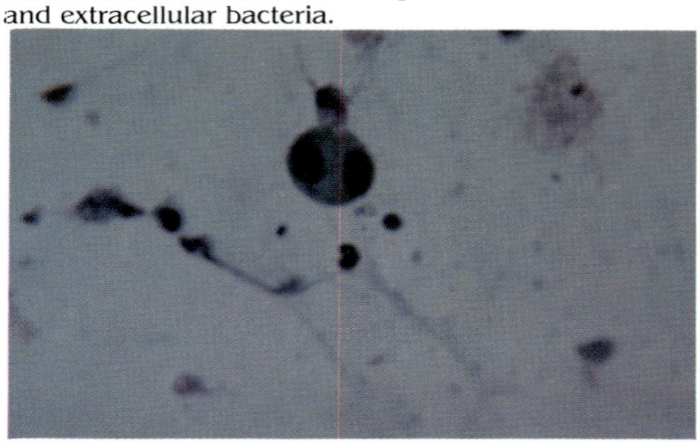

FIGURE 15–13. Macrophage extending a pseudopod.

SECTION ONE

CLINICAL IMMUNOLOGY

Immunology has been a field in which practical application has been ahead and has led to theoretical understanding.

The importance of the immune system is indicated by the fact that the number of cells in our bodies devoted to the immune system is approximately equal to the number of cells in the brain. Only a few years ago, immunologists elicited derision from "hard scientists" by defining an antibody as "a molecule generated by an antigen" and an antigen as "a molecule which reacts with an antibody." That seemingly circuitous reasoning has revealed the most sophisticated molecular and practical applications of any biological system. This field has mysteries still unsolved but it is one in which every step along the path produces some benefit to mankind.

D. E. Koshland, Jr., Ph.D.

Adapted from Editorial: Science 238:1023, 1987.

CHAPTER 1

Structure and Physiology of the Immune System

Bruce S. Rabin, M.D., Ph.D.

The primary role of the immune system is to resist invasive pathogenic microorganisms. Historically, when the immune system failed to function and infection occurred, patients received injections of specific immune serum, which had been produced in animals. The introduction of antibiotics ended the general use of such sera.

During the 20th century, it has become apparent that the immune system is not always directed against extrinsic pathogens. Indeed, on occasion, the immune system fails to differentiate self antigens from foreign antigens and can initiate an immune response against self (autologous) tissue. The result of such an immune response may be autoimmune disease. Autoimmune disease is the result of the immune system's attacking self antigens and inducing disease.

Another example of the immune system's producing responses that are not beneficial is in the allergic diseases. In these diseases, the immune system can bring about the release of vasoactive mediators, resulting in conditions such as asthma or rhinitis.

Transplantation of tissue between genetically identical individuals (i.e., identical twins) takes place with no problems of tissue rejection. However, transplantation of tissue between nonidentical individuals of the species (allotransplantation) is hampered by problems of tissue rejection. Rejection of transplanted tissue is due to an immune response against antigens on the transplant.

Individuals receiving tissue transplants receive immunosuppressive therapy that is designed to allow the transplant to survive by suppressing the immune system. Such individuals are at a high risk of developing a malignancy. Thus, it has become apparent that the immune system plays a role in prevention of malignancy. Indeed, an extensive amount of animal experimentation has shown that the immune system has the potential for eliminating malignant tissue. Attempts are being made in humans to activate the immune system to eliminate malignancies after they develop.

Another area in which it is important to understand how the immune system functions is in individuals who have an immune deficiency disease. This may occur congenitally or be acquired later in life. The result of such deficiency diseases of the immune system is that the individuals are at a high risk of chronic infectious disease, and such infection may prove fatal. Patients with acquired immune deficiency syndrome (AIDS) are an outstanding example.

COMPONENTS OF THE IMMUNE SYSTEM

The immune system is highly intricate and involves communication between its various

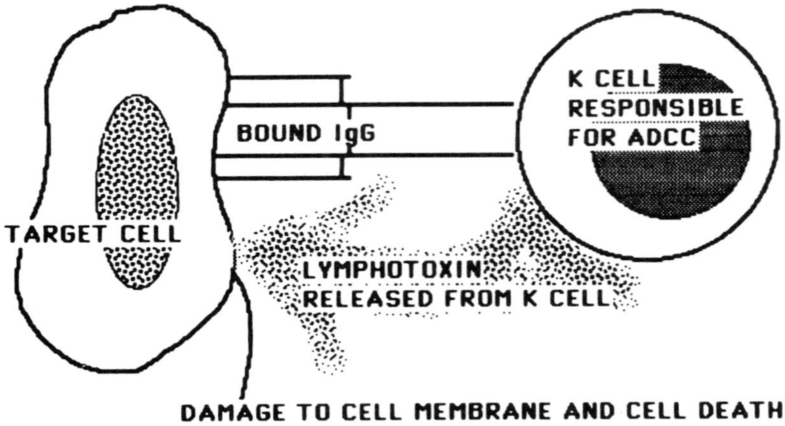

FIGURE 1–1. The reaction of antibody-dependent cellular cytotoxicity involves a K lymphocyte with a receptor for the Fc portion of IgG binding to an IgG molecule that has attached to a target cell. The K cell then releases a toxic factor that will kill the target cell. The K cell is not sensitized to the target cell, but rather binds to antibody that specifically reacts with the target cell.

components. These components involve cells, genes, and secreted molecules.

Two primary types of cells are involved in the immune system: the phagocytic cells and the immunologically reactive cells (lymphocytes and plasma cells). The phagocytic cells are the tissue macrophages and circulating monocytes. The macrophages do not specifically react with an antigen. However, these cells are capable of concentrating antigen on their surface for the presentation of antigen to lymphocytes. Additionally, macrophages release biologically active soluble substances (for example, prostaglandins and interleukins), which may regulate lymphocyte activity. This immunologic activity is not related to the phagocytic function of these cells and their role in clearing foreign microorganisms and dead tissue cells from the body.

Lymphocytes

The specific immunologically reactive cells of the immune system are the lymphocytes. There are two major classifications of lymphocytes, the B lymphocytes and the T lymphocytes. The B lymphocytes are involved with the release of specific immunoglobulin (antibody, humoral immune response) following exposure to an antigen. A primary humoral immune response is what occurs following initial exposure to an antigen. A secondary or anamnestic (memory) response occurs following a second exposure to the same antigen.

The T lymphocyte (thymus-dependent) population is heterogeneous, consisting of lymphocytes with multiple functions. Regardless of the function of the T lymphocyte, it is dependent on the presence of the thymus gland for its maturation. Mature T lymphocytes can function as effector cells in the cell-mediated immune response. These are cells capable of performing such functions as rejection of transplanted tissue and production of the delayed hypersensitivity skin response. Helper T lymphocytes interact with B lymphocytes to allow the B lymphocytes to produce antibody. Those antigens requiring a T helper cell are called T-dependent antigens. Antigens that can directly stimulate B lymphocytes are referred to as T-independent antigens. In addition, helper T lymphocytes interact with other T lymphocytes to allow those T cells to produce cell-mediated immune responses. Suppressor T lymphocytes are a population of cells that inhibit either the humoral or the cell-mediated immune response.

Using monoclonal antibody, it has been found that the different T lymphocyte populations have differing antigens on their surface. There is an antigen that is selectively present on the helper T lymphocytes (CD 4) and another antigen that is present on the suppressor lymphocyte population (CD 8). Other antigens are present on all T lymphocytes (CD 3). Classically, T lymphocytes were identified by their binding of sheep erythrocytes to a receptor for sheep erythrocytes. A monoclonal antibody specifically directed to the sheep erythrocyte receptor can also be used to identify such cells. However, CD 3 antibodies detect all T cells, regardless of their capability of binding sheep erythrocytes.

An additional population of lymphocytes is the null population. These cells are not identifiable as either T or B lymphocytes. The null population is also a heterogeneous population. One type of cell from this population is the K lymphocyte, which is responsible for the phenomenon known as antibody-dependent cellular cytotoxicity (ADCC). The ADCC cell has a receptor for the Fc portion of IgG on its surface. When an IgG antibody is bound to an antigen, its Fc receptor is exposed. ADCC directs a cytotoxic activity against the target cell (Fig. 1–1).

Another lymphocyte of the null cell population is the NK or natural killer cell. These lymphocytes are believed to be capable of eliminating cells that spontaneously become malignant. The mechanism by which they work is unknown. Morphologically they are large, granular lymphocytes and contain a unique antigen that can be identified by an appropriate monoclonal antibody (Leu 11). The functional activity of the NK lymphocyte population is increased by interferon.

Figure 1–2 illustrates critical steps in the development of the immune system. A lymphoid stem cell is present in the bone marrow. This cell gives rise to the various components of the immune system. Under the influence of the thymus gland, the stem cell becomes an immature T lymphocyte. At the immature T cell stage, the reactivity of the cell to self antigens is eliminated when that cell encounters antigens present in the environment of the fetus. This is a critical factor in the development of tolerance to self antigens. Under continued influence of the thymus gland, the immature T lymphocyte matures into the functionally active T cell population. These are the effector cells, the suppressor and the helper cell. Interactions exist between these cell populations. For example, too much suppressor cell function will inhibit the ability of

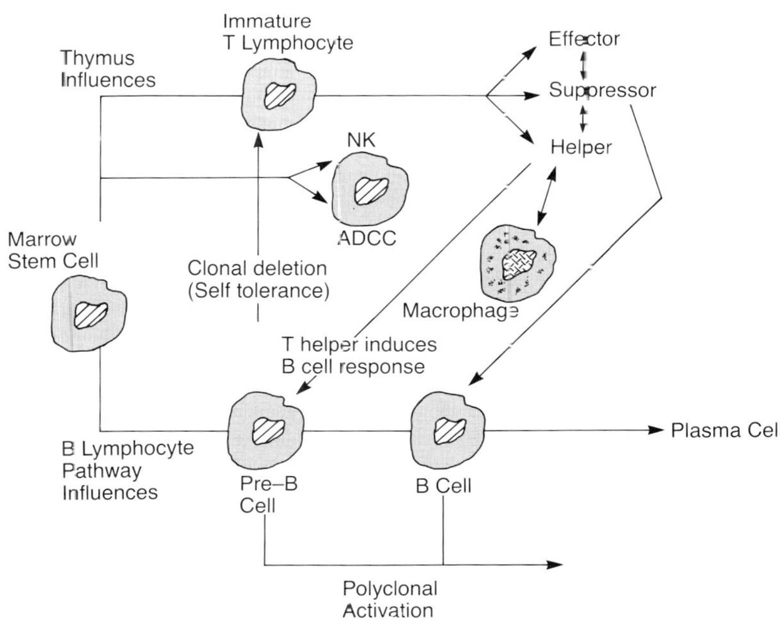

FIGURE 1–2. The bone marrow stem cell is acted upon by hormone-like substances that can influence it along pathways to mature into a T or a B lymphocyte. When the immature T lymphocyte encounters autologous antigen, it may functionally be inactivated so that it cannot react to self antigens; thus, autoimmune disease does not result. The immature T cell matures into an effector T cell that can exert a cytotoxic response to tissue, a suppressor T cell that can impede immunologic responses, or a helper T cell that promotes immune responses. There is regulatory interaction between the various T cell populations. The macrophage is a central cell in the immune response and interacts with helper T lymphocytes and suppressor T lymphocytes. The B lymphocyte is also influenced by the helper T cell and by antigen presentation from the macrophage. In addition, B lymphocytes are regulated by the idiotype network, which is antibody-directed to immunoglobulins present on the surface of B lymphocytes. Such antibody can prevent B lymphocytes from becoming activated, or may actually activate them. If B lymphocytes that have not become tolerant by reaction to autologous antigens are activated by helper T cell or some type of polyclonal activator, autoimmune disease may result. The natural killer and antibody-dependent cytotoxicity cell (K cell) arises from the marrow stem cell and is neither a T nor a B lymphocyte.

helper T lymphocytes to function. Substances released from macrophages, shown below the helper cell, also exert an influence on the T cell populations. The marrow stem cell also gives rise to the NK and ADCC cells. These cells are neither T nor B.

Other influences, as yet undefined, give rise to pre-B lymphocytes, which can mature into fully functional B lymphocytes, which give rise to plasma cells. The pre-B cell may be capable of reacting to self antigen. Possibly, under the influence of a helper cell or a nonspecific polyclonal activator, pre-B cells can mature into autoreactive T lymphocytes. However, this usually does not occur because of the role of suppressor lymphocytes on B lymphocytes.

Considerable information is available regarding the normal development of B lymphocytes. Initial stem cell differentiation takes place within the fetal liver and bone marrow. The first recognizable B lymphocyte in the human liver is present during the 7th week of gestation. These are large, rapidly dividing cells that give rise to small, resting lymphoid cells. Both the large and small lymphocytes contain small amounts of intracytoplasmic IgM but they lack functional surface receptors for antigen, the Fc portion of IgG, and C3. These latter receptors are normally present on mature B lymphocytes. The small pre-B lymphocyte is a precursor for an immature B lymphocyte that possesses surface IgM. Because the large pre-B lymphocytes divide rapidly and lack surface receptors through which clonal abortion could be directed, they may generate clonal diversity by a genetically preprogrammed mechanism. Surface IgM–bearing B lymphocytes first appear in the liver of the human fetus around the 8th week of gestation. These cells can easily be aborted by antibody to IgM determinants or by encountering self antigens to which their surface IgM may be directed. These cells have a paucity or absence of Fc and C3 receptors.

Without the need for antigen or T lymphocytes, immature B lymphocytes mature into B lymphocytes that express all of the surface constituents known to facilitate collaboration with helper T cells and macrophages. Mature B lymphocytes can be induced to proliferate by antigen and to mature into antibody-secreting plasma cells or memory lymphocytes. Small populations of surface IgM–positive lymphocytes begin to express one of the IgG subclasses. Soon after, a few cells with surface IgM and IgA can be detected. Surface IgD is the last surface immunoglobulin to be expressed on the B lymphocyte sublines. Once surface IgD is present, B lymphocytes become tolerant with a great deal of difficulty. The absence of surface IgD on immature lymphocytes may be an essential correlate of their ease of becoming tolerant.

By treatment with an anti-IgM chain antibody from birth, development of all classes of B lymphocytes is inhibited. This would suggest that all B lymphocytes arise from the IgM-bearing cell.

In the human fetus, the proportion of spleen lymphocytes bearing surface IgM, IgG, IgA, and IgD reaches adult percentages at the beginning of the third trimester.

Physiologically important processes mediated by either humoral or cellular immunity are enumerated in Table 1–1. The distribution of the two major lymphocyte populations and the anatomic location of these are given in Table 1–2.

Table 1–1. PHYSIOLOGICALLY IMPORTANT PROCESSES MEDIATED BY HUMORAL AND CELLULAR IMMUNITY

Process	Humoral Immunity	Cell-Mediated Immunity
Environmental	Encapsulated pyogenic bacteria (pneumococci, streptococci, meningococci, *H. influenzae*)	Intracellular pathogenic organisms (many bacteria, viruses, protozoa, and fungi)
Transplantation rejection reactions	Major cause of hyperacute rejection reaction; role in acute and chronic rejection less well defined	Major mechanism for rejecting transplanted organs
Tumor immunity	Immunologic enhancement?	Prime mechanism for eliminating neoplastic cells
Autoimmune disorders	Formed elements of blood; "toxic complex" diseases	Solid organs

Table 1–2. ANATOMIC LOCATION OF T AND B LYMPHOCYTES

	T Cells	B Cells
Peripheral blood	60–80%	20–30%
Thoracic duct	85–90%	10–15%
Lymph nodes	Paracortical regions	Germinal centers, subcapsular region, medullary cords
Spleen	Periarteriolar sheaths	Germinal centers, periphery of periarteriolar sheaths, red pulp

T Lymphocyte Function

When mice are acutely infected with a virus, T lymphocytes arise that are capable of lysing virally infected target cells. The cytotoxic T lymphocytes that arise have specificity not only for the antigens of the infecting virus, but also for the major histocompatibility complex antigens present on the cell surface. This phenomenon is termed MHC restriction. The nature of the cytotoxic T cell antigen receptors—whether one binding site for both antigen and histocompatibility marker, or two—is unknown. The MHC restriction phenomenon can be defined as the requirement for identity of a specific MHC gene product to allow T effector functions to be induced and exerted through interaction with other cells, such as antigen-presenting cells or target cells expressing a foreign antigen.

It was recently recognized that supernatants of mitogen-activated or mixed lymphocyte cultures contain T cell growth factor (now called interleukin-2) that supports the continuous growth and proliferation of human and murine T cells. This has allowed both the expansion of T lymphocyte populations and the cloning of cells belonging to functionally different subpopulations.

Numerous studies have shown that IL–2 does not support growth of nonactivated T lymphocytes. Thus, it has been postulated that a T cell population must be "activated" both to become sensitive to IL–2 and to produce this growth factor in order to proliferate. Due to the well-documented macrophage requirement for mitogen-induced IL–2 production and the observation that IL–1 is a macrophage product, it has been hypothesized that IL–1 may be an essential signal required by IL–2 producer T cells. Although the involvement of IL–1 and the production of IL–2 by stimulated T cells appears unquestionable, the precise mechanisms by which IL–1 functions in this capacity remain unknown (Fig. 1–3).

The salient feature of the IL–2 concept is the observation that T cells require two signals in order to be activated. Signal 1 represents antigen recognition. Upon receptor antigen interaction, the antigen-selected T cell clones become sensitive to the inducive effect (signal 2) of IL–2, which initiates T cell activation.

B Lymphocyte Function

Basically, how B lymphocytes are stimulated to become the antibody-forming cells is not yet fully understood. Certain antigens are capable of reacting directly with the corresponding antibody on the surface of a B lymphocyte to induce it to transform or to proliferate into active antibody-producing cells. Such antigens generally have reappearing antigenic determinants of the same specificity so that they can simultaneously trigger a number of receptors on the surface of the same B lymphocyte. Other antigens, or small quantities of antigen, may have to be taken onto the surface of a macrophage, thus being more readily available for stimulating a B lymphocyte either directly or through the cooperation of a helper T lymphocyte. In this way, a high local concentration of antigen is achieved during cell to cell contact with the B lymphocyte, thereby stimulating a greater number of receptor sites in a given cell than if the antigen were uniformly dispersed throughout body fluid. Once stimulated, that cell undergoes division and produces the antibody for which it is genetically programmed.

TYPES OF IMMUNE REACTIONS AND THEIR RELATION TO HUMAN DISEASE (IMMUNOPATHOLOGY)

There are six types of immune reactions that may damage tissue:

- Type I Anaphylactic (immediate hypersensitivity IgE)
- Type II Cytotoxic antibody (IgG, IgM)
- Type III Immune complex

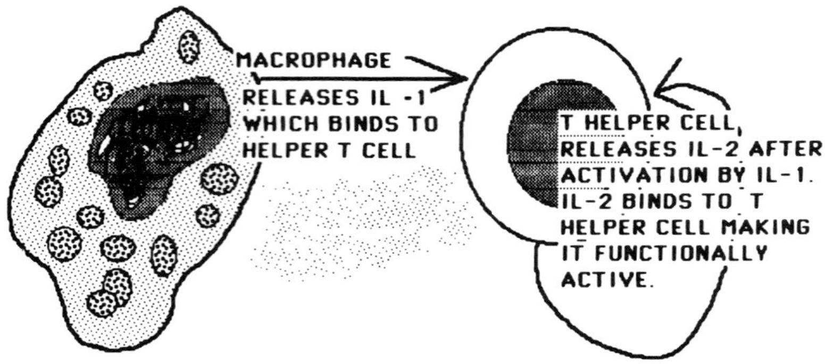

FIGURE 1–3. A macrophage upon interaction with an antigen releases IL–1, which binds to the helper T lymphocyte. The helper T lymphocyte responds by releasing IL–2, which feeds back on the helper T cell, augmenting the binding sites for IL–2 and production of IL–2 by the helper T lymphocyte.

Type IV T cell–mediated (delayed) hypersensitivity
Type V Stimulating antibody
Type VI Antibody-dependent cell-mediated cytotoxicity (ADCC, K cell)

Type I

The IgE antibody binds to mast cells in tissue. When two antibodies of the same specificity are adjacent to each other and encounter the antigen to which they are reactive, changes occur in the membrane of the mast cell, which results in histamine release. Individuals who undergo this type of reaction are termed atopic; a common manifestation of this is asthma. Urticaria is a skin reaction that often develops as a result of absorption of antigen through the intestinal tract. Not all urticaria is caused by an immune reaction. Individuals who are atopic frequently have extremely high levels of serum IgE.

Most of the reactions found in atopic individuals are secondary to the release of histamine, kinins, and other substances that increase capillary permeability.

Type II

An example of a type II reaction is autoimmune hemolytic anemia or antibody that binds to the glomerular basement membrane in patients with Goodpasture's syndrome. Thus, this is a reaction in which antibody binds to the tissue and may damage that tissue or damage the tissue secondary to activation of the complement system.

Type III

Immune complex occurs when a precipitating antibody combines with the antigen either in the circulation or in the tissue. These complexes have the capability of depositing in tissue where they activate the complement system. Once the complement system is activated, an inflammatory reaction (Arthus) is established. Small complexes in antigen excess tend to remain in the circulation. Large complexes formed in equivalence or in antibody excess are rapidly taken up and degraded by phagocytic cells. The intermediate size complexes formed in moderate antigen excess are soluble but large enough to react with complement and are most likely the size complex deposited in the tissue when inflammation is induced. Some tissue may have a receptor for the third component of complement. Thus, the renal glomerulus possesses such a receptor, and this may be a factor in deposition of immune complexes in the kidney.

Type IV

Type IV reactions are the T cell–mediated reactions, such as the delayed hypersensitivity skin test response. The classic example of this reaction is the tuberculin skin test response. Type IV reactions can also occur on the skin from reactions with meals, drugs, or poison ivy.

Type V

There are IgG antibodies that react with tissue receptor sites. One such antibody is the antibody found in patients with Graves' disease, in whom the antibody actually stimulates thyroid hormone production.

Type VI

K cells are capable of exerting a cytotoxic effect on target cells that are coated with antibody. The K cell is not sensitized to the target. The cytotoxic reaction is complement independent and is brought about by the K cell, which has an Fc receptor on it, binding to the Fc portion of the antibody molecule that is on the cell surface. K cell–mediated reactions may be important in a variety of human diseases.

REFERENCES

Bellanti JA: Immunology III. Philadelphia, WB Saunders, 1984.

Joklik WK, Willeth HP, Amos DB: Zinsser Microbiology. 18th ed. Norwalk, Appleton-Century-Crofts, 1984, pp 253–423.

Roitt IM, Brostoff J, Male DK: Immunology. St. Louis, CV Mosby, 1985.

Stites DP, Stobo JD, Wells JU: Basic and Clinical Immunology. 7th ed. Norwalk, Appleton and Lange Medical Publications, 1987.

CHAPTER 2

Immunopathology: Immunologic Deficiency Disease and Evaluation of the Patient with Abnormal Immunity

Bruce S. Rabin, M.D., Ph.D.

Recurrent infection is the classic manifestation of abnormal immunity. However, as our knowledge of the interrelated functions of immunoglobulins, complement, lymphocytes, and phagocytic cells grows, the term immunity might also include the ability to resist autoimmune disease and neoplasia as well. In general, a disorder of one of the components of the immune system results in characteristic clinical manifestations (Table 2–1). Most commonly this is infection. Therefore, the emphasis in this chapter is on the evaluation of a patient with recurrent infection.

It is often unclear which patients deserve an immunologic evaluation. Recurrent infections are a part of a normal childhood, and demarcation between normal and abnormal numbers of infections is not possible. The following reviews the approach to a patient with a possible immune deficiency disease.

Table 2–1. CLINICAL MANIFESTATIONS OF IMMUNE SYSTEM DISORDERS

Immunologic Defect	Characteristic Clinical Presentation
B cell (immunoglobulin)	Recurrent bacterial infections
IgA	Giardia intestinal infestation, sinopulmonary infection
T cell (cell-mediated)	Recurrent viral, fungal, or protozoal infection
Complement	
Early components	Recurrent bacterial infection, SLE, connective tissue diseases
Late components	Neisseria infection, connective tissue diseases
C1 esterase inhibitor	Angioedema
Neutrophil	
Microbial killing	Pseudomonas infection
Chemotaxis	Pyogenic infection (Staphylococcus, Streptococcus, Haemophilus)

IMMUNOLOGIC EVALUATION

History

In the initial evaluation, the history is most important. Several areas must be carefully evaluated. First, the type of infection and the location are quite helpful. Every attempt should be made to isolate and identify the infective agent. In general, recurrent bacterial infection suggests an immunoglobulin or neutrophil defect, whereas viral, fungal, and protozoal infections are common with T cell dysfunction. Certain infections are highly characteristic for some disorders. For example, pneumocystis is commonly seen in patients with a severe T cell defect; candidiasis also suggests a T cell defect. Recurrent Neisseria infections are the hallmark of late complement component deficiency. Intestinal giardiasis is commonly seen in patients with hypogammaglobulinemia.

The location of infection may also yield clues to determine the nature of an immunodeficiency. Recurrent sinopulmonary infections are often the presenting problem in patients with hypogammaglobulinemia or IgA deficiency. If the skin is the primary site of infection, chemotaxis and phagocytosis may require evaluation.

A summary of growth and development in a child should be included in the history. Children with B cell defects will grow normally until 6 to 9 months of age, when maternal immunoglobulins have declined and no longer afford protection; children with T cell defects often show symptoms at an earlier age. Immunizations given and any adverse reactions are important facts to document. Live viral vaccines may cause severe, life-threatening problems in T cell deficient children.

A list of medications, specifically asking about cytotoxic drugs or steroids, should be obtained.

A family history should be taken. Since many immunodeficiency syndromes are associated with autoimmune diseases, the occurrence of diabetes, systemic lupus erythematosus (SLE), rheumatoid arthritis, thyroid disease, or adrenal disease in a family member may be important. Since certain immunodeficiency disorders are inherited, such as X-linked agammaglobulinemia, the importance of a family history of immunodeficiency or of unexplained early death of a family member is obvious. Complement deficiencies are also inherited.

Finally, the history should help exclude nonimmunologic causes for infection, such as diabetes, cystic fibrosis, Kartagener's syndrome, alpha$_1$-antitrypsin deficiency, or mechanical obstruction.

Physical Examination

The physical examination should include a careful study of the skin and throat, abdomen, and joints. The presence or absence of lymphoid and splenic tissue must be documented.

Initial Laboratory Evaluation

Although the clinician should have some indication of the nature of the immune defect from the history and physical evaluation, screening for the integrity of each arm of the immune system (T cell, B cell, complement, and phagocytes) is often needed. This basic laboratory evaluation for immune function is quite simple and is outlined below.

System	Screening Tests
Cell-mediated (T cell)	Total lymphocyte count Delayed hypersensitivity skin tests
Antibody (B cell)	Total protein electrophoresis Quantitative immunoglobulins
Complement	CH_{50}
Neutrophil	Microbicidal assay Chemotaxis

In a normal adult, the total lymphocyte count is greater than 1000/mm^3. Children should have higher counts of 1500 to 1800/mm^3. One should review the blood smear personally, if possible, to exclude the possibility of monocytes being counted as lymphocytes. Lymphocytopenia may be present in 6 per cent of normal patients; however, it is commonly noted in patients with malignancy, acute infections, SLE, Hodgkin's disease, uremia, and congestive heart failure.

Delayed hypersensitivity should be present to at least one antigen in all persons, excepting infants, who may not yet have been exposed to the antigens used for testing.

Serum protein electrophoresis will demonstrate the presence or absence of a normal amount of gamma globulin. Quantitation of individual immunoglobulins is needed to evaluate patients suspected of a deficiency of a single class of immunoglobulin, such as IgA deficiency.

If a CH_{50} test is abnormal, assays for the individual components will determine the exact nature of the defect. Infectious problems are seen in patients with a complete deficiency in a given complement component, which will cause a marked decrease in CH_{50}.

Neutrophil defects are investigated through specialized laboratories. Disorders that would show a deficiency in microbial killing or chemotaxis include chronic granulomatous disease, myeloperoxidase or G6PD deficiency, Chediak-Higashi syndrome, and hyper-IgE syndrome.

Secondary Studies

If a screening study is abnormal, further tests are indicated. These are summarized in the following.

B Cell Studies

1. Quantitation of B cells, either by surface immunoglobulin staining or by monoclonal anti-B cell antibody.
2. Determination of specific antibody production in vivo by one of several methods:
   a. Isohemagglutinins.
   b. Antibody titers to antigens to which the patient has been exposed naturally or by vaccination, such as streptococcal, measles, mumps, tetanus, diphtheria, and rubella antigens.
   c. Schick test.
3. Secretory antibody levels.
4. In vitro antibody synthesis.
5. T cell subpopulations for helper and suppressor cell enumeration.

T Cell Studies

1. Quantitation of total T cells, and of T helper and T suppressor subsets, by monoclonal antibody technique.
2. In vitro T cell stimulation by mitogens (pokeweed, concanavalin, or phytohemagglutinin) or by specific antigen such as candida.
3. Assay for lymphokine production by macrophage inhibition studies.
4. Mixed lymphocyte culture.
5. Lymph node biopsy for determination of architecture and cellular content.
6. Enzyme assays for adenosine deaminase and purine nucleoside phosphorylase content of RBCs.

With information from the history, physical, and specific immunologic tests, the nature of a patient's immune deficiency should be characterized.

Evaluation of B Lymphocytes

The end product of B lymphocyte function is specific antibody in serum. The concentration of serum immunoglobulin does not indicate that B lymphocytes are functioning normally or abnormally. For example, there is an immune deficiency disease in which serum immunoglobulin levels are normal; however, the individual does not respond with specific antibody production following immunization with an antigen. Probably the best way to evaluate B lymphocyte function is by immunization. In this regard, immunization with typhoid vaccine can be used to measure IgG antibody response to the typhoid H antigen and an IgM antibody response to the typhoid O antigen. A recall antigen that can be used for measuring secondary immune responses is tetanus toxoid.

There are various ways in which B lymphocytes can be quantitated using receptors on the B cell surface. B lymphocytes possess immunoglobulin on the cell surface. Such immunoglobulin may serve as a receptor for specific antigen. However, the presence of immunoglobulin can be used to detect and characterize B lymphocytes. This can be done using a fluorescein-labeled anti-immunoglobulin serum. The fluorescein-labeled antiserum will bind to immunoglobulin present on the surface of lymphocytes, and such cells can then be enumerated.

Recently, monoclonal antibody reactive to B lymphocytes has become available (CD 19, CD 20, CD 22). Such antibody can be used to identify B lymphocytes by reacting to a specific antigenic site that is present on B but not on T lymphocytes.

A nonspecific mitogen (an agent that will induce lymphocytes into mitosis without previously having been exposed to the lymphocytes) for B lymphocytes is pokeweed mitogen (PWM). When incubated with PWM, B lymphocytes are induced into mitotic division. Such mitotic activity can be measured by incorporating radioactive thymidine into newly synthesized DNA.

Immunoglobulin release by B lymphocytes can be quantitated in various ways. These in vitro assays allow determination of the function of B lymphocytes in the presence of normal or abnormal T lymphocytes. This type of procedure can be used to determine if B lymphocytes are capable of synthesizing immunoglobulin when obtained from individuals with humoral immune deficiency diseases. Mixing B lymphocytes from a patient with common variable immune deficiency disease with normal T helper lymphocytes reveals that some individuals with this disease have normal B cells, but they are inhibited from functioning owing to T cell abnormalities present in the patient.

T Lymphocyte Evaluation

The easiest way to quantitatively determine the presence of T lymphocytes is by determining the absolute lymphocyte count in the peripheral blood. Assuming a lower limit of normal of 1500 lymphocytes/mm^3 and 80 per cent of peripheral blood lymphocytes being T lymphocytes, an indication of an absolute depression of T lymphocytes is obtained when the absolute lymphocyte count is below 1200/mm^3.

An in vivo functional assay of T cells is the delayed hypersensitivity skin test. The delayed hypersensitivity skin test reaction evolves through an interaction of different cell populations and soluble mediators. An approximation of these interactions is as follows. Following introduction of the antigen into the skin, lymphocytes in their normal passage through that site are exposed to the antigen. Very few of these lymphocytes are actually sensitized to the antigen. However, when one of the sensitized lymphocytes encounters the antigen, it undergoes a series of changes that primarily involve the release of soluble mediators. One mediator has the property of inducing lymphocytes that are not reactive to the antigen into mitosis. Such a factor may be called blastogenic factor. The blastogenic factor induces the nonsensitized lymphocytes into mitosis and, thus, increases the number of lymphocytes accumulating at the site of antigen injection.

An additional factor released from the sensitized lymphocytes is called transfer factor. Transfer factor is capable of converting lymphocytes that are not reactive to an antigen to lymphocytes that are reactive to the antigen. Thus, while lymphocytes are accumulating at the site, they are being converted to lymphocytes reactive to the antigen. In this way, there is an increase in lymphocytes responding to the antigen and releasing soluble mediators.

Further factors released from the sensitized lymphocytes have the capability of attracting phagocytic cells to the site of reaction. Such cells include polymorphonuclear leukocytes, eosinophils, and macrophages. Other factors activate the phagocytic cells, particularly the macrophages, producing a cell population that is capable of injesting and eliminating the foreign antigen at the site. Factors inhibitory to cell migration, such as leukocyte inhibition factor and macrophage inhibition factor, are released.

To allow the accumulating cells out of the vasculature and into the tissue, a substance called skin reactive factor, which has the capability of releasing histamine from mast cells, is released. This results in an increased vascular permeability and migration of the various cell populations into the tissue in an attempt to eliminate the antigen.

The reaction takes approximately 48 to 72 hours to reach its maximum. Following this, the reaction gradually declines. There are many reasons why the reaction declines. Some of these involve the production of substances that neutralize the various mediator factors released from the lymphocytes. These neutralizing substances would then inactivate the various driving factors of the reaction.

The suppressor lymphocyte population also is a factor in shutting off the reaction. Following exposure to an antigen, the suppressor lymphocytes become stimulated and active at a slower rate than does the effector T lymphocyte population. Therefore, the initial reaction is to produce the delayed hypersensitivity reaction, but as the suppressor lymphocytes become activated, they will shut off the reaction.

On occasion, the reaction does not shut off and produces a very severe chronic reaction in an individual. When this occurs, topical steroids have to be used, and on occasion, steroids must be injected into the rejection site.

If an individual fails to respond to a variety of delayed hypersensitivity challenges, the individual can be considered anergic. The state of anergy indicates a likely defective functional T cell system. However, it should be remembered that delayed hypersensitivity skin test reactions are recall reactions, and the individual must have been exposed to that agent before becoming positive to the delayed hypersensitivity skin test. In addition, it is not uncommon to find a patient with malignancy who will produce delayed hypersensitivity skin test reactions to recall antigens. However, such an individual may fail to respond to a newly encountered antigen. The antigen usually used to sensitize an individual for delayed hypersensitivity skin testing is dinitrochlorobenzene.

There are a variety of in vitro functional tests that can be performed to assess the T lymphocyte population. These include their reaction to nonspecific mitogens, which can induce cell division in lymphocytes that have not previously been exposed to that mitogen. Such substances include phytohemagglutinin (PHA) and concanavalin A (con A). These two mitogens probably stimulate different T lymphocyte populations, with con A probably stimulating more suppressor lymphocytes. However, both of these nonspecific mitogens stimulate not only T lymphocytes, but also some B lymphocyte populations.

A specific mitogen is an agent to which T lymphocytes have been previously sensitized. Upon reexposure to this mitogen, the lymphocytes will be induced into mitotic activity. An example of a specific mitogen is candida or tetanus toxoid. Like nonspecific mitogens, the specific mitogens stimulate not only T lymphocytes, but also some B lymphocytes.

The most reliable test for mitotic activity of T lymphocytes is allogeneic stimulation. In this procedure, lymphocytes from the individual being evaluated are incubated with lymphocytes from a normal individual. The normal lymphocytes have been treated so that they cannot be induced into mitosis. If the responding cells see antigens on the stimulating cell population that differ from their own, they will be induced into mitotic activity. The responding cells are only T lymphocytes. The stimulating cell in this reaction is the B lymphocyte.

Other functional tests of T lymphocyte function relate to the ability of the cells to release soluble mediators that influence other cell populations. An example of this is a factor called macrophage migration inhibition factor (MIF) and leukocyte inhibition factor (LIF). The assay most commonly used is the LIF test. In this procedure, lymphocytes from the individual being evaluated are incubated with an antigen to which the individual may have been sensitized. If the lymphocytes are sensitized to that antigen, they will release a substance called LIF. This substance has the property of preventing migration of polymorphonuclear leukocytes on a solid surface. The inhibition of migration of the polymorphonuclear leukocytes is an indication that LIF was released by sensitized lymphocytes. A positive test would indicate that an individual has been sensitized to the antigen being evaluated. The macrophage migration inhibition factor assay utilizes guinea pig macrophages as the indicator system. This test is more difficult to perform and does not correlate as well as the LIF test to positive delayed hypersensitivity skin test responses.

There are, in addition, procedures that allow one to functionally characterize B lymphocytes, T helper cells, and T suppressor cells. Such assays involve the quantitation of the number of B lymphocytes that synthesize antibody and how they are influenced by the presence of T helper or T suppressor cells. In addition, the functional activity of T helper cells or T suppressor cells can be measured by their ability to promote or inhibit various in vitro cellular immune responses of a normal lymphocyte population.

The various lymphocyte populations can be quantitated in blood and tissue using monoclonal antibodies. There are currently available monoclonal antibodies to the total T lymphocyte population, T helper lymphocytes, T suppressor lymphocytes, monocytes, natural killer cells, and B lymphocytes. These antibodies will react with surface membrane markers on the various lymphocyte populations. Using these antibodies, and very sensitive means of identifying to which cells such antibodies are bound, one can identify and quantitate each of the cell populations. This is especially useful if one is examining tissue to determine what type of immune response may be producing tissue disease.

A common procedure is to characterize lymphocyte subpopulations in various immunologically mediated diseases. For example, in autoimmune disease, one tends to find a decrease in the suppressor cell population. One could hypothesize that this is etiologically related to the presence of the autoimmune disease. Whether or not this is true will require extensive investigation. However, as more diseases are studied, interesting lymphocyte population alterations are being detected. For example, some patients with the common variable immune deficiency disease are now known to have an excessive number of suppressor lymphocytes. The suppressor lymphocytes are capable of inhibiting immunoglobulin production by B lymphocytes. The B lymphocyte population is entirely normal in these patients. Previous to these studies, it was thought that all patients with common variable immune deficiency disease had a defect in their B lymphocyte population. Thus, it is possible that diseases that were lumped together can be subcategorized based on a more detailed immunologic investigation.

A review of immune deficiency diseases follows and is outlined in Table 2–2.

B CELL DISORDERS

IgA Deficiency

This is the most common type of immunodeficiency, with a frequency of approximately 1:500. Although many IgA deficient patients are normal, these patients may present at any age with recurrent sinopulmonary infections and may develop chronic pulmonary disease. Treatment consists of antibiotic therapy, since IgA replacement is not feasible and may cause anaphylaxis in patients who have synthesized anti-IgA antibodies.

The cause for this defect is unknown; postulated causes include T suppression specific for IgA-secreting cells, a lack of T help for IgA-secreting cells, or an inability to release IgA from cells.

A patient with serum IgA may lack IgA in secretions owing to a lack of secretory piece, which is essential for IgA transport across epithelial cells. Tests for the presence of IgA and secretory piece in tears are available.

Acquired IgA deficiency has been associated with hydantoin and D-penicillamine therapy.

Common Variable Immunodeficiency

Common variable immunodeficiency (CVI) is characterized by low or absent levels of IgG, IgA, or IgM. It may be noted at any age. As with IgA deficiency, respiratory infections may be prominent; however, conjunctivitis, septicemia, and meningitis are also common. Diarrhea due to *Giardia lamblia* is noted frequently. Autoim-

Table 2–2. IMMUNE DEFICIENCY DISEASES

Disorder	Immunologic Alterations	Etiology	Symptoms
B Cell			
Selective IgA	IgA	Unknown	Recurrent sinopulmonary infection
Common variable	IgG, A, M	Variable	Recurrent bacterial infection at any age
X-linked	IgG, A, M	Absent B cells	Recurrent bacterial infection at 3–6 months
Transient hypogammaglobulinemia	IgG, A, M; specific Ab present	Delayed maturation of B cells	Recurrent bacterial infection at 3–6 months
T Cell			
DiGeorge	T cell function; normal B cell function	Dysgenesis of III and IV pharyngeal pouches	Recurrent viral, fungal, and parasitic infection; hypocalcemia
Nezelof	T cell function; variable B cell studies	Multiple	Infections similar to above, but less severe
AIDS	T cell function; H/S ratio	HTLV-III	Fever, weight loss; candida, CMV, pneumocystis; Kaposi's sarcoma
Mucocutaneous candidiasis	Absent T cell response to candida	Unknown	Progressive candidiasis of skin and nails
Combined Disorders			
Severe combined (SCID)	Severe T and B cell dysfunction	Multiple	Infection with multiple agents; diarrhea
Wiskott-Aldrich	Normal T IgM cell number responses to specific Ag; IgM	Unknown	Recurrent infection; eczema; thrombocytopenia
Ataxia-telangiectasia	IgA; T cell function	? Developmental defect	Sinopulmonary infection; telangiectasia; cerebellar ataxis

mune disorders such as hemolytic or pernicious anemia, alopecia, and arthritis are associated with this disorder.

As CVI appears to have multiple etiologic factors, immunologic studies may determine the defect in an individual patient. Causes include lack of B cells, excessive T cell suppression or inadequate T cell help, or an inability for B cells to secrete immunoglobulins that they synthesize.

A patient with CVI and recurrent infections should receive immunoglobulin therapy in an attempt to prevent chronic pulmonary damage. Patients who develop diarrhea should be tested for giardiasis.

X-linked Infantile Hypogammaglobulinemia

This was the first immune deficiency recognized, being described by Bruton in 1952. Male infants become symptomatic with chronic bacterial infections at about 5 to 6 months when maternal IgG has declined. Patients respond well to antibiotic therapy, but become reinfected when therapy is discontinued.

Hypogammaglobulinemia will be apparent on serum protein electrophoresis (SPE). Total immunoglobulin levels are less than 250 mg/ml. B cells are absent in blood and markedly decreased in lymph nodes. Specific antibody responses are also absent. T cell functions are present.

Treatment consists of antibiotic therapy and gamma globulin replacement.

Transient Hypogammaglobulinemia of Infancy

In young children, immunoglobulin deficiency may be temporary owing to delayed maturation of the B cell system. Recurrent respiratory or ear infections begin at 3 to 6 months when maternal IgG in the infants has been catabolized. Differentiation between X-linked gammaglobulinemia and transient hypogammaglobulinemia of infancy is not always easy. The presence of isohemagglutinins and antibody levels to specific antigens (such as diphtheria and tetanus toxoid, to which most infants have been immunized) are felt to favor the diagnosis of transient hypogammaglobulinemia. Also, B cells may be present in the circulation, as opposed to X-linked hypogammaglobulinemia. Patients generally do not require immunoglobulin replacement, although this would be indicated in patients with severe infection or growth retardation. Therapy should be discontinued periodically to allow determination of endogenous immunoglobulin levels. Most often, normal immunoglobulin synthesis begins by 24 months of age.

T CELL DISORDERS

DiGeorge's and Nezelof's Syndromes

These disorders are felt to be secondary to an isolated T cell defect; however, B cell function may be partially disordered because of a lack of T cell cooperation.

DiGeorge's syndrome is the result of abnormal development of the III and IV pharyngeal pouches, with resulting dysgenesis of the thymus gland and parathyroids. Patients present in the newborn period with tetany secondary to hypocalcemia. The thymic shadow on the chest radiograph is absent. Abnormalities of the face, including hypertelorism and low set ears, and of the trachea, esophagus, heart, and great vessels are also criteria for DiGeorge's syndrome. As one might predict, fungal, viral, and parasitic infections predominate. T cell numbers are low, and functional tests are abnormal. B cells are present and immunoglobulins are usually normal.

Nezelof's syndrome is similar to DiGeorge's syndrome but does not have the associated features of hypocalcemia or physical abnormalities. These patients generally are not as ill as are patients with DiGeorge's syndrome, but fail to thrive and have thrush, chronic diarrhea, viral illnesses, and pneumocystis pneumonia. T cell numbers and functions are again decreased; immunoglobulins may be normal, increased, or slightly decreased. B cell numbers are normal.

Some cases of T cell deficiency have been attributed to deficiency of the enzyme purine nucleoside phosphorylase (PNP), which catalyzes the conversion of inosine to hypoxanthine and of guanosine to guanine. This causes an accumulation of deoxyguanosine, which is postulated to be toxic to T cells, therefore causing a selective T cell deficiency.

Treatment for these disorders is imperfect. Reconstitution of T cell immunity by thymus transplantation has been successful in some cases; graft versus host disease has also been reported in these patients. Some cases of PNP have been treated with RBC transfusions, which contain the deficient enzyme.

Chronic Mucocutaneous Candidiasis

Unlike more severe immunodeficiency syndromes, chronic mucocutaneous candidiasis (CMC) is secondary to a restricted defect in T cells that is limited to an inability to fight infection due to candida. Patients may present from childhood to young adulthood with thrush, followed by progressive candidal infection of the skin and nails. A high incidence of endocrine abnormalities such as hypoparathyroidism, Addison's disease, diabetes, and hypothyroidism is noted in these patients.

Patients are immunologically normal excepting a negative delayed skin test to candida and negative lymphocyte stimulation to candida. The most specific test for this disorder is failure of lymphocytes stimulated with candida to produce macrophage inhibitory factor (MIF).

Treatment with antifungal medication, while not curative, can check the patient's disease. Life span for these patients is normal.

COMBINED T AND B CELL DISORDERS

Severe Combined Immunodeficiency

The diversity of features of patients with severe combined immunodeficiency (SCID) reflects the diversity of causes, many of which are probably yet unknown. This syndrome consists of severe T and B cell dysfunction and generally causes death by 2 or 3 years of age if untreated. Infection with pneumocystis or candida, intractable diarrhea, and disseminated reaction to live vaccines are common. Patients are agammaglobulinemic and lymphopenic with an absence of lymphoid tissue.

Bone marrow transplantation for stem cell reconstitution is the most successful therapy for most cases of SCID. About 60 per cent of transplants are successful if an HLA-matched donor is available. Transplantation with cultured or fetal thymic cells or with fetal liver has also been reported to be successful. RBC transfusions may be successful in treating some cases of adenosine deaminase (ADA) deficiency.

Wiskott-Aldrich Syndrome

This disorder is characterized by a triad of thrombocytopenia, eczema, and recurrent infection. Petechiae due to the low platelet count are often noted in the neonatal period. Eczema and recurrent infection of a progressively severe nature are commonly seen within the first year.

Immunoglobulin levels are abnormal, often with a pattern of elevated IgA and IgE levels and decreased or normal IgM and IgG. Immunoglobulin production, especially to polysaccharide antigens, is abnormal, although B cells are present. Lymphocyte numbers and proliferation to mitogens are apparently normal, but lymphocyte responses to specific antigens are often absent.

The pathogenesis of Wiskott-Aldrich syndrome is as yet unknown. Treatment is aimed toward controlling infections with antibiotic and platelet support for periods of bleeding. High-dose immunoglobulin replacement has been helpful in some cases. An increased incidence of lymphoid malignancy has been observed.

Ataxia-Telangiectasia

Characteristic features of ataxia-telangiectasia include recurrent sinopulmonary infection, oculocutaneous telangiectasia, and progressive cerebellar ataxia. Immunoglobulin levels are variable, but IgA deficiency is noted in over 50 per cent of the cases. B cells, including IgA-staining B cells, are normal or only slightly decreased. T cells may be decreased, and only a small number of patients respond to delayed hypersensitivity skin tests. Lymphoid tissue mass is decreased; the thymus appears arrested in an immature state.

The cause of this disorder is obscure. It has

been postulated that abnormal tissue development is present, as evidenced by persistent alpha-fetoprotein in the sera of many of these patients. A defect in DNA repair is also noted.

Treatment is limited to antibiotic therapy for the recurrent respiratory infections. An increased incidence of malignancy is a major cause of death in this syndrome.

Acquired Immune Deficiency Syndrome (AIDS)

Recently, a virus has been identified that has been termed the immunodeficiency virus (HIV), which primarily infects T helper lymphocytes and produces their destruction. These patients have an immunologic deficiency disease in which they cannot produce an adequate immune response to infectious agents requiring T cell–mediated reactions. They may also have immunologic suppression due to the relatively high number of T suppressor cells present in their circulation. This disease is primarily confined to male homosexuals, hemophiliacs, and intravenous drug users. However, it has been detected in females and some individuals who have been in close contact with individuals with the disease.

REFERENCES

Bellanti JA: Immunology III. Philadelphia, WB Saunders, 1984.

Stites DP, Stobo JD, Wells VJ: Basic and Clinical Immunology. Vol 6. Norwalk, Appleton and Lange, 1987.

Wedgwood RJ, Rosen FS, Paul NW: Primary Immunodeficiency Diseases. Birth Defects: Original Article Series. Vol 191. New York, Alan R Liss, 1983.

CHAPTER 3

Immunopathology of Autoimmune Disease

Bruce S. Rabin, M.D., Ph.D.

AUTOIMMUNITY

One of the more perplexing problems in both medicine and immunology concerns the immunologic differentiation of "self" from "non-self." Why should anyone develop a pathologic immune response to his or her own tissue antigens? Alternatively, why does not everyone react to his own antigens? Unfortunately, there are no simple or unified answers to these questions. However, recent studies have led to the theories that may, in certain circumstances, explain the development of autoimmunity. Further, these concepts of disease pathology suggest potential new approaches to therapy of patients with autoimmune diseases.

We will define autoimmune disease as "pathologic processes that are either *caused by* or *associated with* the action of an immune response (either cellular or humoral) against self antigens." The critical factors in this definition are the terms "caused by" and "associated with." In the former, the pathologic processes are initiated by a self-directed immune response. In this case, the disease cause is immunologic. In the latter circumstance, the primary event is tissue damage due to nonimmunologic processes. However, the injury elicits an immune response that may perpetuate the pathologic state. Such a condition may be viewed as a disease associated with an autoimmune response.

The criteria for classifying a disease process as involving autoimmune processes, as delineated by Milgrom and Witebsky,[1] are (1) the presence of either a circulating antibody or cell-mediated immune reaction that is directed at antigens of the target organs; (2) the identification of a specific antigen within the involved organ that is the target of the immune response; (3) the immunization of experimental animals with this specific antigen must elicit an immune response; (4) the disease must be produced in an experimental animal; (5) the disease can be transferred from an immunized animal to a normal recipient by serum and/or immunologically competent lymphocytes.

IMMUNOGENETICS

The predisposition to develop an autoimmune disease may partially be determined by genetic factors. For example, it is well known that most autoimmune conditions show a higher occurrence rate within families with one affected individual,[2] and females are more frequently affected than are males.[3] Recently, it has been shown that the sex difference associated with the spontaneous occurrence of autoimmune disease in experimental animals can be altered by castration.[4] Normally, in autoimmune prone strains of animals, the female develops the disease earlier and more severely than does the male. Castration of the male converts the disease course to the female pattern. In animal models, such as New Zealand mice, genetic factors clearly determine disease susceptibility. The New Zealand black (NZB) mouse develops an autoimmune hemolytic anemia, whereas the offspring of an NZB/NZW mating (F1 hybrids) develop a lupus-like glomerulonephritis.[5]

A large number of human autoimmune diseases have been found to be significantly correlated with certain HL A antigens. Table 3–1 lists a number of these and expresses the association in terms of the "relative risk," defined as the risk of getting a disease when a specific HL A antigen is present versus when it is absent. The most striking disease association is that of ankylosing spondylitis and HL A–B27. Approximately 90 per cent or more of individuals with ankylosing spondylitis are positive for HL A–B27.

Environmental factors have been found to have an important role in the development of autoimmune disorders, as monozygotic twins frequently show discordance for HL A-associated diseases. In addition, there is no simple mendelian mode of inheritance. However, familial transmission is noted in many of the HL A-associated diseases, and family studies of ankylosing spondylitis probands have suggested that susceptibility to this disease demonstrates a pattern of inheritance consistent with an autosomal dominant trait.

A significant number of autoimmune diseases are associated with the HL A–A1, B8, and DR3 haplotype. These include Sjögren's disease, idiopathic Addison's disease, Graves' disease, and insulin-dependent diabetes mellitus. In general, the associations with HL A–DR3 demonstrate greater relative risks than with HL A–A1 or B8, suggesting that the D-linked genes may be exerting a greater influence. As the HL A–D locus is analogous to the I region of the murine major histocompatibility complex (MHC), which controls the immune response gene products, it has been postulated that specific HL A–D types may be associated with immunoregulatory dysfunctions.

Knowledge in the area of HL A and disease has been rapidly expanding and will continue to increase as other HL A markers such as DP and DQ are studied in relationship to disease associations. In addition to providing us with information on both the histocompatibility complex and mechanisms of genetic predisposition to disease, additional associations may be found that will be of diagnostic and clinical value.

Table 3–1. ASSOCIATIONS BETWEEN HL A ANTIGENS AND SELECTED DISEASES

Condition	HL A	Relative Risk
Congenital adrenal hyperplasia	B47	15.4
Ankylosing spondylitis	B27	87.4
Reiter's disease	B27	37.0
Acute anterior uveitis	B27	10.4
Subacute thyroiditis	B35	13.7
Psoriasis vulgaris	Cw6	13.3
Dermatitis herpetiformis	DR3	15.4
Celiac disease	DR3	10.8
Sicca syndrome (Sjögren's disease)	DR3	9.7
Idiopathic Addison's disease	DR3	6.3
Graves' disease	DR3	3.7
Insulin-dependent diabetes	DR3	3.3
	DR4	6.4
Myasthenia gravis	DR3	2.5
Systemic lupus erythematosus (SLE)	DR3	5.8
Idiopathic membranous nephropathy	DR3	12.0
Multiple sclerosis	DR2	4.1
Optic neuritis	DR2	2.4
Rheumatoid arthritis	DR4	4.2
IgA nephropathy	DR4	4.0
Hydralazine-induced SLE	DR4	5.6
Hashimoto's thyroiditis	DR5	3.2
Pernicious anemia	DR5	5.4

IMMUNE ACTIVATION

The concept of T-B lymphocyte cooperation is essential to an understanding of how some autoimmune diseases occur. The exact mechanisms involved in T-B cooperation are not known, but it appears that with complex antigens, the T cell reacts with one portion of the immunogenic molecule, whereas the B cell reacts with another region.[6] For example, the T helper cell may react with a carrier protein, whereas the B cell responds to a hapten (Fig. 3–1).

The response is determined by the ability of both the T and B cells to respond to antigenic determinants on the same molecule. This concept is essential to the understanding of the theories of autoimmunity to be presented.

In a genetically susceptible individual, five theories have been proposed to explain the development of immune responses directed at self antigens. These include: (1) sequestered antigen theory; (2) antigenic similarity between

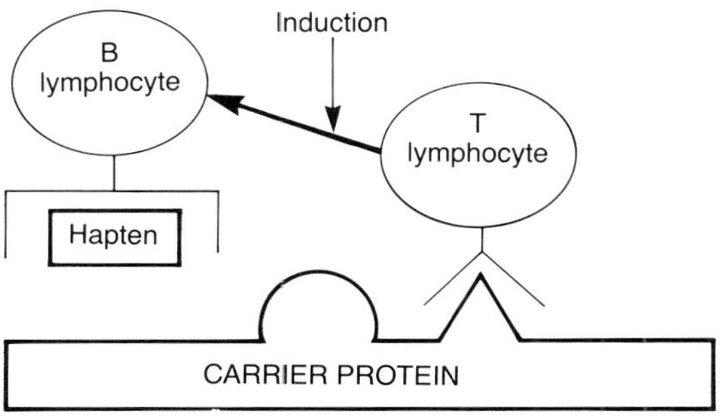

FIGURE 3–1. Interaction of T and B lymphocytes with an antigen. For a B lymphocyte to react to a hapten, it must be induced by a helper T lymphocyte. In this figure, the T lymphocyte is reacting to an antigenic site on the carrier protein. Note that the B lymphocyte and T lymphocyte do not have to interact with the same antigenic site for the B lymphocyte to produce antibody.

tissue constituents and exogenous antigens; (3) breakdown of tolerance by alteration of self antigens; (4) alteration of lymphocytes controlling the immune response; and (5) polyclonal B lymphocyte activation.

Sequestered Antigen

The sequestered antigen theory states that during embryogenesis, certain antigens are shielded or hidden from lymphoid cells. As such, these antigens do not elicit a tolerant state (self-tolerance). If the sequestered antigens are released into the circulation and contact competent lymphocytes, the immune system cannot distinguish these antigens from foreign immunogens and responds as if they were of exogenous origin. The disease sympathetic ophthalmia is believed to result from this mechanism. Normally, the lens of the eye is a hidden antigen. However, a traumatic injury to an eye can expose lens antigens. As a result, lymphocytes reactive to the individual's own lens can develop. In some, these autoreactive cells can cause opacification of the noninjured lens.

It appears that the sequestered antigen theory has limited applicability. In most circumstances, host antigens are not hidden from the immune system. Rather, other mechanisms appear to prevent the development of autoreactive cells.

Cross-Reacting Antigen (Antigenic Similarity)

A second theory of autoimmunity involves antigenic similarities between self antigens and those of an exogenous agent. An immune response directed at foreign antigens elicits an antibody response that can cross-react with self antigens. Antibodies elicited by certain strains of beta-hemolytic streptococci may react with myocardial antigens.[7] The sera of approximately 55 per cent of patients with rheumatic fever contain an antibody to beta-hemolytic streptococci that reacts with myocardial but not other tissue. The pathogenesis of acute rheumatic fever is considered to be as follows: a beta-hemolytic streptococcal infection elicits an immune response that, in susceptible individuals, is capable of cross-reacting with myocardial tissue and thus inducing an autoimmune carditis. Another example of cross-reacting antibodies are those elicited by *Mycoplasma pneumoniae*, which also react with the I antigen of human red cells.[8] These cross-reacting antibodies can cause a transient autoimmune hemolytic anemia of the cold-agglutinin type.

In order for cross-reacting antibodies to interact with self antigens, there must be a breakdown of tolerance to the self antigen. Experimentally, this can be shown to occur in mice rendered tolerant to bovine serum albumin (BSA). By definition, after tolerance has been established, these animals will not respond to BSA challenge. However, if challenged with a closely related protein, horse serum albumin (HSA), the mice will develop an antibody response to both BSA and HSA (Fig. 3–2).

Alteration of Self Antigen

By employing a cross-reacting antigen, naturally occurring autoreactive B lymphocytes can be activated.[9] This has been shown in rabbits. Thyroglobulin alone will not elicit an immune response. However, if thyroglobulin is coupled to a chemical hapten, immunization will stimulate T lymphocytes to react with the hapten portion of the complex. These helper cells can then induce a B lymphocyte response, which includes cells elaborating antithyroglobulin antibodies. The thyroglobulin is a self antigen; the hapten is foreign. The T lymphocytes stimulated

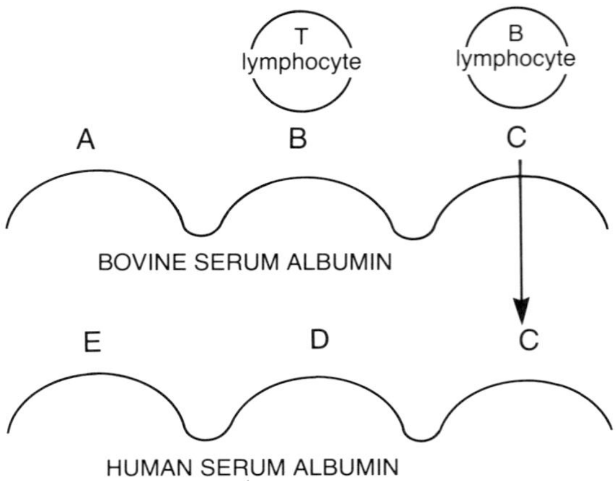

FIGURE 3–2. Bovine serum albumin containing antigenic sites A, B, and C. The antigenic site C is also present on serum albumin. The cross-reacting antigen (bovine serum albumin) allows the T lymphocyte to react with antigenic site B, thus inducting the B lymphocyte capable of reacting to site C. When the B lymphocyte reacts to site C on bovine serum albumin, it can also cross-react to the identical site C on human serum albumin. Thus, an immune response can occur to a self antigen.

to react to the hapten can serve to activate B lymphocytes capable of synthesizing antibodies to self antigens.

This theory of autoimmunity also postulates a breakdown of tolerance. However, in this instance, the breakdown is a consequence of an alteration in a self antigen rather than a response to a cross-reacting antigen.

In order to maintain tolerance, an antigen must be present in the natural or unaltered state. If structurally changed, it will elicit an immune response. This can be accomplished by physical, chemical, or biological factors. Physical changes, such as those found in areas of inflammation, may lead to aggregation and/or other changes in the structural integrity of an antigen. If chemicals combine with antigens, the foreign substances may then function as a hapten and, by stimulating an appropriate population of T cells, activate autoreactive B cells.

Several biological agents may alter self antigens. The most commonly implicated agents are the myxoviruses.[10] The mechanisms for viral breakdown of tolerance are not fully known. In part, they may be related to the viral enzymes, which include neuraminidase, an enzyme capable of splitting sialic acid from proteins and thus exposing new antigen sites. Alternatively, at some point during its life cycle, the virus may be represented on the cell membrane of an infected cell. This can provide the antigenic stimulus needed to induce activation of T helper cells, which in turn could stimulate a response by autoreactive B cells.

There is evidence that tolerogens can induce lasting changes in mature B cells themselves. Mice injected with deaggregated heterologous immunoglobulins do not respond to subsequent challenge with the antigen in an immunogenic form. B cells from such mice remain unresponsive even after transfer to recipients given supplemental T cells. It is unlikely that these B cells are refractory to stimulation by antigen merely because their surface receptors are already occupied by tolerogen. However, only a few antigens are known to induce this form of tolerance. Tolerance induced by most foreign protein antigens seems to exist primarily in T cells rather than B cells. By contrast, many autologous protein antigens, some of which are immunogenic for mature B cells, appear to have induced the deletion of the corresponding B cells.

It has become clear that this hypothesis for self-tolerance is an oversimplification. Normal animals show evidence of autoimmunity, including circulating autoantibodies and autoantigen-binding B cells.[11–13] These are found even when the autoreactive lymphocytes are known to have been exposed to the corresponding autoantigen from early life.

At some stage in the differentiation of B lymphocytes from stem cells to mature antibody-forming precursor cells, B lymphocytes go through a phase during which contact with antigen induces tolerance. The tolerant state induced in differentiating cells is independent of suppressor cells, and appears to result from inhibited maturation. This is probably how most self-reactive lymphocytes are functionally eliminated. In addition, this type of tolerance exhibits specificity; for instance, B cells reactive with the trinitrophenol hapten are unaffected by the elimination of clones reactive with dinitrophenol.

Obviously this system is not fail-safe, since autoreactive B lymphocytes exist in the adult. Possibly, some autoantigens are not expressed until after the B cells complete their differentiation or because the concentration of autoantigen is too low.

Regardless of how the immune system gets activated by antigenic alteration, the overall effect would be damage to tissue. Such damage may lead to profound physiologic abnormalities as, for example, when associated with a loss of insulin-producing cells of the pancreas. Many autoimmune diseases may result from these types of etiologic processes.

Alteration of Lymphocytes

This theory of autoimmunity is based on alterations in the immune apparatus rather than in the antigenic environment. In normal individuals, development of self-reactive clones of immunologically competent lymphocytes is suppressed. However, if the integrity of the immune system is compromised, such cells may arise and thereby initiate reactions directed at endogenous self antigens. In the present form, this theory represents a modification of Burnet's original postulates regarding "forbidden clones."[14]

There are various experimental indications that the immune system is held in check by a population of lymphocytes commonly referred to as suppressor cells. Immunization of an animal with pneumococcal polysaccharide leads to antibody production. If the animal has its thymus gland removed prior to immunization, there is a marked increase in the amount of antibody produced. This would indicate that a loss of suppressor lymphocytes leads to increased antibody synthesis. In humans with various immunodeficiency diseases, excessive numbers of suppressor lymphocytes are found that inhibit the synthesis of antibody. Depletion of suppressor lymphocytes from peripheral blood in humans leads to the generation of autoreactive B lymphocytes. These observations suggest that as long as the balance between suppression and responsiveness is maintained, normal immunologic function exists. However, once an imbalance occurs, either an immune deficiency disease or an autoimmune disease results.

Suppressor activities have been attributed to a population of thymic-dependent lymphocytes, and therefore abnormal thymic function may be a primary cause of defective regulatory mechanisms. This activity appears to be separable from the other activities of T lymphocytes, i.e., mediators of cellular immunity, "killer" function, and "helper" activity. The role of the suppressor activities of the thymus in autoimmune diseases has been shown to be important in certain strains of mice. Thymectomy in the NZB/W strain accelerates the autoimmune renal disease,[15] whereas adoptive transfer of normal T lymphocytes can retard its progression. This suggests that defective T lymphocyte suppressor activities may be an important facet in the expression of autoimmunity.

Experimental allergic encephalomyelitis (EAE) has provided important additional insights into the regulatory role of T lymphocytes in the genesis of autoimmune diseases. This disease can be produced in several experimental animals by immunization with a myelin protein antigen in complete Freund's adjuvant. By several criteria, it appears that the disease is due primarily to activation of cellular immunity. Although serum antibodies to spinal cord antigens can be demonstrated, it is believed that these are of minor importance in the pathogenesis of EAE.

The route of antigenic administration is essential to the development of EAE. Although it can be regularly produced by suspensions of antigen in complete Freund's adjuvant, it does not occur in animals immunized either intravenously or with incomplete Freund's adjuvant. The latter animals do manifest both humoral and cellular responses to spinal cord antigens in vitro, even though they do not have disease. Thus, in both groups, sensitized lymphocytes of both the T and B cell type are present. However, only those animals that have received the complete adjuvant develop the disease. These differences may be due to the regulatory activities of the immune system. It appears most likely that the resistance to EAE in the group immunized with incomplete adjuvant is due to suppressor factors elicited by this method of immunization. These factors, which may involve a population of thymic-dependent lymphocytes, appear to prevent sensitized T cells from manifesting their activity in vivo.

Further evidence supporting the importance of suppressor T cells has been derived from studies of spontaneous autoimmune thyroiditis in the genetically susceptible obese chicken. In chickens, the production of T or B cells can be controlled by surgically extirpating either the thymus or the bursa of Fabricius. Thymectomized chickens develop autoimmune thyroiditis at an accelerated rate; bursectomy tends to ameliorate the disease. This implies that the thymus or the T lymphocytes derived from this

Table 3–2. ANTIBODIES DETECTED IN THE SERUM OF PATIENTS WITH AUTOIMMUNE DISEASE

Antigen Reactivity of Antibody	Disease Associations
Antinuclear	Systemic lupus erythematous (90–98%)
	Scleroderma (60%)
	Sjögren's syndrome (88%)
	Dermatomyositis (45%)
	Chronic active hepatitis (75%)
	Primary biliary cirrhosis (46%)
	Cryptogenic cirrhosis (38%)
	Rheumatoid arthritis (25%)
Anti-mitochondrial	Primary biliary cirrhosis (94%)
	Chronic active hepatitis (28%)
	Sjögren's syndrome (occasionally)
	Viral hepatitis (67%)
	Cryptogenic cirrhosis (40%)
Anti–smooth muscle	Lupoid hepatitis (75%)
	Primary biliary cirrhosis (50%)
	Alcoholic cirrhosis (50%)
	Chronic active hepatitis (70%)
	Infectious mononucleosis
	Malignant tumors
Anti-thyroid	Pernicious anemia (55%)
	Myasthenia gravis (35%)
	Thyroid autoimmunity states (85%)
Anti–glomerular basement membrane	Glomerulonephritis (Goodpasture's syndrome) (80%)
	Chronic active hepatitis
Anti-adrenal	Addison's disease (50%)
Anti–parietal cell	Pernicious anemia (90%)
	Atrophic gastritis often in conjunction with iron deficiency anemia (in women)
Anti–striated muscle	Myasthenia gravis (30%)
	Myasthenia gravis and thymoma (95%)
	Thymus tumors (some)
Anti–pancreas islet cell	Newly diagnosed insulin-dependent diabetes (80%)
Anti-skin	Intercellular
	Pemphigus vulgaris
	Pemphigus foliaceus
	Linear at basement membrane
	Bullous pemphigoid

central organ may exert a suppressor role in the production of this autoimmune disease.

Polyclonal B Cell Activation

The activation of B lymphocytes by a polyclonal activator may lead to autoimmune disease. Those B lymphocytes with the capability of producing autoantibody can be activated, and an autoimmune disease results.

When self antigen is present in low concentrations, B cells with low receptor reactivities escape tolerance induction and are competent to interact with autologous antigen. However, the affinity of the B cell receptors for self antigens is often too weak to trigger differentiation and antibody synthesis. Polyclonal B cell activators may trigger such B cells to produce antibody of low avidity.

Microbial products are capable of causing polyclonal B cell activation in vivo. Injection of bacterial lipopolysaccharide (LPS) into mice causes the production of circulating anti-DNA antibody.[16] LPS has been used to induce B cells to secrete antibody directed against both syngeneic and allogeneic thymocytes either in vitro or in vivo. This response was of the IgM class and occurred in a variety of murine strains.[17]

These findings suggest that B cells capable of producing autoantibody exist in normal mice and can be activated with polyclonal stimulants such as LPS. It has also been reported that LPS-activated murine spleen cells appear to produce antibodies of the IgM class with specificity for autologous serum albumin.[18]

Clinically, it is commonly recognized that individuals with various immune deficiencies are prone to develop autoimmune diseases. Patients with hypogammaglobulinemia (either the congenital sex-linked form or the acquired type) develop an arthritis similar to rheumatoid arthritis. Although the pathophysiologic processes in this disorder are not fully known, it may result from either chronic viral infections, disordered cellular immunity, and/or deficiencies in T suppressor cells. Evidence has been presented to indicate that deficient T suppressor cell function is of importance in the lupus-like syndromes seen in the NZB mice, and it has been postulated that deficiencies in T cell function are of prime importance in the genesis of autoimmune disease. Although defective T suppressor cells may be one important factor, spontaneous B cell activation may also play a pathogenic role.

As our knowledge of immunology expands, an increasing number of pathologic conditions have been found in which immunologic mechanisms assume an important role in the disease pathogenesis. Even in a disease in which an immunologic change is secondary to tissue alteration, immunopathologic findings are extremely helpful as either diagnostic or prognostic indicators. Table 3–2 lists various autoantibodies and the diseases with which they are associated.

SUMMARY

There is no single definitive explanation that can account for the genesis of all autoimmune diseases. In all probability, no one theory can apply to this spectrum of diseases, and most autoimmune diseases can be viewed as the end result of an interaction involving several factors or different diseases having different etiologic factors. Genetic susceptibility is of prime importance; yet, additional factors are required in order for a disease to manifest itself in a susceptible population. The breakdown of tolerance to self antigens through either exposure to cross-reacting material or alterations of self antigens themselves may be important in many diseases. It appears that these conditions depend on generation of a population of T helper cells that can recognize antigens and stimulate responses by autoreactive B cells.

It is noteworthy that therapy of autoimmune diseases in clinical situations is principally directed at suppressing the activities of effector cells. All currently available treatments can basically be grouped into agents that interfere with the inflammatory response resulting from an immune reaction or those that suppress the initiation of the response. Yet, the currently tenable theories of autoimmunity suggest that in most diseases, the aim of treatment should be directed at (1) eliminating cross-reacting or altered self antigens, or (2) increasing the activities of suppressor cells.

REFERENCES

1. Milgrom F, Witebsky E: Autoantibodies and autoimmune diseases. JAMA 181:706, 1962.
2. Lachmann P: Auto-allergy in Clinical Aspects of Immunology. (Cell PGH, Coombs RPA, eds.) Philadelphia, FA Davis, 1968, pp 597–610.
3. Hooper BA, Whittingham S, Mathews JD, et al: Autoimmunity in a rural community. Clin Exp Immunol 12:79, 1972.
4. Roubinian JR, Papoian R, Talal N: Androgenic hormones modulate autoantibody responses and improve survival in murine lupus. J Clin Invest 59:1066, 1977.
5. Holmes MC Burnet FM: The characteristics of F1 and backcross hybrids between "high leukaemia" (AKR) and "autoimmune" (NZB) mouse strains. Aust J Exp Biol Med Sci 44:235, 1966.
6. Katz DH, Benacerraf B: The regulatory influence of activated T cells on B cell responses to antigen. Adv Immunol 15:1, 1972.
7. Zabriskie JB: Mimetic relationships between group A streptococci and mammalian tissues. Adv Immunol 7:147, 1967.
8. Thomas I: Circulating autoantibodies and human disease with a note on primary atypical pneumonia. N Engl J Med 270:1157, 1964.
9. Roberts IM, Whittingham S, Markay IR: Tolerance to an autoantigen thyroglobulin. Lancet 2:936, 1973.
10. Isacson P: Myxoviruses and autoimmunity. Prog Allergy 10:256, 1967.
11. Elson CJ, Naysmity JD, Taylor RB: B cell tolerance and autoimmunity. Int Rev Exp Pathol 19:137, 1979.
12. Clagett JA, Weigle WO: Roles of T and B lymphocytes in the termination of unresponsiveness to autologous thyroglobulin in mice. J Exp Med 139:643, 1974.
13. Penhale WJ, Farmer A, Irvine WJ: Thyroiditis in T cell depleted rats. Clin Exp Immunol 21:362, 1975.
14. Burnet FM: Autoimmune disease. H. Pathology of the immune response. Br Med J 2:720, 1959.
15. Roubinian JR, Papoian R, Talal N: Effects of neonatal thymectomy and splenectomy on survival and regulation of autoantibody formation in NZB/NZW F_1 mice. J Immunol 118:1524, 1977.
16. Izui S, Lambert PH, Fournie GJ, et al: Features of experimental lupus erythematosus in mice injected with bacterial lipopolysaccharides. J Exp Med 145:1115, 1970.
17. McHugh YE, Bonavida B: Autoreactive antibody forming cells directed against thymocytes and thymus derived lymphocytes. J Immunol 121:1090, 1978.
18. Primi D, Smith CIE, Hammarstrom L, Moller G: Polyclonal B cell activators induce immunological response to autologous serum proteins. Cell Immunol 34:367, 1975.

CHAPTER 4

Clinical Use of Monoclonal Antibodies

Bruce S. Rabin, M.D., Ph.D.

One of the most exciting developments in medicine during the past few years has been the development and clinical application of monoclonal antibodies. Physicians are familiar with the concept of monoclonal immunoglobulin as this is associated with patients with multiple myeloma. In such patients, there is a homogenous or monoclonal immunoglobulin present in the gamma globulin region when a patient's serum is electrophoresed. Many people have wondered what the monoclonal immunoglobulin did in patients with multiple myeloma. The answer always was "nothing," because it was an antibody directed to an antigen that had not been identified. The current excitement about monoclonal antibodies has resulted from the production of these monoclonal immunoglobulins to an antigen that has been selected to have a monoclonal antibody produced to it. In other words, the specificity of the monoclonal immunoglobulin can now be at the discretion of the laboratory producing it.

PRODUCTION OF MONOCLONAL ANTIBODIES

Multiple myeloma is a disease in which there is the malignant proliferation of immunoglobulin-producing plasma cells. All of the plasma cells produce the identical immunoglobulin, since the malignant subpopulation arises from a single cell and is therefore considered to be a clone of cells. The current technology regarding monoclonal antibody production uses malignant plasma cells that will proliferate continually. To have the cells produce the desired monoclonal antibody, they are fused with lymphocytes obtained from animals that have been immunized to the desired antigen. The cell resulting from the fusion is called a hybridoma.

Briefly, monoclonal antibodies are produced in the following manner. A mouse is immunized with the desired antigen, and then a suspension of spleen lymphocytes is fused with malignant plasma cells that are maintained in tissue culture. Tissue culture conditions are utilized so that lymphocytes that have not fused with plasma cells do not proliferate and die. In addition, the plasma cells that have not fused with lymphocytes die in culture. Thus, the only surviving cells are the hybridoma cells. The hybridoma cells have chromosomes from both the lymphocyte and plasma cell. Many of the chromosomes are then extruded from the hybridoma so that a normal number of chromosomes remain.

Not all of the hybridoma cells will be useful. For example, some of the hybridomas may extrude the chromosomes that are responsible for immunoglobulin synthesis. Other hybridomas may produce antibody, but not to the antigen to which the lymphocyte donor animal was immunized. Many of the antibodies represent the normal repertoire of gamma globulin being produced by the immunized animal. Of course, some of the hybridomas will be producing antibody to the desired antigen. The problem is to select those hybridomas for continued growth.

The selection process involves isolating single hybridoma cells in small tissue culture vessels. The individual cells are allowed to proliferate, and the secreted immunoglobulin is then evaluated for its specificity. In this way, only those proliferating hybridomas producing the desired monoclonal antibody are retained. These can then be grown so that large quantities of the desirable antibody are obtained. A diagrammatic representation of the hybridoma process is given in Figure 4–1. Monoclonal antibodies have been developed that may have usefulness in patients with malignancy. For example, monoclonal antibodies can be used to detect antigens associated with tumors in the serum of patients and, thus, provide a means of tumor diagnosis.

Monoclonal antibodies can be produced that will react with malignant tissue and, if the antibodies carry a radioactive marker, may allow the localization of tumor in a patient. In addition, if antibodies can be produced that bind to a tumor, they can be used to carry chemotherapeutic agents to the tumor. These various areas of usefulness of monoclonal antibodies will be reviewed.

MONOCLONAL ANTIBODIES TO DETECT MALIGNANCY

Some tumors release hormones or antigens that are present only during fetal development. Highly sensitive procedures are needed to detect the substances in the serum, and these procedures must be reliable to provide accurate quantitation. Monoclonal antibodies can be produced to these substances and, because of their high degree of specificity, they will have no reactivity to other substances. Thus, only the material that is meant to be measured will actually be detected. Examples include the measurement of carcinoembryonic antigen, which may be associated with colonic or pancreatic malignancy; the beta subunit of human chorionic gonadotropin, which may be associated with embryonal carcinoma; and alpha-fetoprotein, which may be associated with the presence of hepatoma. If a patient is known to have a malignancy, the presence of these circulating substances can be used to evaluate the response to chemotherapy or surgery; and if they return to normal levels after treatment of the malignancy, they can be used to determine if recurrences have taken place.

MONOCLONAL ANTIBODIES TO LOCALIZE TUMORS

If monoclonal antibodies can be prepared to antigens present on solid tumors, and if the antigens are fixed to the surface of the tumor cell, radioactively labeled antibodies may be used to identify where metastases are. This would involve a collaboration between nuclear medicine and immunology laboratories for the production and detection of the localized antibody. Such procedures can also be used to determine changes in size of metastases of tumors that do not release a circulating antigen that could be measured.

MONOCLONAL ANTIBODIES AS THERAPEUTIC AGENTS

A most exciting area for the potential use of monoclonal antibodies is in the treatment of malignancies. Ideally, a monoclonal antibody would be prepared to an antigen present on a tumor, the antibody would be infused into the patient, and the tumor would be destroyed by the antibody. However, as is usually the case, the ideal may not easily be achieved.

For example, as was previously mentioned, some tumors release tumor-related antigens from their surface, and these antigens are found in the circulation. If a monoclonal antibody were prepared to one of these antigens and infused into the patient, the antibody would be neutralized in the circulation and not reach the target tissue. In such a case, a means would have to be found to remove the circulating antigen. Possibly, this could be achieved by plasmapheresis or passing the plasma over an insoluble matrix with the monoclonal antibody bound to it to remove the circulating antigen.

Another problem relates to the concept termed antigenic modulation. This occurs when an antibody reacts to an antigen present on a

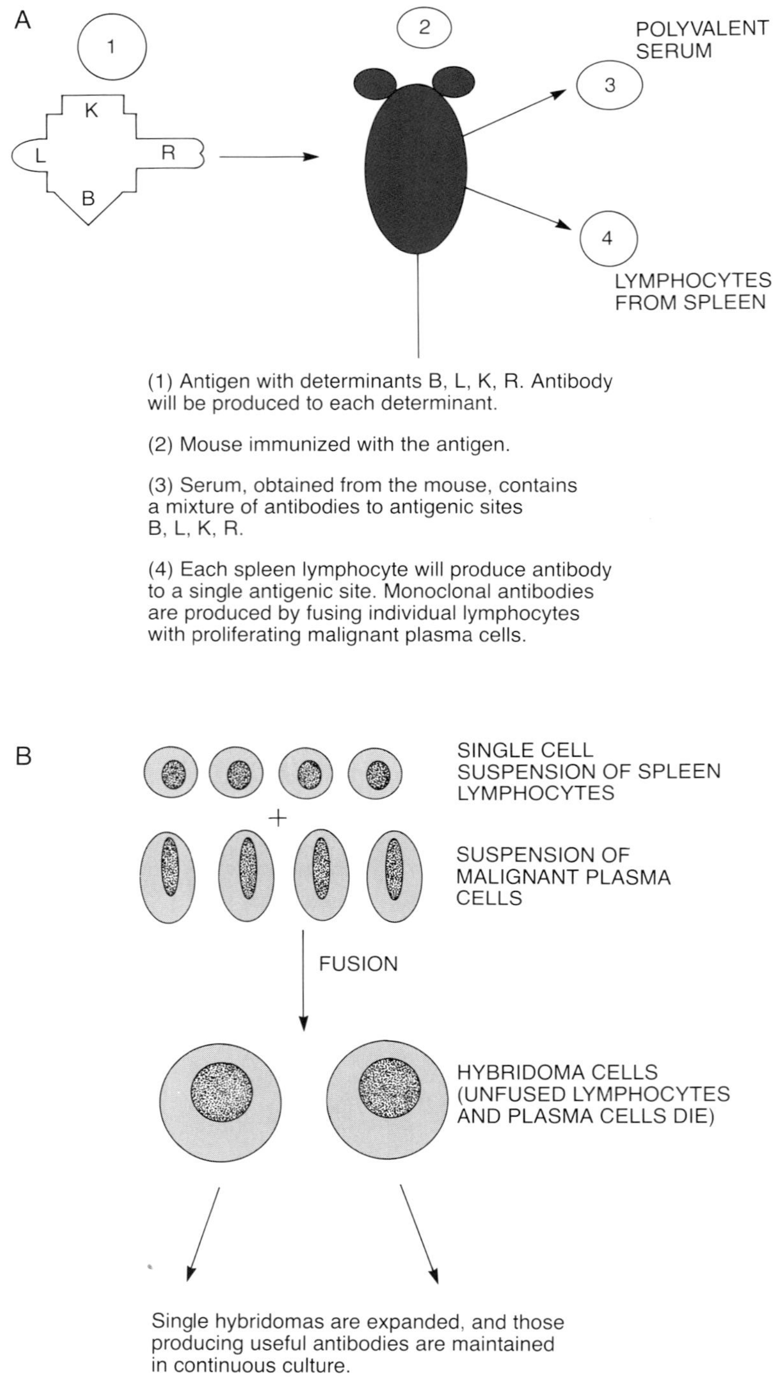

FIGURE 4–1. Schematic representation of production of monoclonal antibody. *A,* Following immunization, each spleen lymphocyte produces antibody to a single determinant on the antigen. A single cell suspension of spleen lymphocytes is fused to malignant plasma cells. The fused cells are called hybridomas. *B,* The fused cells will continue to grow, whereas the individual lymphocytes and malignant plasma cells will die in tissue culture. The hybridoma cells are isolated as single cells in tissue culture. The isolated cells multiply so that large quantities derived from single cells are available. The antibody produced by these clones of cells is then evaluated; those clones producing antibody to the desired antigenic determinant are maintained, and the antibody is used for the purpose for which it was produced.

cell surface. The antigen eventually disappears from the cell surface and does not reappear. Thus, the antibody is no longer useful. Obviously, if this occurs, more than one antibody will be needed. The antibodies will have to react to different antigens present on the cell surface and would be used sequentially.

The vast majority of monoclonal antibodies being made today are mouse immunoglobulin. However, it is possible to produce monoclonal antibodies of human origin. In this case, the plasma cell used for the fusion would be from a human, and the lymphocyte fused to it would be from a human donor. Although this may offer some advantages in that it is less likely to get an antibody produced by the recipient of the monoclonal antibody to human immunoglobulin than to mouse immunoglobulin, it is possible that such human antibodies would not have the same clinical usefulness for treating malignancies. When one species is immunized with tissue from another, the species immunized frequently recognizes many antigens present on the tissue with which it is being immunized. However, if the tissue were injected into a member of the same species from which the tissue was taken, only a few of the antigens would be recognized. Therefore, if a human malignant tissue were immunized into a human, it is unlikely that very many of the tumor-specific antigens would be recognized. Thus, immunization of a mouse with a tumor is preferable. There are various ways in which monoclonal antibodies can destroy the tissue to which they are targeted. One obvious way is by activation of the complement system with a subsequent lysis of the target tissue. However, human complement is not very efficient to produce lysis of solid tissue. A promising approach for the destruction of tissue by monoclonal antibodies is by the coupling of toxins to the antibody. The toxin most commonly used is ricin. Ricin is composed of two subunits, an A chain and a B chain. The A chain mediates the toxic effect, since this is an enzyme capable of irreversible inhibition of ribosomal protein synthesis in the cytoplasm. However, the A chain cannot bind to the cell or penetrate the cell membrane unless it is conjugated to the B chain. By having the toxin bound to a monoclonal antibody, it does not indiscriminately bind to various cells but is, rather, delivered to the target tissue. Other toxins may also be found to be useful in this regard.

MONOCLONAL ANTIBODIES DEFINING LYMPHOCYTE POPULATIONS

A good example of how monoclonal antibodies can be used to obtain information regarding patients with malignancy is provided by studying the use of these antibodies to define different lymphocyte subpopulations. At one time, we thought of lymphocytes as being either small, medium, or large. Then we learned that there were two types of lymphocytes: the B lymphocyte, which produced immunoglobulin; and the T lymphocyte, which was active in delayed hypersensitivity reactions. Subsequently, we learned that T lymphocytes consisted of suppressor lymphocytes, which regulate the immune response; cytotoxic lymphocytes, which are reactive to foreign antigens; and helper lymphocytes, which promote the immune response. Monoclonal antibodies have been developed to define the different T lymphocytes. These monoclonal antibodies can be used to identify the different types of lymphocytes in the circulating blood or in tissue (Table 4–1).

An indirect way in which monoclonal antibodies are being found useful is in bone marrow transplantation between individuals who are not

Table 4–1 MONOCLONAL ANTIBODIES DEFINING LYMPHOCYTE SUBPOPULATIONS

Antibody*	Antigen Cluster Definition	Lymphocyte Population
Leu 4 OKT 3	CD 3	95% of mature T lymphocytes
Leu 3 OKT 4	CD 4	The helper-inducer T lymphocyte subset, 40–60% of mature T cells
Leu 2 OKT 8	CD 8	The suppressor-cytotoxic T lymphocyte subset, 20–40% of mature T cells
Leu 11	CD 16	5–20% of peripheral blood mononuclear cells, including those cells responsible for natural killer activity
Leu 18	—	Labels the suppressor lymphocytes within the Leu 2 population
Leu–DR OKT Ia	—	5–25% of peripheral blood lymphocytes; includes B lymphocytes, monocytes, and activated T cells

*Leu is the designation used by the Becton Dickinson Company. OKT is the designation used by the Ortho Company.

identical for the major transplantation antigen. If bone marrow is transplanted from one individual into another, and the two individuals are not identical for the major transplantation antigens, a graft versus host disease will occur. Monoclonal antibodies can be used to render the transplanted marrow compatible with the recipient.

To accomplish this, all mature T lymphocytes must be removed from the donor bone marrow. Monoclonal antibodies directed to T lymphocytes can be used to accomplish this. This leaves immature T lymphocytes present in the bone marrow. Immature T lymphocytes have not yet developed thymus markers. As the immature T lymphocytes go through various maturation steps in the new host environment, they should become tolerant to the bone marrow transplant recipient. The new marrow will then repopulate the recipient lymphoid system without producing a graft versus host disease.

SUMMARY

Monoclonal antibodies are homogenous immunoglobulin proteins produced to an antigen that has been preselected. These antibodies react to specific sites on the antigen and, if the antigen is part of the cell surface, can mediate a destructive response against that cell. The antibodies may be useful in patients with malignancies to detect tumor-related antigens in patient serum, to localize the presence of metastatic disease, and therapeutically. The technology of monoclonal antibodies is rapidly emerging and will soon be part of our routine procedures in treating patients with malignancy.

REFERENCES

1. Blythman HE, Casellas P, Gros O, et al: Immunotoxins: hybrid molecules of monoclonal antibodies and a toxin subunit specifically kill tumor cells. Nature 290:145, 1981.
2. Dillman RO, Shawler RE, Sobol RE, et al: Murine monoclonal antibody therapy in two patients with chronic lymphocytic leukemia. Blood 59:1036, 1982.
3. Gilliland DG, Steplewski Z, Collier RJ, et al: Antibody-directed cytotoxic agents: use of monoclonal antibody to direct the action of toxin A chains to colorectal carcinoma cells. Proc Natl Acad Sci 77:4539, 1980.
4. Goldberg DM, Deland FH: History and status of tumor imaging with radiolabeled antibodies. J Biol Response Mod 1:121, 1982.
5. Kohler G, Milstein C: Continuous cultures of fused cells secreting antibody of predefined specificity. Nature 256:495, 1975.
6. Miller RA, Maloney DG, McKillop J, Levy R: In vivo effects of murine hybridoma monoclonal antibody in a patient with T-cell leukemia. Blood 58:78, 1981.
7. Miller RA, Maloney DG, Warnke R, Levy R: Treatment of B cell lymphoma with monoclonal anti-idiotype antibody. N Engl J Med 306:517, 1982.
8. Neville DM, Youle RJ: Monoclonal antibody-ricin or ricin A chain hybrids: kinetic analysis of cell killing for tumor therapy. Immunol Rev 62:75, 1982.
9. Ritz J, Schlossman SF: Utilization of monoclonal antibodies in treatment of leukemia and lymphoma. Blood 59:1, 1982.
10. Rogers GT, Rawlins GA, Bagshawe KD: Somatic-cell hybrids producing antibodies against Lea. Br J Cancer 43:1, 1981.

CHAPTER 5

Immunologic Aspects of Aging and Nutrition

Bruce S. Rabin, M.D., Ph.D.

The activity of the immune system changes with aging.[1] Cellular immune mechanisms often decrease, whereas levels of serum immunoglobulin may increase. In addition, humoral immune responses directed to self antigens (autoantibodies) become more frequent in the aged population. The alterations in the aging immune system have been compared to a graft versus host reaction. It has also been suggested that the thymus may be the "aging clock" for the immune system.[2]

Autoreactive changes occurring in the immune system with longevity may produce secondary tissue changes that are lumped together as "aging." Maintenance of the immune components that inhibit the development of age-related autoreactivity may be reflected in an improved quality of health during aging. Regardless of whether the maximum life span is extended, it is possible that maintenance of a normal immune system during aging will lead to less chronic disease in the latter part of the life span. An increase in maximum life span may then be secondary to a decreased incidence of chronic disease.[3] Another way to view this is to consider self antigens as being more than benign bystanders whose only purpose is to elicit antibody production.

It is likely that most self antigens play a role in normal physiologic function. Thus, such antigens may be receptors on cell surfaces or involved with cellular transport mechanisms. Humoral or cellular immune responses directed to these physiologically active antigens may impair their function and lead to biochemical and physiologic changes associated with the aging phenomenon.

It is well established, in experimental animals, that alterations of a normal diet can lead to a depression of immunologic responsiveness. If it can be established that a decrease in immunologic responsiveness results in a decreased propensity to manifest autoimmune disease, this could be considered beneficial. Assuming that autoimmune responses participate in the aging phenomenon, a prolongation of life may result from a decrease in immunologic competency. On the other hand, decreased immunologic system function may produce an increased susceptibility to infectious disease. One of the prime theories of autoimmunity states that antigenic alteration is secondary to infectious diseases and leads to the development of autoimmune disease. In this case, such altered antigens may accelerate the aging phenomenon by promoting the onset of autoimmunity. The primary concern of studies in the immune system, and through this alterations in the aging process, has to be finding a balance in which beneficial effects are not overridden by detrimental effects from another aspect of the immune system.

NUTRITION AND IMMUNITY

A limited number of investigations have been done to study nutritional alteration of the immunologic system and its effect on aging.[4] Strains of animals that show an increased incidence of autoimmunity as they age have a life span shorter than animals that fail to develop autoimmunity during aging. This may be taken to indicate that if the immune system allows the development of autoimmune disease, a decreased life span will result. Indeed, there is abundant evidence in humans that there is an increased incidence of autoantibodies with aging. One could, however, argue that the presence of autoantibodies is protective rather than harmful. Those individuals who do not produce autoantibodies may have a shortened life span in comparison with individuals who produce autoantibodies. The increased frequency of autoantibodies in the aged population is then reflective of their protective effect.

Various nutritional factors have been evaluated for their effect on the immune system. These include the amount of food ingested, the composition of the diet, and the timing and length of dietary manipulation. All have been found to exert an influence on the immune system as manifested by immunologic responses to exogenous antigens and both spontaneous and experimentally induced autoimmune disease.

The effect of protein-calorie malnutrition on immunologic responsiveness has been studied in both mice and rats. In comparison with a control diet, the antibody response to Salmonella was shown to be reduced 50 per cent by feeding mice a diet consisting of 90 per cent of a control diet supplemented with 10 per cent sucrose. A similar reduction of antibody formation to sheep erythrocytes has also been noted by protein-calorie restriction. This reduction can be partially corrected by injection of thymocytes into the protein deficient animals. This suggests that T cell activity is primarily altered by protein deprivation. However, it has also been reported that an increased immunologic responsiveness to sheep erythrocytes may occur in association with protein restriction. The 19S antibody response may be affected more than the 7S antibody response.[5]

Whereas a decreased antibody response has been reported in some experiments, with the suggestion of an increased antibody response in others, cellular immune functions such as graft versus host reactions and skin graft rejection have been consistently reported to be increased in intensity in protein-calorie malnutrition. However, in severely malnourished animals, an increased survival of skin grafts has been reported to occur. Thus, in each experiment, it is important to determine what is meant by malnutrition. The duration of the diet, concentration of each component, strain of animal, age when the animal is started on the experimental diet, and source of protein in the diet must be noted.

It is possible that protein-calorie malnutrition selectively affects lymphocyte subpopulations. A decrease in suppressor lymphocyte activity following injection with sheep red blood cells or polyvinylpyrrolidone has been reported in mice receiving a protein-restricted diet. It is possible that such observations are influenced by the extent of protein reduction and the duration of time the animal is on the diet.

NUTRITION AND AUTOIMMUNITY

A striking amelioration of severity and a delay in onset of spontaneously occurring systemic lupus erythematosus in the NZB/NZW mouse have been produced by a protein-calorie malnutrition. The concentration of circulating immune complexes is reduced in the serum of the NZB/W mice, and this may be a prime factor in the altered clinical course of disease in the protein-calorie malnourished animals. Interestingly, calorie restriction has been shown to decrease the concentration of serum thymic factor. The relationship of decreased serum thymic factor to the ameliorated disease course in NZB/W mice needs to be investigated. Serum thymic factor concentration can also be decreased by either a zinc or pyridoxine deficiency.[6, 7]

An example of altering an experimentally induced immunologic disease by dietary manipulation is suggested by a model of alloxan-induced diabetes. This disease fails to develop in animals maintained on a protein deficient diet. It has been suggested that this experimentally induced disease results from an immune response directed against alloxan-damaged beta islet cells. Animals lacking T cell function fail to develop the disease. Thus, protein-calorie malnutrition, which is known to alter cellular immunity, may be influencing the T lymphocyte population in preventing developing disease.

Another example of an immunologically induced disease that is altered by nutritional factors is adjuvant-induced arthritis. This disease does not develop in animals that have been deprived of copper, magnesium, or zinc.

Several reports have indicated that mineral concentration can induce an effect on the immune system. The element that has been most extensively studied is zinc. Zinc deficiency leads to a depression of both cellular immunity and antibody production in experimental animals. The weight of the thymus and lymph nodes is usually decreased in zinc deficiency. There is a discrepancy regarding the activity of natural killer cells, with one report indicating increased activity and another indicating decreased activity in zinc deficiency.

As with protein-calorie malnutrition, the immune response to sheep erythrocytes in zinc deficient animals can be restored by injecting thymocytes into the animals prior to immunization. This suggests that zinc deficiency primarily affects the T helper cell population. In zinc deficiency, IgG antibody production to sheep erythrocytes is more markedly affected than is IgM antibody production. It has also been shown that zinc deficiency does not exert its immunosuppressive effect by causing the adrenal glands to secrete increased amounts of steroids.[8]

One experiment has been reported that indicated an effect of zinc deficiency on autoimmunity and, potentially, the aging phenomenon. Autologous rosette formation was determined in C57LBL mice. These cells have been reported to be lymphocytes that are capable of manifesting autoimmune responses. In the presence of zinc deficiency, there was an increase in the number of autorosette-forming lymphocytes present in the spleen. Animals fed an increased concentration of zinc did not have a depression of autologous rosette-forming cells in comparison with animals fed a normal diet. Thus, an inadequate amount of zinc in the diet may predispose to the development of autologous rosette-forming cells and, potentially, cells that can manifest autoimmune responses.

It has been well established that a decreased amount of food intake is associated with an increase in the life span of experimental animals. A decreased intake of protein or various minerals alters the functional capacity of the immune system. It has been suggested that a primary factor in the aging phenomenon is an autoimmune response directed to self antigen. Thus, if altered nutrition is capable of suppressing autoimmune responses, the result may be an increase in life span.

REFERENCES

1. Makinodan T: Retrospect and prospect. *In* Biology of Aging. New York, Plenum Press, 1977, p 1.
2. Kay MMB: An overview of immune aging. Mech Ageing Dev 9:39, 1979.
3. Walford RL: Immunology and aging. Am J Clin Pathol 74:247, 1980.
4. Gerbase-Delima M, Meredith P, Walford RL: Immune function and survival in a long-lived mouse strain subjected to under-nutrition. Gerontologia 21:184, 1975.
5. Mathur M, Ramalingaswami V, Deo MG: Influence of protein deficiency on 19S-antibody forming cells in rats and mice. J Nutr 102:841, 1972.
6. Fernandes G, Yunis EJ, Good RA: Influence of diet on survival of mice. Proc Natl Acad Sci USA 75:1279, 1976.
7. Chandra RK, Heresi G, Au B: Serum thymic factor activity in deficiencies of calories, zinc, vitamin A and pyroxidine. Clin Exp Immunol 42:332, 1980.
8. DePasquale-Jardieu P, Fraker P: Further characterization of the role of corticosterone in the loss of humoral immunity in zinc deficient A/J mice. J Immunol 124:2650, 1980.

CHAPTER 6

Stress and the Immune System

Bruce S. Rabin, M.D., Ph.D.
Donald T. Lysle, Ph.D.
Joan E. Cunnick, Ph.D.

The interrelationship between the central nervous system and the immune system is both obvious and subtle. As early as the 19th century, physicians observed a relationship between melancholia and the incidence of cancer in women.[1]

More recent evidence of an interaction between the central nervous and immune systems was obtained through studies of conditioning.[2] Exposing rodents to a conditioned stimulus that had been paired with an immunomodulating agent, such as cyclophosphamide, produced changes in humoral and cellular immunity. Such conditioning can be biologically relevant, as has been demonstrated by substituting conditioned stimuli for immunosuppressive agents in NZB mice, an animal model of autoimmune disease.[3]

The interaction between the central nervous system and the immune system does not appear to be unidirectional. For example, multiple sclerosis and Guillain-Barré syndrome are diseases whose pathogenesis is related to immune reactions in either central or peripheral nervous tissue. However, the relationship between the immune system and other central nervous system diseases is less well established. This chapter examines in detail the possible mechanisms for a connection between the central nervous system and the immune system.

CNS–IMMUNE SYSTEM PATHWAYS

The autonomic nervous system and the hypothalamic-pituitary axis are two pathways that must be considered when examining the interaction between the CNS and the immune system. There is extensive evidence implicating an immune connection for both of these pathways.

There have been direct demonstrations of lymphoid tissue innervation by sympathetic and parasympathetic nerves. There is evidence of innervation of the thymus, bone marrow, spleen, lymph nodes, and gut-associated lymphoid tissues.[4] These findings suggest a direct interaction between the central nervous and immune systems.

Using chemical sympathectomy,[5] it has been shown that the number of antibody-producing cells in the spleen of rats is increased following injection of sheep erythrocytes. Surgical sympathectomy of the superior cervical ganglion has also been shown to enhance the immune response to sheep erythrocytes. There are also studies indicating that mice subjected to sympathectomy have reduced antibody responses following immunization.[6] These differences, along with other research, indicate that the species of the animal, the age, sex, and strain of the animal, and the antigen being used are just some of the factors that may influence the effect of sympathectomy on immunologic function. Regardless of these complexities, it is clear that immunomodulation can occur by modification of the sympathetic innervation of lymphoid tissue.

A direct functional connection between the central nervous system and the immune system has been demonstrated by the production of lesions in the CNS. Destruction of posterior or anterior parts of the hypothalamus of rodents leads to decreased immune reactivity,[7, 8] whereas electrical stimulation of the hypothalamus leads to an increase in antibody production.[9, 10] In an immunized animal there is an increase in electrical activity of neurons of the hypothalamus at the peak of the immune response.[11] In humans who have brain tumors, a tumor affecting the left side of the brain leads to an impairment of in vitro phytohemagglutinin (PHA) responsiveness, but right-sided cerebral tumors do not affect PHA responses.[12]

HORMONE MEDIATORS

The cells of the immune system possess receptors for various hormonal mediators, which can bind to the lymphocyte surface. Many of these hormones are produced by the nervous system and thus allow the immune system to react to neural regulation. Such hormones can functionally alter lymphocytes and are important in the determination of how the brain influences immunologic function.

Endorphins are a group of endogenous brain polypeptide hormones. It has been found that naturally occurring peptides can exert opiate-like effects in the brain by interacting with opiate receptors on cell membranes. Enkephalins are pentapeptides that are also classified as endorphins. Both beta-endorphin and enkephalin may bind to lymphocytes and have been found to both enhance and suppress immune function.[13, 14] Whether there is enhancement or suppression of immune function may depend on the concentration of the neuropeptide, the cell population being assayed, and the species studied.[15, 16]

The effect of the opiate-like hormones on the function of the immune system has been evaluated both in vitro (using rodent and human lymphocytes) and in vivo. Alpha-endorphin inhibits the primary, in vitro, antibody response of human peripheral blood lymphocytes to ovalbumin when present in low concentration (5.0 μg/ml), but does not interfere with the response when present at 10 μg/ml.[17] Alpha-endorphin can also inhibit the in vitro antibody response of mouse spleen lymphocytes to sheep erythrocytes.[18] Both leu- and met-enkephalin inhibit the response to sheep erythrocytes, but are less effective than is alpha-endorphin. Beta-endorphin, from which alpha-endorphin is split, can decrease the response of human peripheral blood lymphocytes to PHA in vitro when present at concentrations of 10^{-7} to 10^{-9} M.[19] Leu-enkephalin has also been reported to decrease the mitogenic response of human lymphocytes to PHA.[20]

Some reports indicate that enhancement of in vitro reactivity of lymphocytes occurs by incubation with hormones such as beta-endorphin or leu- and met-enkephalin. Human, mouse, and rat lymphocytes have been studied. Responses such as increased proliferation to PHA, enhancement of the plaque-forming cell response to ovalbumin, and increased natural killer cell activity have all been reported. However, the mechanism of enhancement or supression of immune reactivity by brain-related hormones has not been well characterized. It is known, however, that beta-endorphin does not work by binding to the IL–2 receptor.[21, 22]

Other hormones, such as adrenal steroids, have been implicated in immunomodulation. In regard to the effect of adrenal steroids on immunologic function, a variety of conflicting results have been published. Part of this problem may be due to the varying response of different species to the effect of adrenal steroids. Some species are extremely sensitive to corticosteroids (rat, mouse, rabbit), whereas other species are relatively resistant to these effects (human, monkey, guinea pig). Species that are sensitive to corticosteroids have lymphocytes that are lysed by pharmacologic levels of the hormone. Thus, in any studies, species must be considered.

Clinical observations of increased susceptibility to infection with elevated adrenal hormone levels have been extensive.[23–26] A variety of experimental approaches, which use a stressor and quantitate adrenal cortical hormone production, indicate that elevated levels of the hormone produce immunologic suppression. In addition, in vitro studies and in vivo situations in which adrenal hormone levels are experimentally elevated indicate the immunosuppressive effects of adrenal hormones. These studies showed impairment of neutrophil migration and lymphocyte function.[27–29] Moreover, adrenal cortical steroid hormones have been found to increase the absolute number of neutrophils in the peripheral blood of a patient and decrease the number of lymphocytes.[30]

Although there is substantial evidence to indicate that adrenal cortical hormones induce suppression of the immune system, the relationship is extremely complex. The influence of adrenal cortical hormones on the immune system seems to depend on the species, type of assay, and concentration of adrenal cortical hormone as well as the subpopulations of lymphocytes assayed. Thus, more research is needed to clarify the relationship among the adrenal corticosteroids and the immune system.[30–34]

Several other hormones may be involved in the regulation of the immune system. The possibility that prostaglandin E_2 (PGE_2) participates in the immunologic suppression associated with stress has been suggested.[22]

Interestingly, there is evidence that lymphocytes produce hormones such as ACTH and endorphin, which may themselves regulate immune function.[35] Thus, there is considerable interaction between the central nervous and immune systems, and possibly even internal control loops of neuropeptides that are produced by the immune system to regulate its function.

STRESS AND DISEASE

Stress is believed to be capable of influencing disease susceptibility. It is of interest that many of the diseases whose onset or exacerbation is associated with the presence of a stressful condition are believed to have immune reactivity to tissue as part of their pathogenesis. Thus, it is possible that the influence of stress on functioning of the immune system may have clinically relevant sequelae.

Obviously, clearly defined etiologic relationships between stressful life events and the onset of disease are difficult to causally relate to each other. However, considerable epidemiologic data show that such a relationship does exist.

The onset of Crohn's disease has been associated with the patient's undergoing stressful life events.[36, 37] Examples of stressors associated with Crohn's disease include bereavement, pregnancy, marriage or divorce, and relocation. The analysis of pooled studies comprising over 150 patients has found that stress is related to both the onset of disease and relapse.

The onset of insulin-dependent diabetes, a disease with an immune pathogenesis, is frequently associated with stress.[38, 39] Death of a child's parent, divorce, and separation correlate with disease onset. Those environmental factors, in addition to immunologic factors, are believed to be associated with the onset of insulin-dependent diabetes.

The onset and severity of rheumatoid arthritis has also been reported to be associated with stress.[40] Female patients with rheumatoid arthritis are found to be more nervous, tense, worried, and moody than their healthy female siblings. One factor affecting the course of disease may be related to the integrity of the patient's psychological defenses. Those patients who experience emotional decompensation are more likely to have a rapidly progressing disease with more incapacitation and a poor response to medical therapy.[40]

Recurrences of uveitis are seen in individuals who have recently lost spouses or who undergo other stresses such as divorce, business losses, or failure to pass an examination.[41] There are also indications that the course of malignant disease may be related to the presence or absence of stress.[42, 43]

Extrapolation of these observations suggests that stress influences the pathogenesis of many disease states and has some direct effect on immune system function.

STRESS

What is meant by stress? The term "stress" has been used in a variety of ways, and consequently it has acquired various meanings. For our purposes, there are two aspects to a stressful experience. First, it involves the presentation of an aversive or nonpreferred stimulus that is referred to as a stressor. A stressor may be either physical or psychological. Examples of physical stressors are prolonged heat or exertion. A psychological stressor is bereavement or the expectation of adversity. Second, the stress response refers to the physiologic and psychological changes induced by a stressor. The combination of a stressor and a stress response is what we refer to as stress.

The processing of a psychological stressor by the central nervous system may differ from the processing of a physical stressor. The psychological stressor must be perceived as a stressor by the brain, whereas a physical stressor may exert its effect without cortical processing. It has not yet been determined whether the changes induced in response to a stressor are the same for psychological and physical stressors or for two different types of physical or emotional stressors.

The release of hormones by various organs of the body is a well-documented response to a stressor. The hormonal response may be derived from the hypothalamus, pituitary, adrenal gland, or lymphocytes.[44] The effect of the stress-related hormones may alter function of a variety of endocrine organs, produce changes in the vasculature, alter functioning of the sympathetic or parasympathetic neurons, or produce changes in immunologic function.

A variety of animal species have been studied in experiments designed to determine the effect of stress on immune system function. In evaluating such studies, a number of variables that can influence the results must be considered. Among these are the type of stressor, the chronicity of the stressor, the way in which the stressor is administered, the species of animal, the strain of animal, the age of the animal, the compartment of the immune system evaluated, and the sex of the animal. In addition, nonregulated factors related to housing, such as the temperature of the animal room, the frequency and care with which cages are cleaned, and extraneous noise in the room, may all serve as stressors that influence the immune responsiveness of the animal in addition to the actual stressor being measured.

Sex differences in mortality have been well documented for a wide range of vertebrate and invertebrate species, including humans.[45–47] For example, the life span of females exceeds that of males for 12 of 17 strains of in-bred and outbred mice in which data have been reported. A significant contributor to the mortality differences is a sex difference in susceptibility to infection and disease, which may reflect, at least in part, differential responsiveness of the immune system. Although numerous exceptions exist with regard to species, age, and specific disorder, there is a clear general trend toward greater male vulnerability.

These findings point out the difficulty in generalizing in regard to how stress may affect the immune system. Without considering species, strain, and sex, inappropriate conclusions may be reached.

STRESS AND IMMUNITY

Studies in monkeys and humans have indicated that stress may have an influence on immunologic parameters. Monkeys that experienced early separation from their mothers or peers had reduced in vitro responsiveness to both T and B cell nonspecific mitogens.[48] Likewise, nonspecific T cell responsiveness in vitro declines in humans whose spouses die and who are undergoing bereavement.[49] The stress of a pending examination for first-year medical students produces decreased natural killer (NK) cell activity and serum IgA in individuals who score low on tests that measure social adjustment and high on tests assessing loneliness.[50]

An emotional state of well-being has been found to influence immunologic parameters in geriatric patients and individuals with malignancy. In a study of 45 geriatric individuals who received relaxation training, there was an increase in T lymphocyte responsiveness to PHA[51] in comparison to matched individuals who did not receive such training. It has been found that NK cell activity correlates with the spread of cancer to axillary lymph nodes in patients with primary breast cancer.[42] Patients who have high levels of NK activity are generally well adjusted to their illness, whereas patients who have lower NK activity are viewed as distressed or maladjusted.[42]

These findings are consistent with studies in animals showing an enhanced tumor growth for animals undergoing stress as compared to nonstressed animals.[52] It has been suggested that the effect of stress on tumor growth in animals is related to the production of endogenous opiates. It has not yet been determined if this mechanism is responsible for the immunosuppression in humans.

STUDIES IN DEPRESSION

A number of studies of immune function have been carried out in depressed patients. Findings have included decreased T helper cells,[53] decreased responsiveness of lymphocytes to nonspecific mitogens,[54, 55] and decreased natural killer cell activity.[56] Most of these changes, however, could be secondary to the depression, since they are fairly similar to the changes that have been recorded in nonspecific stress.

The response of lymphocytes to mitogens in patients with depression has been negatively correlated with the severity of depression.[55] This may suggest that the immune changes are related to the underlying biologic processes in depression. However, this assertion remains unsupported by experimental evidence at this time.

Another study of depressed patients that looked at corticosteroids and immunologic responses presented some interesting observations.[57] Depressed patients who were resistant to the cortisol-suppressing effect of dexamethasone also showed nonsuppression of their PHA response by dexamethasone. This suggests that in depression, there is a cellular (including lymphocytes) nonsensitivity to the effects of corticosteroids. Once again, it is not clear whether this is simply an "effect" of depression or whether this may be involved in the pathogenesis of some symptoms of the disease.

The effects of stress on the immune system have been demonstrated using various species of animals in combination with various stressors. These effects consist of a measurable decrease of immune responsiveness, an increased susceptibility to infection, and an enhancement of tumor growth. These findings appear to have important implications for health. However, the health implications are probably restricted more to maintaining good quality health in healthy individuals than to treating disease. It is likely that the message passed down from grandparents, "stop worrying so much, you'll get sick," is valid and should be heeded.

REFERENCES

1. Sklar L, Anisman H: Stress and cancer. Psychol Bull 89:369, 1981.
2. Ader R, Cohen N: Behavior and brain. Science 8:379, 1985.
3. Ader R, Cohen N: Behaviorally conditioned immunosuppression and murine systemic lupus erythematosus. Science 215:1534, 1982.
4. Bullock K: Neuroanatomy of lymphoid tissue: a review. *In* Guillemin R, Cohn M, Melnechuk T (eds): Neural Modulation of Immunity. New York, Raven Press, 1985, p 111.
5. Besedovsky HO, del Ray A, Sorkin E, et al: Immunoregulation mediated by the sympathetic nervous system. Cell Immunol 48:346, 1979.
6. Hall NR, McClure JE, Hu SK, et al: Effects of 6-hydroxydopamine upon primary and secondary thymus dependent immune responses. Immunopharmacology 5:39, 1982.
7. Cross RJ, Markesbery MR, Brooks WH, Roszman TL: Hypothalamic immune reactions. I. The acute effect of anterior hypothalamic lesions on the immune response. Brain Res 196:79, 1980.
8. Roszman TL, Jackson JC, Cross RJ, et al: Neuroanatomical and neurotransmitter influences on immune function. J Immunol 135:769, 1985.
9. Korneva EA: Neurohumoral regulation of immunological homeostasis. Fiziol Chel 2:469, 1976.
10. Tsypin AB, Malstev VH: The effect of hypothalamic stimulation on the serum content of normal antibodies. Patol Fiziol Eskp Ter 11:83, 1972.
11. Besedovsky HO, Sorkin E, Felix D, Haas H: Hypothalamic changes during the immune response. Eur J Immunol 7:323, 1977.
12. Blomgren H, Blom V, Ullen H: Relation between the site of primary intracranial tumors and mitogenic responses of blood lymphocytes. Cancer Immunol Immunother 21:31, 1986.
13. Risch SC, Janowsky DS, Judd LL, et al: The role of endogenous opioid systems in neuroendocrine regulation. Psychiatr Clin North Am 6:429, 1983.
14. Weber RJ, Pert CB: Opiatergic modulation of the immune system. *In* Muller EE, Genazzani AR (eds): Central and Peripheral Endorphins: Basic and Clinical Aspects. New York, Raven Press, 1984, p 35.
15. Wybran J: Enkephalins, endorphins, substance P, and the immune system. *In* Guillemin R, Cohn M, Melnechuk T (eds): Neural Modulation of Immunity. New York, Raven Press, 1985, p 157.
16. Shavit Y, Lewis JW, Terman GW, et al: Opioid peptides mediate the suppressive effect of stress on natural killer cell cytotoxicity. Science 223:188, 1984.
17. Heijnen CJ, Bevers C, Kavelaars A, Ballieux RE: Effect of endorphin on the antigen-induced primary antibody response of human blood B cells in vitro. J Immunol 136:213, 1986.
18. Johnson HM, Smith EM, Turres BA, Blalock JE: Regulation of the in vitro antibody response by neuroendocrine hormones. PNAS 79:4171, 1982.
19. McCain HW, Lamster IB, Bozzone JM, Grbic JT: Beta-endorphin modulates human immune activity via nonopiate receptor mechanisms. Life Sci 37:1619, 1982.
20. Wybran J: Enkephalins and endorphins as modifiers of the immune system: present and future. Fed Proc 44:92, 1985.
21. Farrar WL: Relationship between lymphokine and opiatergic modulation of lymphocyte proliferation in en-

kephalins and endorphins. *In* Plotnikoff NP, Faith RE, Murgo AJ, Good RA (eds): Stress and the Immune System. New York, Plenum Press, 1986, p 241.
22. Qui-Shi L, Gui-Zhen Y: Influence of surgical stress on cellular immunity and the induction of plastic adherent suppressor cells of spleen in mice. Immunol Invest 15:419, 1986.
23. Christie BM, Pierson RE, Braddy PM, et al: Efficacy of corticosteroids as supportive therapy for bronchial pneumonia in yearling feedlot cattle. Bov Pract 12:115, 1977.
24. Davies DH, Carmichael LE: Role of cell-mediated immunity in the recovery of cattle from primary and recurrent infection with infectious bovine rhinotracheitis virus. Infect Immun 8:510, 1973.
25. Martin WB, Scott FMM: Latent infection of cattle with bovid herpesvirus 2. Arch Virol 60:51, 1979.
26. Stockdale PHG, Niilo L: Production of bovine coccidiosis with Eimeria zuernii. Can Vet L 17:35, 1976.
27. Crabtree GR, Munck A, Smith KA: Glucocorticoids and lymphocytes. II. Cell cycle–dependent changes in glucocorticoid receptor content. J Immunol 125:13, 1980.
28. Onsrud M, Thorsby E: Influence of in vivo hydrocortisone on some human blood lymphocyte subpopulations. I. Effect on natural killer cell activity. Scand J Immunol 13:573, 1981.
29. Robbins DL, Gershwin ME: Identification and characterization of lymphocyte subpopulations. Semin Arthritis Rheum 7:245, 1978.
30. Johnson LK, Longenecker JP, Bacter JD, et al: Glucocorticoid action: a mechanism involving nuclear and non-nuclear pathways. Br J Immunol 107:6, 1982.
31. Black S, Humphrey JH, Niven J: Inhibition of Mantoux reaction by direct suggestion under hypnosis. Br Med J 346:1649, 1963.
32. Gillis S, Crabtree GR, Smith KA: Glucocorticoid induced inhibition of T cell growth factor production. II. The effect on the in vitro generation of cytolytic T cells. J Immunol 123:1632, 1979.
33. Pierpaoli W, Kapp HG, Bianchi E: Interdependence of thymic and neuroendocrine functions in ontogeny. Clin Exp Immunol 24:501, 1976.
34. Riley V: Psychoneuroendocrine influence on immunocompetence and neoplasia. Science 212:1100, 1981.
35. Blalock JE, Smith EM: A complete regulatory loop between the immune and neuroendocrine systems. Fed Proc 44:108, 1985.
36. Rahe RH: Subjects recent life changes and their near-future illness susceptibility. Adv Psychosom Med 8:2, 1972.
37. Gerbert B: Psychological aspects of Crohn's disease. J Behav Med 3:41, 1980.
38. Leaverton DR, White CA, McCormick CR, et al: Parental loss antecedent to childhood diabetes mellitus. J Am Acad Child Psychiatry 19:678, 1980.
39. Vialette B, Ozanon JP, Bernard D, et al: Stress, immunity and type-I (insulin-dependent) diabetes. Diabetologia 29:A604, 1986.
40. Solomon GF: Emotional and personality factors in the onset and course of autoimmune disease, particularly rheumatoid arthritis. *In* Ader R (ed): Psychoneuroimmunology. New York, Academic Press, 1981, pp 159–182.
41. O'Connor GR: Factors related to the initiation and recurrence of uveitis. Am J Ophthmol 96:577, 1983.
42. Levy SM, Herberman RB, Malvish AM, et al: Prognostic risk assessment in primary breast cancer by behavioral and immunologic parameters. Health Psychol 4:99, 1985.
43. Justice A: Review of the effects of stress on cancer in laboratory animals: importance of time of stress application and type of tumor. Psychol Bull 98:108, 1985.
44. Blalock JE, Bost KL, Smith EM: Neuroendocrine peptide hormones and their receptors in the immune system. J Neuroimmunol 10:31, 1985.
45. Hamilton JB: Role of testicular secretions as indicated by effects of castration in man and by studies of pathological conditions and short life span associated with maleness. 3:257, 1948.
46. Preston SN: Mortality Patterns in National Populations. New York, Academic Press, 1976, pp 136–179.
47. Waldron I, Johnston S: Why do women live longer than men? J Human Stress 2:19, 1976.
48. Laudenslager M, Capitanio JP, Reite M: Possible effects of early separation experiences on subsequent immune function in adult macaque monkeys. Am J Psychol 142:862, 1985.
49. Stein M: Bereavement, depression, stress, and immunity. *In* Guillemin R, Cohn M, Melnechuk T (eds): Neural Modulation of Immunity. New York, Raven Press, 1985, p 29.
50. Kiecolt-Glaser JK, Garner W, Speicher C, et al: Psychosocial modifiers of immunocompetence in medical students. Psychosom Med 46:7, 1984.
51. Kiecolt-Glaser JK, Glaser R, Williger D, et al: Psychosocial enhancement of immunocompetence in a geriatric population. Health Psychol 4:25, 1985.
52. Borysenko JZ: Behavioral-physiological factors in the development and management of cancer. Gen Hosp Psychiatry 4:59, 1982.
53. Krueger RB, Levy EM, Cathcart ES, et al: Lymphocyte subsets in patients with major depression: preliminary findings. Advances 1:5, 1984.
54. Schleifer SJ, Keller SE, Myerson AT, et al: Lymphocyte function in major depressive disorder. Arch Gen Psychiatry 41:484, 1984.
55. Schleifer SJ, Keller SE, Sirsis SG, et al: Depression and immunity. Arch Gen Psychiatry 42:129, 1985.
56. Kronfol Z, Schwartz S: NK-cell activity in depressive illness: preliminary findings. Presented at Society of Biological Psychiatry Annual Meeting, Chicago, May 7, 1987.
57. Lowy MT, Reder AT, Antel JP: Glucocorticoid resistance in depression: the dexamethasone suppression test and lymphocyte sensitivity to dexamethasone. Am J Psychiatry 141:1365, 1984.

CHAPTER 7

Interface: Immunology-Allergy-Otorhinolaryngology

Helen F. Krause, M.D., F.A.C.S.

Many diseases seen by the otorhinolaryngologist, including allergy, recurrent infection, and tumors, are immunologic in origin. A number of their mysteries have already been probed by scientific and clinical research clarifying, for instance, the relationship between immunology and the complex of symptoms called allergy. Also, new scientific data and innovative technology have permitted development of methods for the diagnosis and treatment of such problems in otolaryngic patients. In presenting postgraduate courses in allergy and immunology, it is apparent that students have variable levels of knowledge of immunology. Therefore, this chapter briefly reviews basic elements in immunology as they relate to allergy and to otolaryngology.

Immune responses evolved in vertebrates as an adaptation to the increasing complexity of the environment. As more foreign materials (complex antigens such as bacteria, viruses, tumor cells) challenged the early vertebrates, their immune systems developed commensurate complexity in order to repel the pathologic invaders and to protect the host.

Several special classes of proteins, the antibodies or immunoglobulins, eventually evolved. In addition to their primary protective function, some also play a role in allergic reactions. Allergenic sensitivity involves a multitude of cells, chemical mediators, and immune processes; in fact, defects in the homeostatic system can be elicited at a number of levels.

The primary purpose of the immune system was historically understood to be protection against infection. Later, as studies were extended, it became apparent that the immune system is also implicated in other modes of ensuring homeostasis. In particular, it was found to be involved in what we now call allergy, or hypersensitivity to foreign protein. Further, we have learned that autoimmune disease is produced when the patient reacts to his or her own protein as if it were foreign. In modern medicine, transplantation of organs between nonidentical individuals has been hampered by problems of tissue rejection initiated by the immune system, although drugs designed to suppress the system usually permit it to succeed. Immune deficiency diseases, congenital or acquired, have also been recognized. Some patients, such as those with hypogammaglobulinemia, are treated by transfusions of the deficient immunoglobulin (IgG), whereas others, such as those with AIDS, cannot yet be immunologically corrected. Reported developments in tumor immunology, both in diagnosis and therapy, are increasing in recent literature and symposia. Some of these processes are well understood; others are now being explored.

Perhaps it would be helpful to think of the intact immune system as a roadmap, with multiple paths and highways leading to one main destination, resistance to disease. However, there are many intermediate destinations to explore, most of which are interesting, some exciting, and some devastating. Allergy is one such destination, and the routes to it are determined by the host's immune system responses. These responses are under genetic control, and just as with most genetically controlled systems, the end result—the reaction that we see in the patient—may be modified by the degree of dominance or penetrance of the genes as well as by environmental factors.

The immune system is intricate, involving communication between a number of component parts. As described in Chapter 1, there is a complex interplay of cells and the chemical mediators secreted by them. Of these cells, the most primitive are the phagocytes, which are tissue macrophages and circulating monocytes. These cells transport an antigen via surface receptors to a second set of cells, the lymphocytes. The macrophages are also capable of releasing chemical mediators that regulate various lymphocyte activities. Whereas this is the immunologic function of these cells, their primitive function, their primary role, is phagocytosis of foreign organisms and cells.

LYMPHOCYTES: KEY TO THE IMMUNE SYSTEM

The specific and most important cells of the immune system are the lymphocytes. The B cells form the humoral or immediately reactive cellular system of antibodies; T cells form the specifically reactive memory cell complex that controls the humoral system and regulates cell-mediated delayed sensitivity. Null cells are another lymphocyte group interacting with thymic hormones to develop additional immune capabilities.

Lymphatic stem cells move from the yolk sac to the fetal liver and spleen to begin differentiation, then pass into the marrow of the long bones. They may remain in the marrow from birth into the teens. As the immune system matures and develops its special needs, the stem cells may produce any of the lymphatic cells described—B cells, T cells, or null cells. Cells that travel by way of the thymus, stimulated by the hormone thymosin, are designated T cells. Depending on how they were marked in the thymus, they become specialized as helper or suppressor cells or as null cells. Stem cells destined to become B cells migrate to an unknown point of activation, perhaps in the intestinal epithelial system. There must be constant interaction between the two systems, the humoral (B) and cellular (T), to ensure normal protection and homeostasis. Abnormal reactivity may occur when the two systems are out of balance; illness or disease then results.

All lymphocytes travel by way of the lymphatic and hemopoietic systems to the peripheral lymph nodes. The T cells migrate to the medulla of these lymph nodes, and the B cells into the follicular and deep cortical portions. The B cells mature there until stimulated to become plasma cells that produce immunoglobulins. Using monoclonal antibody technology, it is now possible to differentiate the various types of lymphocytes and to identify what are called subset population levels in an individual patient.

The newly identified null cells, described in Chapter 1, are neither a true T nor a B lymphocyte. One type is involved in antibody-dependent cellular cytotoxicity (ADCC). This particular cell reacts with IgG when it is bound to an antigen, causing cytotoxic activity against the target cell. Another, the NK or natural killer cell, has receptor sites on its surface for eliminating spontaneously occurring malignant cells.

In order to combat some antigens that are presented to the body, a T helper cell is required; hence, they are called T-dependent antigens. Antigens that can directly stimulate B lymphocytes are referred to as T-independent antigens.

An early protective function of the immune system is the development of tolerance to self antigens. T cells with self antigens are eliminated during embryogenesis; therefore, autoimmune disease later in life is forestalled. T cells that survive are those already discussed. B cells are not clonally aborted as are T cells; rather, they are controlled by suppressor T cells to prevent autoimmune reactions.

ANTIBODIES: HISTORY

The term "allergy" was coined by Clemens von Pirquet in the early 1900s to describe a hypersensitivity state acquired through exposure to a specific substance foreign to the body. This term is valid today, for we know that the allergen (or antigen) may, after one or more exposures, stimulate the development of reactive antibodies. In 1921, Prausnitz and Küstner described a "skin sensitizing antibody." Their PK test was developed to identify the presence of a factor in serum that can be transferred to the skin of a nonsensitive patient, conferring sensitivity to a test of the original antigen. We now know that factor to be antibody. Coca and Cooke in 1923 proposed the term "atopy" to describe the types of symptoms we recognize today as allergy, and also coined the terms "reagin" and "reaginic antibody."

Over 40 years passed, during which many attempts were made to identify this reaginic antibody. However, it was not until the middle 1960s that two groups, working independently, were able to do so. Drs. Teruko and Kimishige Ishizaka in Denver, Colorado, knew about mast cells, which had been described in 1877 by Paul Ehrlich; but these were not related to allergy until the 1940s when they were found to release chemicals (especially histamine) when stimulated by allergens. Using themselves and known sensitive patients as experimental subjects with the PK test procedure and serum testing, in 1966 they finally identified the biologic properties of a substance they called gamma E globulin.

Concurrently, Hans Bennich and S.G.O. Johansson in Sweden identified a peculiar protein biochemically in a multiple myeloma patient. This protein, called ND after the patient's initials, was revealed by radioimmunoassay done with the help of L. Wide to be also elevated in patients with allergic disease, but occurred in very low levels in the normal patient. These two groups met in 1968 in Switzerland. There, a World Health Organization agreement concluded that the two substances in question were the same immunoglobulin, to be identified thereafter as IgE. Other groups of immunoglobulins, G, M, A, and D, had previously been identified, yet the riddle of the skin sensitizing antibody was not solved until the two groups identified it.

Also in the middle 1960s, Gell and Coombs described the release of vasoactive amines from mast cells in sensitized target organs as well as four classes of allergic, inflammatory, or hypersensitivity reactions. A Type I reaction is immediate or anaphylactic, involving IgE. Type II is cytotoxic or cytolytic, involving IgE or IgM. Type III involves immune complex reactions. Type IV is the cell-mediated or delayed hypersensitivity reaction (Table 7–1). Recent additions have been Type V, a stimulating antibody reaction, and Type VI, antibody-dependent cell-mediated cytotoxicity involving null cells (see Chapter 1).

IMMUNOGLOBULINS

All immunoglobulins consist of two identical heavy chains linked by disulfide bonds to two identical light chains (Fig. 7–1). The Fab portion is the combining site for antigen; the Fc portion is the site to which complement attaches. IgG is the simplest form of immunoglobulin; IgM is a pentamer; IgA is a dimer in secretions, but a monomer in serum. In secretions, a secretory component attaches by disulfide bonding to the IgA. The J chain (a small, specialized polypeptide chain) is required to link the individual structures to form the polymers of both IgM and IgA. Each immunoglobulin is composed of multiple amino acids, each in a specific order. Like all proteins, each immunoglobulin is composed of many amino acids in a specific order, the

Table 7–1. CLASSIFICATION OF IMMUNE REACTIONS

Type I	Immediate or anaphylactic IgE—histamine, kinins, etc. Allergy—atopy Rhinitis, asthma, urticaria
Type II	Cytotoxic or cytolytic IgE or IgM Antibody binds to tissue, activating complement Hemolytic anemia Goodpasture's syndrome
Type III	Immune complex formation IgG Precipitating antibody + antigen bind and activate complement Produce tissue inflammation
Type IV	Cell-mediated hypersensitivity (delayed) T cells Tuberculin skin test Poison ivy, drug, or food sensitivity reactions
Type V	Stimulating antibody IgG reacts with tissue receptor sites Graves' disease
Type VI	Antibody-dependent cell-mediated cytotoxicity ADCC or K cells + complement + target cell receptor

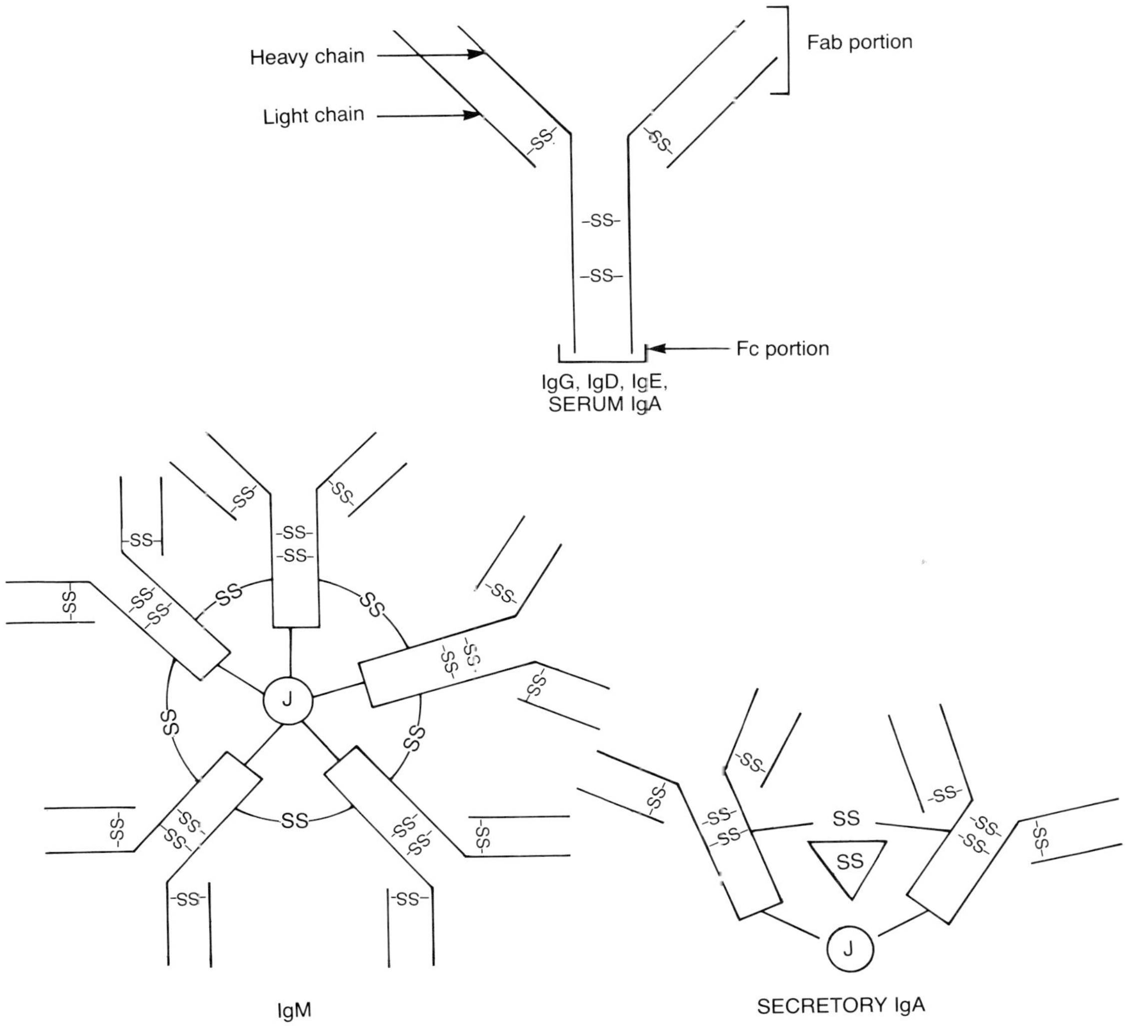

FIGURE 7–1. Basic structure of immunoglobulins. IgG, IgD, IgE, and serum IgA are monomers; IgM is a pentamer; and secretory IgA is a dimer with a secretory component. IgM and secretory IgA also contain J chains.

folding or crinkling of the immunoglobulin molecule producing an antibody-combining site.

Specific antibodies combine with their antigens in a special relationship under genetic control. Previously the relationship was depicted as a lock and key binding. In the early 1980s, research groups identified "hot spots" on various regions of antigens, which appear to be protein portions that antibodies recognize—that is, the antigenic determinants. The antigenic determinants most accessible to antibodies appear to be areas with greater motility in their molecular structure. And, instead of the antibody and antigen binding in a lock and key pattern, this new research suggests that they may be envisioned as two clouds interpenetrating; their fit need not be perfect.

Immunoglobulins, the antibodies, are divided into five classes. Three, IgG, IgA, and IgM, which constitute 85 to 95 per cent of human antibodies, protect normal individuals against bacterial and viral invaders. They may activate complement, producing various other types of reactions, including opsonization, that render invaders more susceptible to phagocytosis, precipitation, agglutination, lysis, or viral neutralization.

IgA is called the secretory immunoglobulin because it is present in mucus membrane secretions, that is, tears, nasal mucus, saliva, bronchial mucus, and vaginal secretions. It is also found in amniotic fluid and colostrum. There are immunoglobulins in vaginal secretions that may be related to infertility. Further, a woman may develop sensitivity to proteins in semen, and anaphylaxis can even result if the semen contains antigens to which the woman is hypersensitive. Increased amounts of IgA are found, along with IgM and IgG, in secretions of the gastrointestinal and respiratory tract of atopic patients. The still-mysterious IgD is found in patients with various collagen and autoimmune diseases, although its actual function is unknown.

Complement is a highly important and fascinating system of nonspecific chemical factors required for interaction with specific antibodies; it operates both in health and in the presence of cellular damage. Complement comprises at least 11 proteins associated with the beta globulin fraction of blood plasma. The sequence of complement activity is reminiscent of a spiral staircase having a few twists and turns, with each step producing only one type of effect (Fig. 7–2). Complement enters the immune system in two pathways, the classic and the later-discovered alternative, or properdin, pathway (Fig. 7–2). It also interacts with other systems in the body to produce a complex of interreactive systems well described in a number of immunology texts.

IgE: HALLMARK OF ALLERGY

On first exposure to an allergen, the reaction is slow. On subsequent exposure, the reaction is faster owing to clonal reproduction of sensitized lymphocytes produced during the first reaction. This, called the anamnestic response, is a specific response resulting in the production of immunoglobulins. It must be differentiated from the nonspecific and more primitive reaction of inflammation called phagocytosis.

Immunoglobulin E is the one of primary concern in the diagnosis and treatment of allergy, although IgG is also of vital importance. Present in skin, respiratory secretions, and serum, IgE can fix to tissue mast cells. When two IgE molecules are bridged by the appropriate antigen (Fig. 7–3), ensuing physiochemical events lead to the degranulation of the cell and release of multiple preformed (granular and eluted) and newly formed chemical mediators that are frequently referred to as vasoactive amines (Table

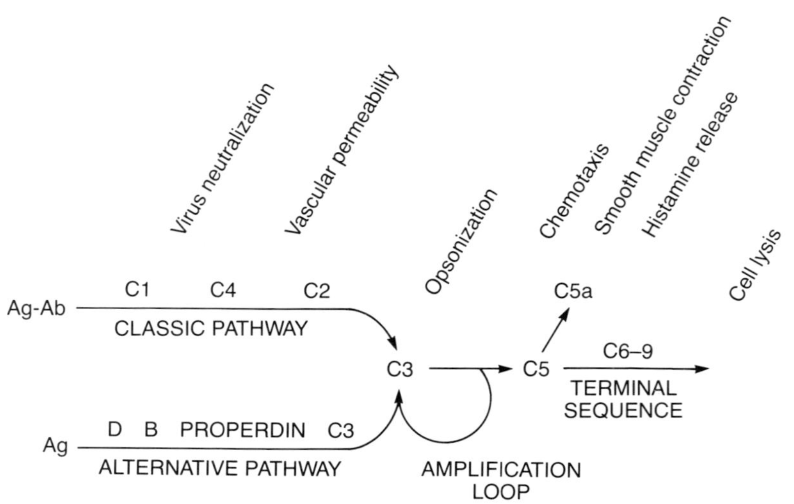

FIGURE 7–2. The complement system. Two pathways for activation are demonstrated. The classic pathway: C1 binds to the Fc portion of antibodies (Ab) that have linked to appropriate antigens (Ag) to form immune complexes. The alternative pathway: antigens on the surface of certain microorganisms permit activation of factors D, B, C3, and properdin in the absence of antibodies. At C3 the two pathways join. An amplification loop provides a positive feedback mechanism to increase the activation of later components. Factors C5 through C9 are then activated in a cascade fashion to release C5a, damaging cell membranes and resulting in cell lysis. The fragments and complexes formed during complement activation have multiple roles in inflammation and host defense. The major actions of complement are listed diagonally at the top of the figure. (After Korenblat and Wedner.)

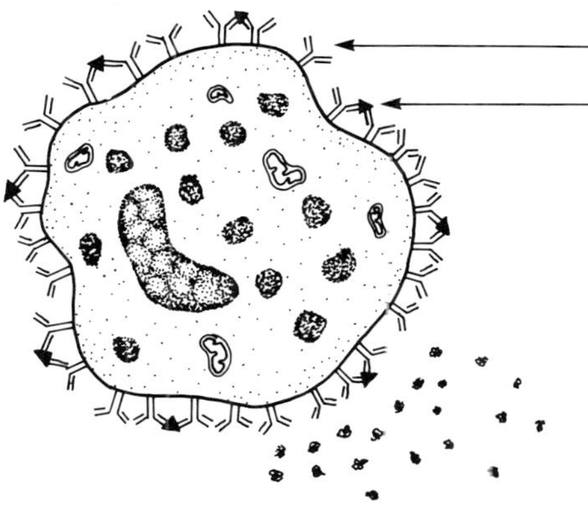

FIGURE 7–3. Mast cell with bridging of antigen and antibody-producing degranulation and release of chemical mediators (vasoactive amines).

7–2). Additional mediators continue to be identified. These chemicals actually produce the physiologic changes we recognize as allergy: increased vascular permeability; smooth muscle contraction, in both respiratory and gastrointestinal tracts; and local increases in eosinophils. Symptoms such as sneezing, rhinorrhea, and increased bronchial secretions then develop. Even low levels of antigen-antibody complex may cause destruction of mast cells, with widespread release of toxic amines into the target organ.

Immunoglobulin E synthesis is a normal immune response, especially in infants; it may be protective rather than pathologic. However, overproduction of this immunoglobulin occurs in various disease states, allergy among them. The level of IgE varies with age. It is normally absent at birth, rising measurably between the ages of 9 months and 2 years. The increase then continues into adolescence and gradually levels off. In a nonallergic normal patient, the total IgE remains stable into the sixth or seventh decades, following a familial pattern. It may then show a gradual decline. Levels in atopic individuals also decrease with age.

Table 7–2. ALLERGIC MEDIATORS

Preformed
- Histamine
- Platelet activating factor (PAF)
- Eosinophil chemotactic factor of anaphylaxis (ECF-A)
- Neutrophil chemotactic factor (NCF)
- Serotonin

Newly synthesized
- Arachidonic acid metabolites
  - Cyclo-oxygenase pathway
    - Prostaglandins
    - Thromboxanes
  - Lipo-oxygenase pathway
    - Leukotrienes

Overproduction of IgE is a hallmark of allergy, at least if no other disease such as parasite infestation is present. An elevated IgE at birth or shortly after is considered predictive of allergy, even before symptoms are evident. The IgE antibody response is primarily genetically determined, and thus the predisposition toward allergy is inherited; but its expression is influenced by a number of environmental factors, such as the amount of allergen exposure, viral infections, smoking, and other chemical and irritating factors. If a potentially ragweed-sensitive patient—for instance, living in Europe—is never exposed to the allergen, he or she will never develop hay fever.

The levels of IgE produced appear to be related to the development of clinical symptoms that we see in otolaryngic allergy. However, evidence now indicates that overproduction of IgE is probably not the primary defect, but rather that there may be a defect in the T cell suppressors controlling the production of IgE. Studies with monoclonal antibody production have permitted identification of subsets of T lymphocytes, as previously described, and the balance between T helper and T suppressor lymphocytes can now be determined with great certainty.

The basic defect in allergy is probably cell mediated. Evidence for this has been found in experimental animals in which a cytotoxic drug (cyclophosphamide) was used to inhibit normal T cell–mediated suppression, and in the elevated levels of IgE in immune deficiency disease whose expression is in T cell deficiency.

SYMPTOM PRODUCTION

Ongoing studies of the cell membrane are introducing new concepts regarding the steps leading to degranulation and release of chemical mediators that produce symptoms of the allergic response. Calcium is necessary for degranulation. The drug cromolyn sulfate has been effective in preventing it. By stabilizing the cell membrane, it prevents release of mediators so that allergic inflammatory responses do not occur. The symptoms produced depend on which target organs of the body are involved in a particular process. It is not known what factors determine the portions of the body that are affected in atopic individuals, although they are most likely under genetic control.

A mucosal theory of atopy has been described, attributing increased IgE levels and allergy symptoms to mucosal damage done by chemical pollutants and other environmental factors in our changing technological world. Many years ago, Hansel described the allergic load: if multiple factors—allergens or irritants—are sequentially introduced into a limited space (that is, the body), and an additional allergen is then introduced, symptoms result. If the contributing or loading factors are reduced, the level of IgE secreted and the resulting cascade of inflammatory effects may also be diminished.

Allergens may enter the body by way of the respiratory tract, the gastrointestinal tract, and the skin (Fig. 7–4)—all areas producing symptoms of concern to the otolaryngologist. Nasal congestion, rhinorrhea, sneezing, wheezing, gastrointestinal disturbances, headaches, middle ear effusion, lower respiratory tract changes, and dermatologic changes in the head and neck may all be produced by allergens, but also, of course, may be produced by nonantigenic causes such as temperature changes, hormonal influences, and stress. The otolaryngic allergist must be aware that these symptoms can also be effected by chemical, physical, and mechanical irritants, by structural abnormalities, or by neurologic stimulation caused by infection, drugs, or other unknown factors.

All these routes to mediator release may produce chemotaxis (Fig. 7–4), which is possibly the cause of the late phase of the allergic reaction that occurs four to six hours after a single assault by an antigen. This delayed reaction, which may be more severe and less easily controlled therapeutically than the immediate reaction, consists of the invasion of phagocytic and other cells that produce active amines and a severe inflammatory reaction in the target organ, be it the lungs or the nose or the skin. The cells and chemicals must be neutralized in order to restore homeostasis. Some allergists believe that chronic allergic problems are due to the merging of repeated immediate (early) and delayed (late) reactions after long exposure to allergen and that immunotherapy is especially effective in controlling the late phase.

Allergy may also be described by the symptoms it elicits, such as allergic rhinitis; by the type of immunologic incident it produces, such as the Gell and Coombs types I through VI; or by the causative trigger, such as pollenosis or exercise-induced asthma.

THERAPY

The relation of immune system alterations to the expression of allergy determines the mode of treatment. The simplest method is the elimination of the allergen and other irritants to decrease the stimulation of IgE production. Medication, such as theophylline, some beta-adrenergic and anticholinergic drugs, and cromolyn, which prevent release of mediators from the mast cells, may be used first. Other medications, for instance the H_1 and H_2 antihistamines, interact with released mediators, preventing them from reaching the target organ. Still others, for example, the decongestants, counter the effects once the target organs have been reached.

In 1935 Cooke described a blocking antibody. It has been determined that this blocking antibody is the immunoglobulin, now called IgG. The practicing physician and researcher may now monitor immunotherapy by observing the IgG levels. The total IgG and its subsets, IgG_1, IgG_2, IgG_3, and IgG_4, have been studied in relationship to immunotherapy as well as to the production of food allergy and to specific subclass deficiency problems related to recurrent infections. With immunotherapy, the level of total IgG rises slowly and levels out in the normally responsive patient. A related pattern is frequently seen in the initial rise and subsequent lowering of the IgE. It appears that patients who react strongly, showing initial high levels of IgE, will respond well, developing high levels of IgG. High-dose immunotherapy regimens appear to

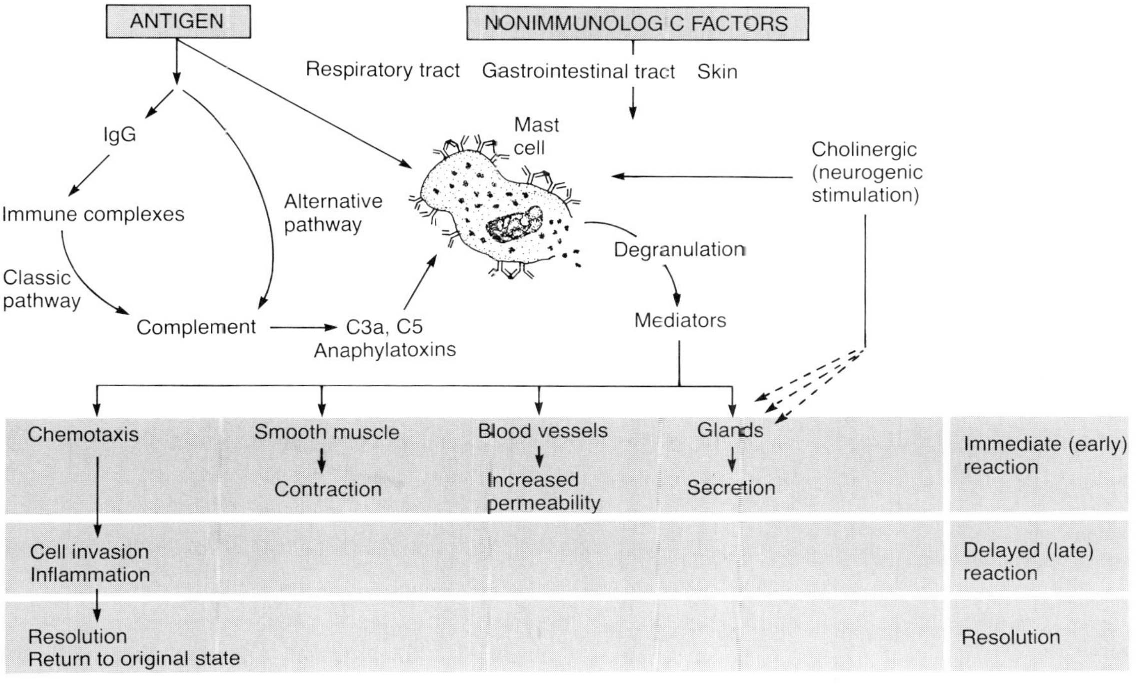

FIGURE 7–4. Development of the immediate and delayed (late) allergic reactions and their resolution.

stimulate the blocking antibody, whereas lower doses may stimulate production of IgE. Therefore, high-dose or maximally tolerated levels of immunotherapy appear to be efficacious in the treatment of the atopic patient.

The pattern of IgG/IgE changes appears to be directly related to the dose schedule of immunotherapy. Therapeutic needs vary with the severity of the symptoms and the ability to determine specific inciting factors. There is a seasonal rise in IgE with respect to pollenosis and insect stings that is blunted by immunotherapy.

Abnormal function of the immune system results in the symptoms otolaryngologists frequently see in their offices. The ability to care for these patients rests on understanding the development of allergic diatheses, and this in turn involves appreciation of the intricacies of the immune system as well as of a major expression of dysfunction, allergy. In addition, as the basic science of the immune system is unraveled, finer understanding of tumor oncology and immunologic therapy may lead to better treatment of head and neck cancers. Autoimmune diseases of the ear and aging as expressed in presbycusis may also succumb to improved techniques.

The next sections of this book discuss the diagnostic techniques currently available to identify patients with allergy and recommend a therapeutic approach for providing the safest, most economical control of this abnormal immune system response.

REFERENCES

Bellanti JA: Immunology III. Philadelphia, WB Saunders, 1985.

Fadel RG, Nalebuff DJ (eds): RAST in Clinical Allergy. Chicago, Year Book Medical Publishers, 1981.

International IgE Symposium. Ann Allergy 48:6, 1982; 49:1, 2, 1982.

Johansson SGO (ed): Diagnosis and Treatment of IgE Mediated Diseases. Amsterdam, Excerpta Medica, 1981.

Kjellman M: Immunoglobulin E and Atopic Allergy in Childhood. Linkoping Univ. Med. Dissertations, No. 36. Linkoping, Sweden, 1976.

Mygind N: Essential Allergy. Oxford, England, Blackwell Scientific Publications, 1986.

Pediatric allergy. Pediatr Clin North Am 22:1, 1975.

Veldman JE, McCabe BF, Huizing EH, Mygind N (eds): Immunobiology, Autoimmunity, Transplantation in Otorhinolaryngology. Amsterdam, Kugler Publications, 1985.

SECTION TWO

OTOLARYNGIC ALLERGY: INHALANT AND EPIDERMAL

PART I

Symptoms

CHAPTER 8

Diagnostic Patterns of Otolaryngic Allergy: Symptoms

Helen F. Krause, M.D., F.A.C.S.

Allergy, which should be considered in the differential diagnosis of many problems in medicine and surgery, holds a particularly important position in otorhinolaryngology. Unfortunately, however, it has been described as a great masquerader, with symptoms mimicking a myriad of other diseases. Like the peaks of an iceberg, various symptoms may surface at different times, so apparently unrelated that they go unrecognized as a form of allergy. Symptom recurrence or chronicity often signals allergy. Yet recurrence (particularly after surgical treatment) that is not recognized as possibly due to allergy frequently sends patients from one doctor to another, desperately seeking help. Wider understanding of allergy as a causative factor may therefore change both the concept of disease and its management.

There are several general features suggestive of allergy.[1] First, it should be appreciated that any body system may become involved, and that some forms of allergy affect more than one body system. A common symptom is fatigue. Chronically ill patients often describe overwhelming fatigue, whereas healthier ones may describe gradually increasing tiredness, "draggy feelings," and restlessness during sleep. These symptoms are usually associated with more specific complaints.

Pruritus—generalized itching or itching limited to a specific body area such as the palate, the back of the throat, the inner or outer canthus of the eye, the ears—is another typical feature of allergy. This may occasionally have consequences of its own. For instance, a patient with throat itching may develop a ticlike pharyngeal action with a clicking sound or bruxism (grinding the teeth) in an attempt to relieve the unpleasant sensation.

Typically, allergy shows intermittence with respect to both frequency and severity, often with diurnal variations. It has also been observed that patients with chronic allergic diseases tend to become more susceptible to infections in the target organs, such as the upper respiratory tract. Thus, the complaint of "a cold all winter long" might represent either true viral respiratory disease or dust, mite, or mold allergy with secondary intermittent infection.

Allergic symptoms may be infrequent, transient, and minimal, requiring no testing and little treatment; or they may be constant, massive, and overwhelming, requiring extensive evaluation. Some symptoms are seasonal; others are perennial, sometimes with seasonal exacerbations.

Allergy may play a role in diseases of each system of the head and neck. The following groups signs and symptoms typical of these systems.

OTOLOGY

In otology, allergy may play a significant role from the auricle to the labyrinth. For example, it must be considered in both acute and chronic otitis externa. Chronic otitis externa may develop from an allergic eczema of the auricle and the external auditory canal, originating in a fungus infection and sensitivity or in food allergy with secondary excoriations (Fig. 8–1). Such an external canal may eventually become stenotic, completely obscuring the allergic basis. Persistent dermatitis of the auricle, and even perichondritis, may develop as complications.

Allergy must also be considered in otitis media, especially in chronic or recurrent cases with effusion. The exact role of allergy in middle ear disease is not yet known. Shambaugh[2] believes that allergic management will prevent 75 per cent of ventilation tube insertions, especially if attention is paid to food allergies. Lim et al.[3] and Kraemer et al.[4] assert that persistent otitis media with effusion may be due in part to allergy, especially from altered eustachian tube function and persistent nasal congestion. Bernstein,[5] observing that few of the cases he re-

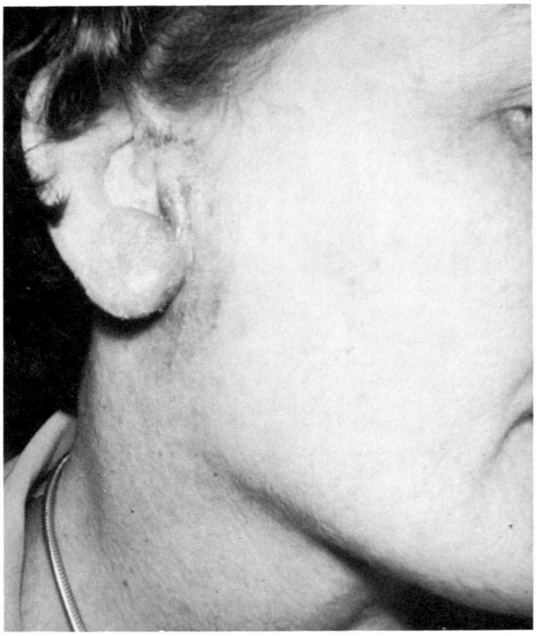

FIGURE 8–1. Eczema of external auditory canal with early perichondritis.

viewed were due to IgE-related disease, is now studying the possible role of food allergy, especially the significance of elevated food-specific IgG and food immune complexes (e.g., related to cow's milk in otitis prone children). Elevations of food immune complexes were present in both serum and middle ear fluid, being higher in the latter in some cases.

It should be noted here that not all researchers necessarily consider "allergy" as the same entity. For instance, this author believes that allergy is a hypersensitivity reaction to a foreign allergen and that it need not be defined as an IgE-induced process. Therefore, food allergy, whatever the mechanism, may well be implicated in otitis media.

Otic polyps may grow in chronically obstructed middle ears (Fig. 8–2). In such patients, it is always wise to evaluate the possibility of allergy.

Nocturnal bruxism has been described as a habit developed to relieve intermittent eustachian tube obstruction, especially in children. The molars may be flattened by this constant grinding (Fig. 8–3), which is of great concern to the orthodontist and to the family.

Ménière's disease, as well as recurrent labyrinthitis without the full syndrome, has been de-

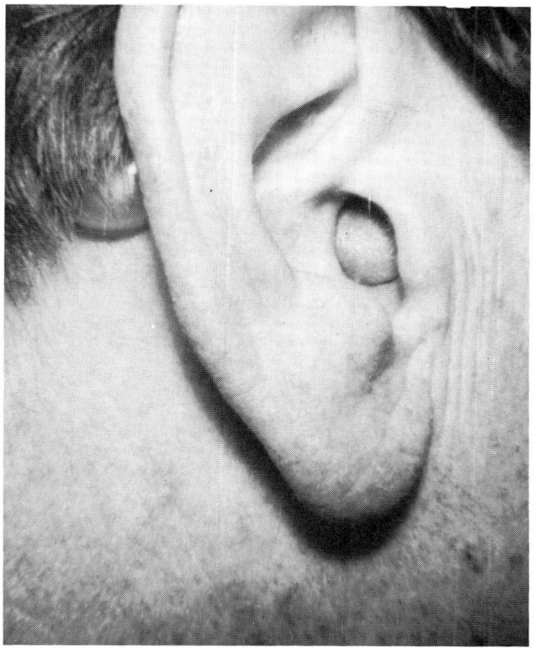

FIGURE 8–2. Otic polyp in highly allergic 50-year-old woman.

scribed in some cases as related to both inhalant and food allergies.

CASE HISTORY: D.R., a 44-year-old nurse and physician's wife, had severe Ménière's disease with hearing loss and debilitating vertigo. A unilateral labyrinthectomy was performed, temporarily relieving the symptoms However, within a year, progressive changes developed in the other ear; the vertigo again became disabling and the hearing again fluctuated. The specter of total hearing loss—the anticipated price of controlling the vertigo—persuaded the patient and her husband to seek other medical causes, and food allergies were found to be significant. With diet management, the woman's hearing stabilized, her vertigo was controlled, and the tinnitus decreased. Dietary indiscretions have been observed to cause the vertigo, tinnitus, and hearing loss to recur.

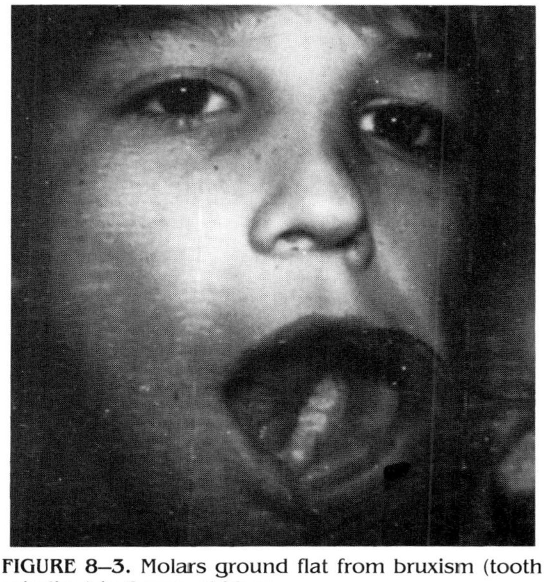

FIGURE 8–3. Molars ground flat from bruxism (tooth grinding) in 8-year-old boy.

Despite considerable research interest in progressive sensorineural hearing loss with labyrinthine dysfunction, there are as yet no clear answers. There are data that suggest an autoimmune basis,[6] although some investigators believe that this problem is primarily allergic, probably food-induced, in origin.[7]

RHINOLOGY

In rhinology, the symptoms of perennial and seasonal allergic rhinitis are the most common presenting complaints. Over 10 per cent of the world's population is believed to have symptoms of allergic rhinitis, with one or more complaints of congestion, rhinorrhea, pruritus, and sneezing. Chronic postnasal drainage may be part of the syndrome of allergic rhinitis, or it may appear alone. In either case, it must be differentiated from vasomotor (or nonallergic) rhinitis, subacute sinusitis, and structural deformities severe enough to alter the normal function of the nasal mucosa.

Allergic rhinitis, whether caused by pollens, dust, mites animal danders, or food, may involve a variety of symptoms as indicated previously. Some may predominate at a given time, owing to a particular reaction to an individual allergen. There may be "stuffiness," "congestion," or "a blocked feeling" due to mucosal edema. If there is no stasis of the material or secondary infection, increased secretion production usually manifests as a clear, watery rhinorrhea with postnasal drainage. The drainage, in addition, may cause repeated throat clearing, leading to pharyngeal irritation or even a sore

Table 8–1. HALLMARKS OF UPPER RESPIRATORY ALLERGY

"Allergic salute"
Linea nasalis (nasal crease)
Nasal and mouth grimacing
Gingival hypertrophy
Pale, boggy, wet nasal mucosa
Nasal cytology: eosinophils and goblet cells
"Allergic shiners"
Dennie's lines

throat, especially if it becomes thick and tenacious or more acidic. There is often reflex sneezing and occasionally itching of the nasal mucosa and palate. Frequently these symptoms are accompanied by allergic ocular complaints, and there may be generalized fatigue and even malaise.

Most often, patients develop symptoms of allergic rhinitis very shortly after exposure to the offending allergen, especially if it is a pollen. However, some experience the brunt of their nasal symptoms hours after exposure—a late or delayed response. Delayed symptoms may be more severe and more difficult to control than those of an immediate response.

There are several hallmarks, sometimes called stigmata,[8] of upper respiratory tract allergy (Table 8–1). The "allergic salute" (Fig. 8–4) represents an attempt to alleviate itching in and about the nose. Repeated "saluting" in a small child may cause the development of thickening and scarring on the supratip area of the nose—the linea nasalis or nasal crease (Fig. 8–5). It is commonly believed that two years' rubbing the nose is necessary to develop this line, but it has been recognized in less time. Adolescents with acne lesions (Fig. 8–5) often complain of particular involvement in this area. Experience in correcting such a scar during nasal reconstruction has revealed it to be dense but shallow; and it may be partially obliterated by dissection of the dermal layers from below.

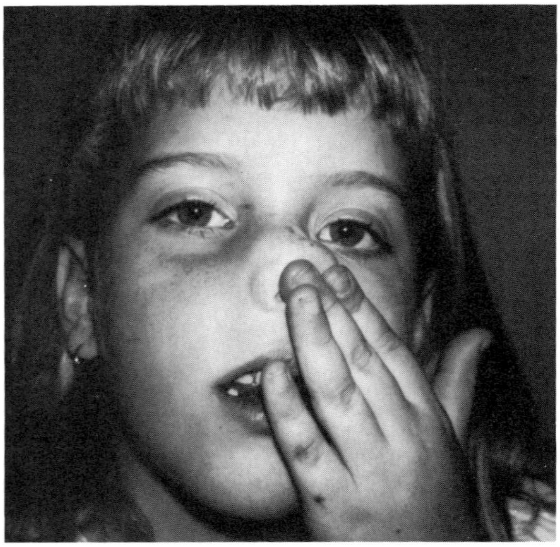

FIGURE 8–4. The "allergic salute."

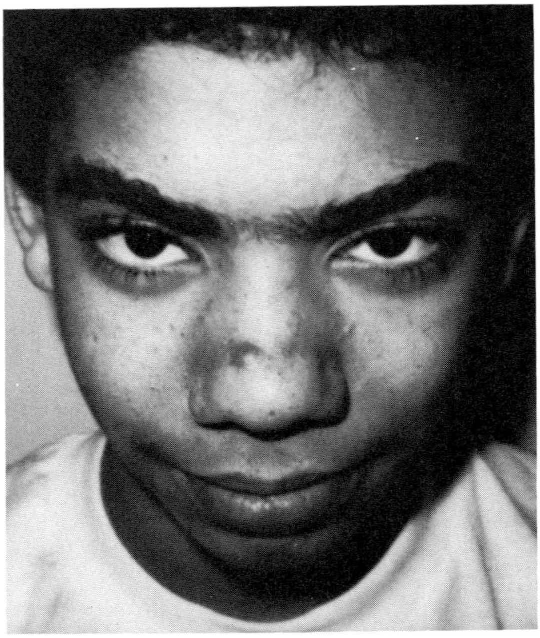

FIGURE 8–5. Nasal crease with acne lesions.

Also, because allergic nasal or palatal mucosa itches, the patient may twist the nose and mouth (allergic grimacing) to relieve the irritation. (Your author was sent to the principal's office in the third grade for "making faces at the teacher"—an action that was recognized, in retrospect, as an effort to relieve allergic discomfort.)

Other hallmarks include gingival hypertrophy or even secondary infection due to persistent mouth breathing.[9] Further, the nasal mucosa may be pale, boggy, and wet with marked edema, although on occasion it may not appear remarkably abnormal. Cytologic studies of nasal secretions or scrapings of mucosa may be helpful if they reveal high numbers of eosinophils and goblet cells.

Allergic shiners, the "black eyes of allergy," are puffy, discolored lower (and occasionally upper) eyelids (Fig. 8–6). These changes result from venous stasis due to edematous upper

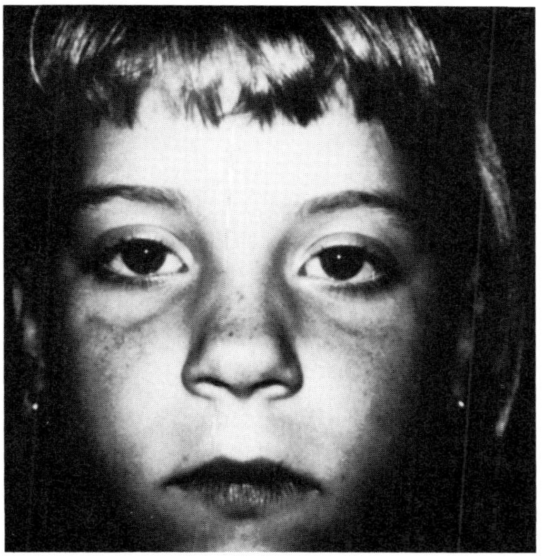

FIGURE 8–6. Allergic "shiners" are the black eyes of allergy in this 7-year-old girl.

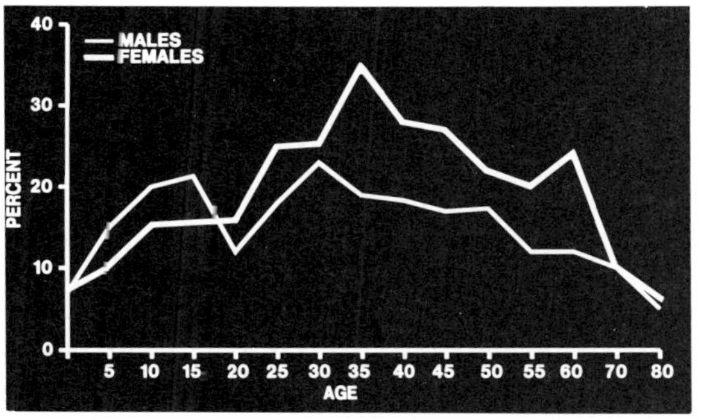

FIGURE 8–7. Incidence of upper respiratory allergy.

respiratory tract tissues and conjunctiva. The thin skin of the lids may actually become stained with hemosiderin. (Before diagnosis, caution is necessary: Ascertain, by the history, that the discoloration is not a familial trait in a nonallergic patient.) Dennie's lines, horizontal grooves below the lower lashes, also result from vascular congestion that induces spasm in the muscle of the lower lid. Discoloration and edema of the eyelids may be accompanied by scaling and secondary lid infection.

Because of the typical age of onset, allergic rhinitis is often classified as a disease of the young (Fig. 8–7). In one third of patients with allergic rhinitis, the onset is before the age of 15 years; in one half, before the age of 25 years; and in three quarters, before the age of 45 years.

Seasonally produced allergic rhinitis affects over 20 per cent of the population of the United States, with pollens (especially ragweed) leading the list of allergens. Perennial allergic rhinitis, on the other hand, occurs year-round, although some patients experience seasonal exacerbations from exposure to pollens or molds. As with seasonal allergic rhinitis, the symptoms are usually itching, sneezing, congestion, or rhinorrhea, most often related to dust, dust mites, molds, or animal proteins. The nasal secretions may be more tenacious, and "sinus" headaches of a vacuum type may be present. Cytologic examination of the secretions often reveals significant eosinophilia in both forms of allergic rhinitis, as well as in the rare nonallergic eosinophilic rhinitis. Edema and its attendant complaints of congestion, stuffiness, or blocking may predominate; or symptoms due to increased, thickened, or more irritating secretions may be more prominent. It may be worthwhile to identify "blockers" versus "runners" for therapy direction.

Allansmith[10] reported that various allergic ocular disorders occur in 8 out of every 10 patients with allergic rhinitis. The most common is allergic or atopic conjunctivitis, characterized by marked itching and redness. Molds may increase the itching at the medial canthus, whereas foods may cause itching at the lateral canthus. The conjunctival vessels become large and promi-

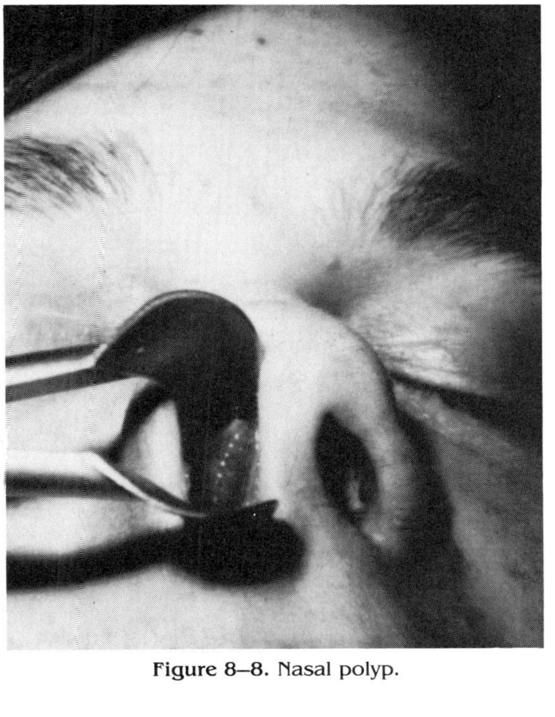

Figure 8–8. Nasal polyp.

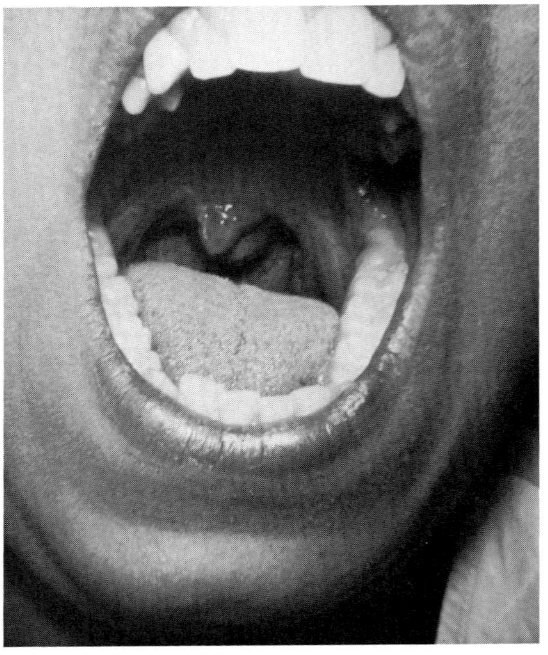

FIGURE 8–9. Choanal polyp in an 11-year-old boy.

nent, and there is increased tearing. Other allergic eye disorders include atopic keratoconjunctivitis, often associated with atopic dermatitis, and vernal keratoconjunctivitis. A more recently described problem is giant papillary conjunctivitis due to contact lens intolerance.

Prolonged allergic rhinitis may be complicated by secondary infection, polyposis, or sinusitis. Allergic polyposis (Figs. 8–8 to 8–10) may occur in the nasal cavity, the choanae, or the sinuses; in fact, all of these areas may be involved simultaneously. These polyps must be differentiated from those due to chronic infection, cystic fibrosis, or the aspirin-sensitivity syndrome associated with asthma. English,[11] in reviewing studies of nasal polyposis, reported that the incidence of associated allergy ranged from 10 to 64 per cent (Table 8–2). The studies varied with respect to techniques for determining the presence or absence of allergy. Some used patient history alone; others used a variety of skin tests. The highest percentages of allergic involvement were found in the studies using skin tests, especially those conducted with intradermal testing—and probably these were the most reliable studies. Chronic or persistent upper respiratory tract infections (with or without polyps), which suggest an underlying allergic mechanism, probably contribute to polyp formation. Polyps, whatever the cause, are usually multiple, often very large, and flattened by prolonged pressure.

Sinusitis may develop as a consequence of allergic edema of the sinus mucosa. It is sterile initially, but secondary infection may supervene. Sinusitis may also result from chronic obstruction of the ostia by allergic edema of the mucosa or by polyps. Subacute sinus involvement, which can be present for a long time without many symptoms, often becomes evident during or after an upper respiratory tract infection. The allergic cause is thus obscured.

In children, sinusitis is frequently missed unless the infection is very obvious. There may be no clear-cut symptoms such as the pain and pressure seen in adults, but signs are apparent

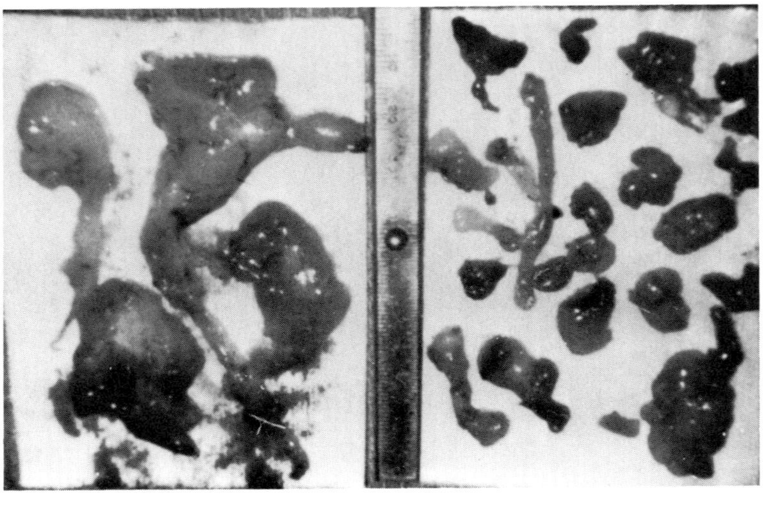

FIGURE 8–10. Sinus and nasal polyps—surgical specimen.

Table 8–2. INCIDENCE BY STUDY OF ALLERGY IN PATIENTS WITH NASAL POLYPS

Author of Study	Year of Publication	Number of Patients Studied	Technique Used	Number of Patients with Allergy	Percentage of Patients with Allergy
Blumstein and Tufft	1957	160	Positive history	86	54
Lanoff et al.	1973	9*	Positive history	2	22
Delaney	1976	100	Positive skin test	10	10
Moloney	1977	42	Positive skin test	27	64
Busuttil et al.	1978	54	Positive skin test	24	44
Holopainen et al.	1979	109	Positive history and skin test	18	17
Schramm and Effron	1980	120*	Positive history	21	17.5
Totals		594		188	32

*Children.

After English GM: Nasal Polyposis in Otolaryngology. Philadelphia, Harper & Row, 1985. Used by permission.

if carefully sought. For example, the child may constantly clear the throat or cough, the breath may be foul, or lower respiratory symptoms may appear or persist. A single Water's view may reveal opacification or a fluid level. Children (and, less often, adults) may rapidly progress to complications, especially orbital cellulitis (Fig. 8–11).

Adults are more frequently symptomatic if the sinuses are involved, complaining of pressure, pain, intense headaches, and purulent drainage. As the infection is treated, it should be kept in mind that allergy may be the original cause. It is also recognized that a patient's asthmatic status may be improved following medical or surgical correction of concurrent sinus disease.

Mucoceles of the paranasal sinuses sometimes develop in the allergic patient, although no statistics have been reported regarding the frequency. They are most often seen in the maxillary and frontal sinuses. Their cause is obscure, as is that of nasal polyps; however, in patients with progressive mucocele formation, allergies should be investigated.

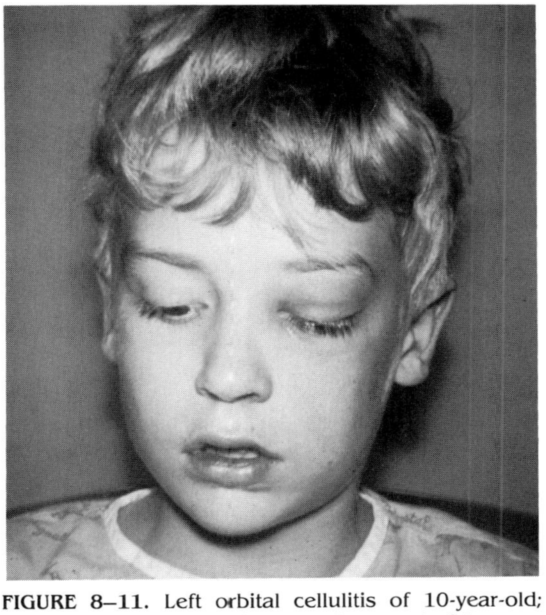

FIGURE 8–11. Left orbital cellulitis of 10-year-old; early resolution stage 14 hours after onset of therapy.

CASE HISTORY: M.C., a 58-year-old woman, presented with a history of childhood asthma and adult seasonal allergy. She was referred by an ophthalmologist for right eye pain and progressive lid swelling that were followed by proptosis, visual disturbances, and frontal headaches. Sinus radiographs (Fig. 8–12) and tomograms revealed a huge right frontal mucocele as well as destruction of the roof of the orbit. There was also opacification of the right antrum. After surgical removal of the mucocele (which extended to the optic nerve), followed by institution of allergic management, the antrum showed rapid clearing. No further sinus surgery was necessary (Fig. 8–13).

Headaches are a common and sometimes mysterious complaint in many branches of medicine. However, although headache symposia discuss every imaginable cause, rarely is allergy mentioned. The fact is, severe headaches may be caused by vacuum sinusitis secondary to closure of the ostia by allergic edema. Also, although headaches from food allergy have been rarely recognized, until recently, they may be intense, overwhelming, and poorly responsive to common headache therapy. Neurologic research in the past three years suggests that as many as 80 per cent of migraine headaches

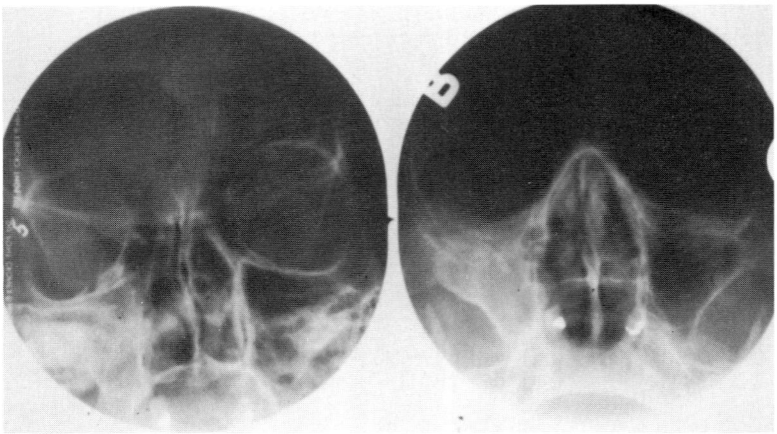

FIGURE 8–12. Preoperative radiographs of patient with left frontal mucocele.

may be allergic (especially related to food sensitivity) in origin.[12, 13]

ALLERGY IN THE PHARYNX AND MOUTH

In the pharynx and mouth, allergy plays another major role in symptoms. The so-called adenoid facies—the sad-looking face with an open mouth, flattened malar eminences, and drooping eyelids—can be seen in children with huge tonsils and adenoids as well as in those with small tonsils and adenoids who have nasal obstruction from allergic edema. In the latter group, the appearance may more realistically be termed "allergic facies" (Fig. 8–14). Many of these children develop high-arched palates (Fig. 8–15) early in life and should undergo early palatal expansion by an orthodontist or pedodontist while the airway obstruction is being treated.[14] In children with both obstructing adenoids and allergies, proper treatment of the allergies may solve both problems, effecting a gradual reduction in the adenoid size (Fig. 8–16) as well as clearing of the rhinitis. No explanation is yet available for this phenomenon, except that perhaps the reduction of the inflammatory component of the rhinitis decreases lymphoid reactivity.

Among other problems involving this region is chronic pharyngitis with lymphoid hyperplasia, often described as a "cobblestoned" posterior pharyngeal wall. The patient with a "lump in the throat" may not have globus hystericus, but may have hypertrophied lingual tonsils or lateral bands of lymphoid tissue on the inflamed nasopharyngeal wall (Fig. 8–17). These pharyngeal mucosal changes, accompanied by hyperemia and often by burning discomfort, may be the result of irritating postnasal drainage or of the drying effects of persistent mouth breathing.

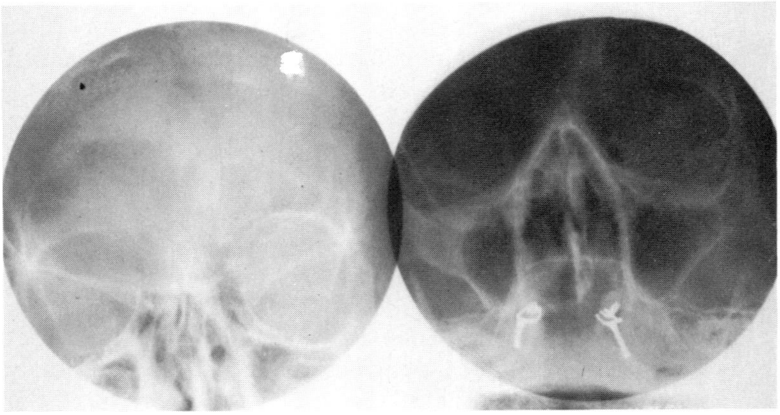

FIGURE 8–13. Postoperative radiographs of patient in Figure 8–12.

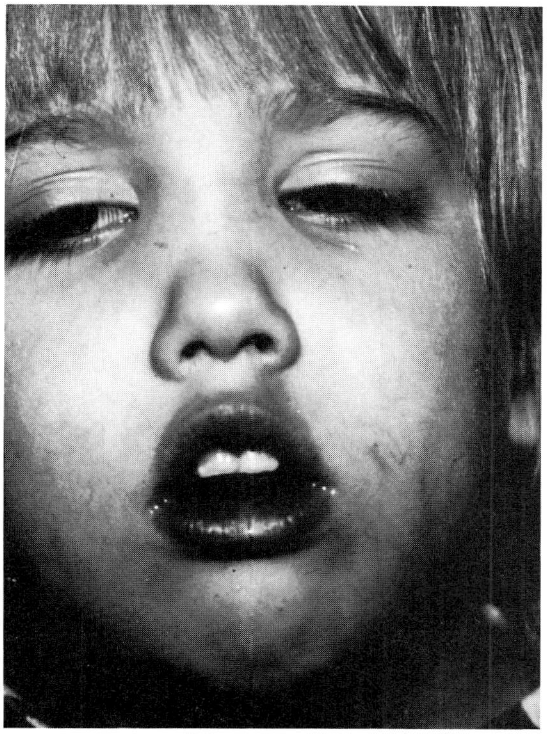

FIGURE 8–14. "Allergic facies" of 5-year-old girl.

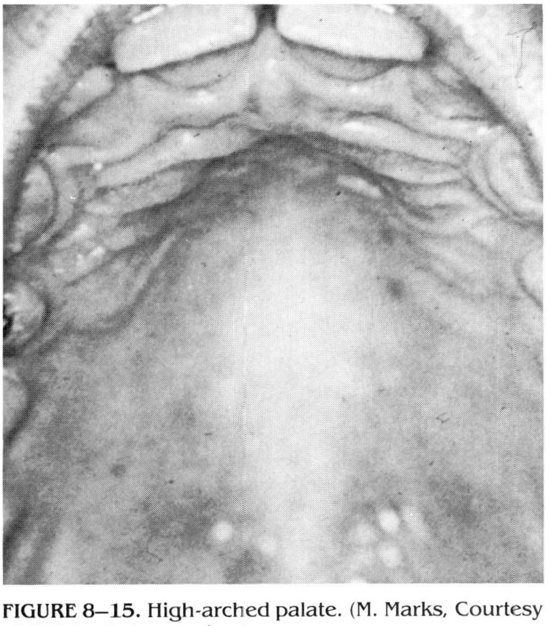

FIGURE 8–15. High-arched palate. (M. Marks, Courtesy of Upjohn Laboratories.)

Further, the pharyngeal tonsils may hypertrophy or become chronically inflamed in the presence of continuing postnasal drainage (Fig. 8–18). Chronic glossitis has been described in association with allergies and with geographic tongue, which occurs in a higher incidence in the allergic population (Fig. 8–19).

Although not commonly recognized, salivary glands sometimes develop acute or chronic allergic edema;[15] most often the parotids are affected, causing a variant parotitis. Mucus plugs and secondary infection may obscure the allergic element. Smears of the duct secretions taken early in the episode will show heavy eosinophil concentrations.

A chronic cough may be related to allergy in both children and adults.[16] Although often secondary to postnasal drainage, it may also be related to an irritable or "twitchy" larynx or trachea or to asthma. In the last case, the condition is considered a laryngeal asthma equivalent with an allergic cause.

LARYNGOLOGY

The larynx, poised as it often is between the allergic upper respiratory tract and the asthmatic lung, may be equally involved in the pathophysiology of allergy. Laryngeal changes of an allergic cause were well described by Dr. Francis Davidson[17] a number of years ago. Acute supraglottic edema due to allergy may present with the same clinical picture seen in acute epiglottitis, whereas allergic subglottic edema is described as "spontaneous croup" of sudden onset (in contrast to infectious laryngotracheobronchitis). In patients with these disorders, the laryngeal examination will reveal pale, watery edema of the laryngeal or subglottic tissues. Edema restricted to the glottis may be mild, moderate, or even occasionally severe (Fig. 8–20).

The acute laryngeal edema of anaphylaxis, resulting from insect bites or drugs, may be a terrifying emergency requiring immediate recognition and treatment. (Rarely, with appropriate emergency care, should a tracheostomy be necessary.) However, to avoid such a crisis, patients at risk, as soon as they are identified, must be instructed to administer self-help in the form of injectable epinephrine as provided by Anakit or EpiPen.

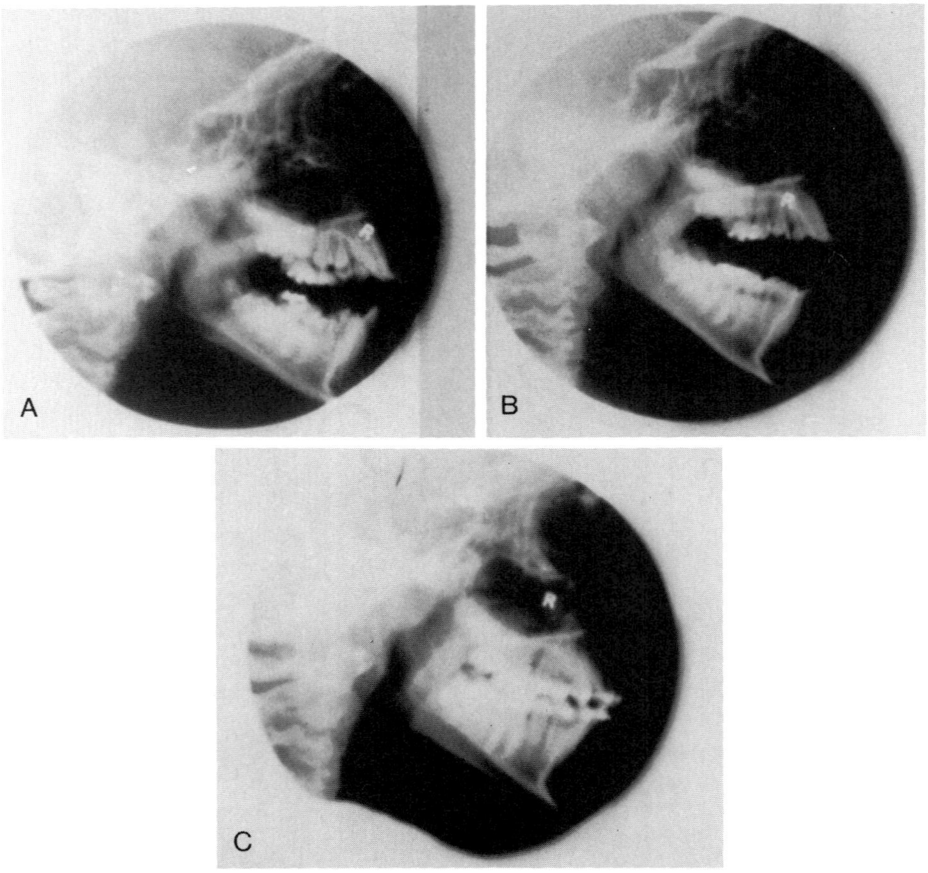

FIGURE 8–16. Radiographs of a 9-year-old boy. *A*, Initial examination: large, partially obstructing adenoids; *B*, 6 months after intensive immunotherapy, adenoids decreasing in size; *C*, 12 months after start of immunotherapy, marked shrinking of adenoids.

Asthma, which is discussed in detail in Chapter 9, should be suspected and recognized by the history, physical examination, and pulmonary function tests. Patients with asthma may have complaints in the upper respiratory tract and larynx that bring them to an otolaryngologist for diagnosis and therapy, often on referral by a pulmonologist or family practitioner. The otolaryngologist should be apprised of the management of this disease even if the patient is being treated for it by a primary care physician. Children or adults may develop a barrel chest, seen in association with dramatic radiographic changes of hyperaeration. The wheezing may fluctuate and may even be absent at a particular examination. Asthmatic patients whose pulmonary symptoms are well controlled by pharmacologic agents without immunotherapy may still develop considerable distress from recurrent rhinitis, requiring allergy care. Also, asthmatics taking steroids may develop allergic rhinitis if the steroids are eliminated; these new symptoms will require therapy.

ALLERGY IN OTHER SYSTEMS

In the practice of otolaryngic allergy, the problems most frequently presented are in the head and neck region. However, these areas are intricately connected with the rest of the body, which comprises a number of other systems that may be affected by allergy. These are briefly reviewed here to make the reader aware of the scope involved. It is important to be cognizant of such relationships in considering the diagnosis and treatment of allergic patients.

Cardiac symptoms may reflect high numbers

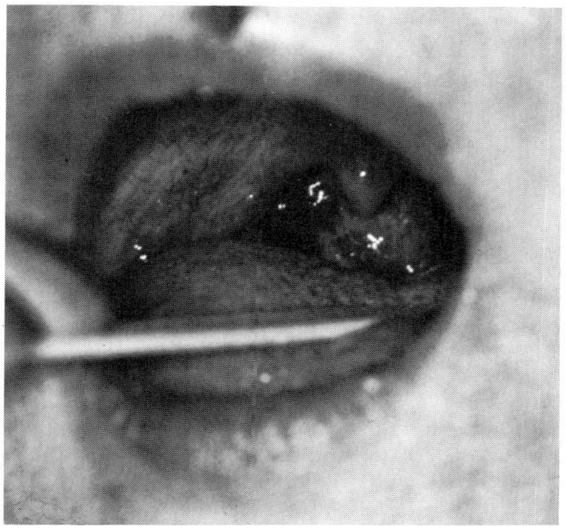

FIGURE 8–17. Inflamed posterior pharyngeal tissue and herpetic lip lesion.

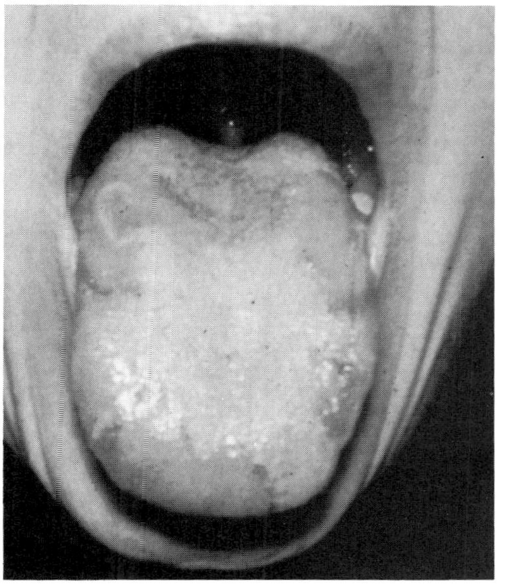

FIGURE 8–19. Typical geographic tongue.

of mast cells in the heart. Researchers at Cornell University have suggested that heart attacks and sudden cardiac death may result if the heart becomes a target organ of systemic allergic reactions.[18–21] True anaphylaxis may develop after an antigen-antibody reaction to a common allergen as the mast cells release histamine, a reaction comparable to bronchoconstriction during an asthma attack. Arrhythmias and rate alterations, especially tachycardia, sometimes occur as a primary allergic reaction or as part of a general allergic response.

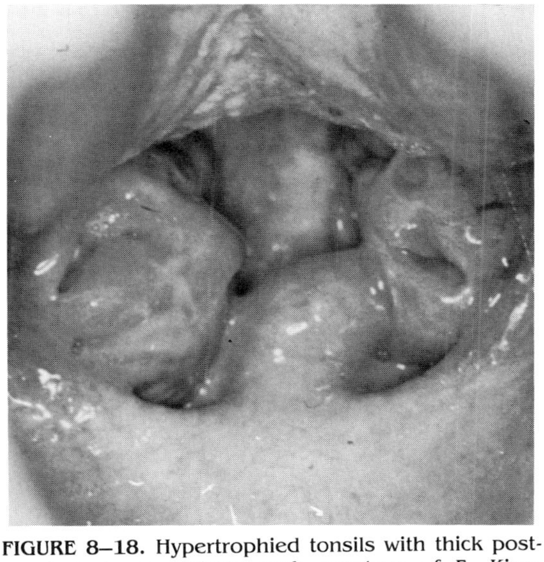

FIGURE 8–18. Hypertrophied tonsils with thick postnasal drainage. (Photograph courtesy of E. King, D.M.D.)

Vascular lesions appear as evidence of vasomotor instability;[1] blotching of the skin and occasionally blanching or blushing may occur. There may also be increased capillary fragility, with easy bruising and even petechiae. The blood pressure may vary, but hypotension is seen more often than is hypertension.

The gastrointestinal tract is often affected by food allergy (or, as it is sometimes called, "food sensitivity"), but it may also be stimulated by inhalant allergies. Nearly every gastrointestinal symptom may be produced; but most often allergy manifests in the mouth as stomatitis and extends to the esophagus to produce heartburn. Gastrointestinal reactions, occurring as the acute IgE type or, more often, as delayed responses, can mimic most abdominal diseases; they are more often due to ingestants. Some researchers have experimentally attempted immunotherapy by nasal inhalation[22] and by ingestion[23] of an allergen. Both routes have resulted in provocation of local symptoms in doses high enough to give any significant alteration in the respiratory tract.

Symptoms have even been recognized in the genitourinary tract,[24] for example, enuresis due to the irritating effect of an allergen in the bladder, or intermittent diuresis. These disorders are most often due to ingestants. Problems of infertility and sensitivity to semen protein con-

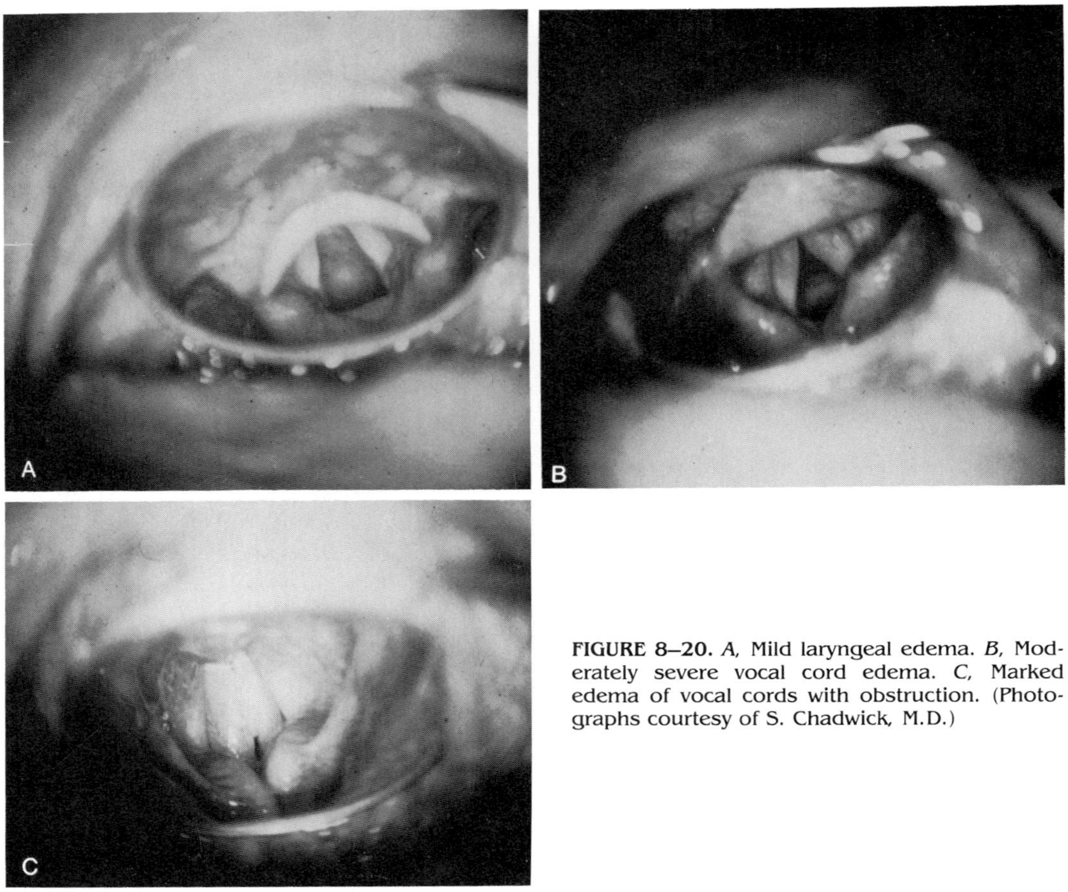

FIGURE 8–20. *A*, Mild laryngeal edema. *B*, Moderately severe vocal cord edema. *C*, Marked edema of vocal cords with obstruction. (Photographs courtesy of S. Chadwick, M.D.)

tinue to be studied.[25] The uterus, containing many mast cells, may be another site of acute reactions to allergens.

Nonspecific lymphedema may occur as a reflection of an allergic diathesis in the reticuloendothelial system.[1] Most often this affects the submandibular and anterior and posterior cervical nodes, although occasionally it appears in the axillary or inguinal areas. Node swelling, especially in the neck, may be a result of chronic inflammation or a direct reflection of an allergic phenomenon.

The skin is often a mirror of allergy.[1, 26] It is not uncommon to see eczema of the face and auricles, often due to foods and sometimes to the presence of multiple inhalant allergies. Angioedema of the lips (Fig. 8–21) and eyelids may also be allergy-related if nonallergic hereditary angioedema is not present. Patients having nut and shellfish allergies are occasionally seen with this entity, which may extend to the tongue and oral mucosa.

Cutaneous disorders of any portion of the body may be allergic in cause, with inhalants, contactants, or ingestants responsible. The vascular system of the skin is affected, and most, but not all, skin involvement is pruritic. Eczema—the classic atopic dermatitis—may appear alone or associated with allergic rhinitis or asthma. Most commonly it first appears in childhood or even infancy, and it often disappears with maturity.

Eczema is classically pruritic, presenting initially with erythematous papules and vesicles (Fig. 8–22). It is characterized in infants and children by facial (Fig. 8–23) and extremity extensor involvement and in adults by chronic (even lichenified) changes, especially on flexor surfaces. In adults, molds appear to cause eczema or hives to develop on extensor and

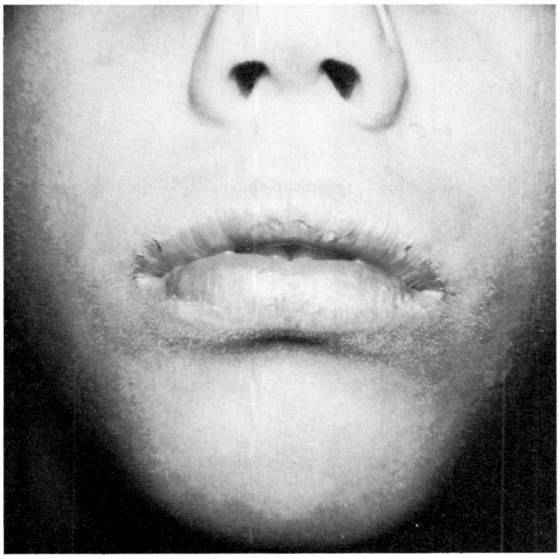

FIGURE 8–21. Angioedema of the lips secondary to allergy to nuts in an 11-year-old boy.

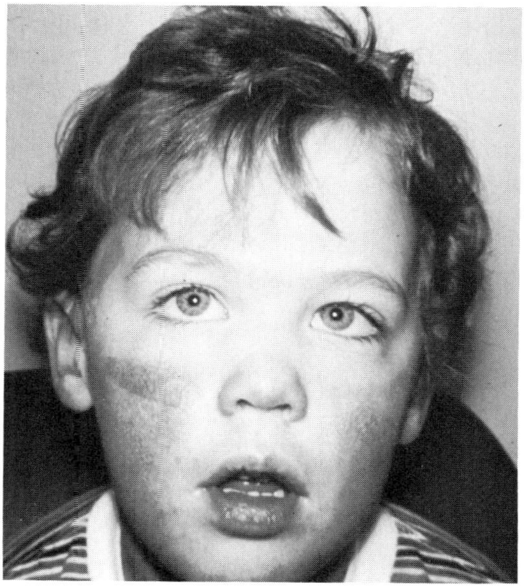

FIGURE 8–23. Facial eczema of 3-year-old boy due to inhalant and milk allergy.

lateral surfaces, whereas foods produce more flexor eczema. However, this dermatitis may develop over the entire body, as may hives (Fig. 8–24). Chronic urticaria cannot be discussed in detail here, but may well be an extension of such a phenomenon, often due to delayed allergic reactions.

The "id reaction" is described as a distant skin sensitivity reaction to a mold infection; it most often appears on the hands, fingers, and feet as minute vesicular lesions that tend to peel (Chapter 12). The lesions usually resolve as both the infection and sensitivity are treated.

Central nervous system involvement may produce the fatigue,[27] lassitude, irritability, and

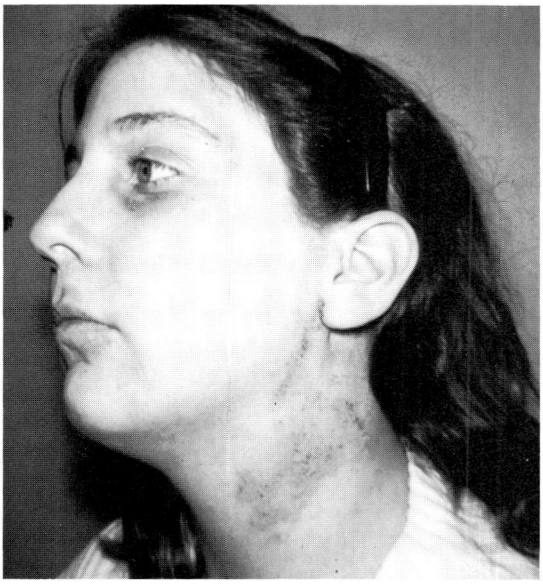

FIGURE 8–22. Recurrent eczema of 18-year-old girl especially marked on face and neck, but also present on arms and legs; resolving with therapy for inhalant and food allergies.

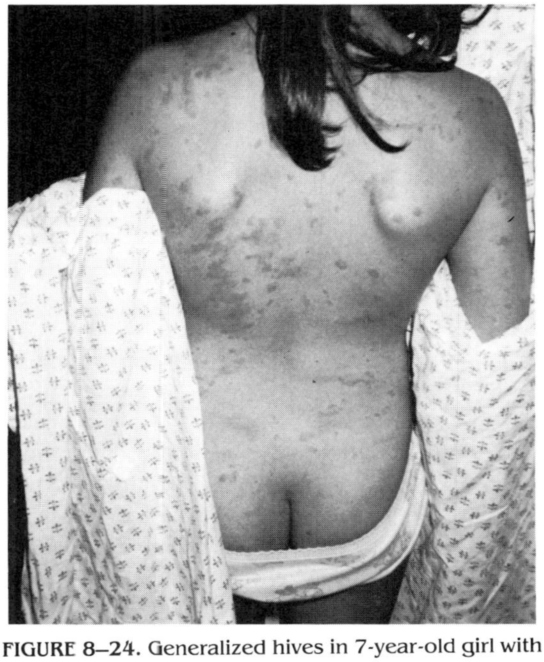

FIGURE 8–24. Generalized hives in 7-year-old girl with inhalant and food allergies.

depression that are such frequent complaints of allergic patients, as well as difficulty in concentration, memory problems, and sleep disturbances. These symptoms may be due to cerebral edema associated with the allergic reaction, although this has not been proved. Severe reactions may even produce seizures. Headaches, as already discussed, are often due to sinusitis but may be directly related to central nervous system involvement.

ANAPHYLAXIS

All body systems are potential targets of anaphylaxis,[28] an immunologically mediated reaction that develops rapidly and is potentially life-threatening. Histamine is most certainly involved in its expression, but other yet-unidentified chemical mediators may also contribute. Anaphylaxis may be stimulated by an immunologic reaction precipitated by an antigen that is inhaled, ingested, injected, or touched. Injected materials may include drugs, insect or snake venom, blood and immunization products, and allergen extracts—all potentially antigenic agents.

Type II allergic reactions (the cytotoxic) and type III (involving immune complexes and complement) may also cause anaphylaxis. Early treatment of these is essential to prevent what may appear to be a minor reaction from rapidly progressing.

Anaphylactoid reactions[29] are not true immunologic phenomena, but they may involve the same body systems and be just as lethal. They most often result from drug injections, such as of radiopaque dyes used in contrast studies.

In both types of reactions, several systems may become target organs. Cutaneous involvement usually produces flushing, itching or urticaria, and/or angioedema. Involvement of the respiratory system may be the most dangerous. The reaction begins with sneezing, rhinorrhea, and nasal obstruction, and may then progress to edema of the tongue, lips, palate, and pharyngeal wall and further to the epiglottis, laryngeal tissues, and trachea, producing a respiratory emergency. The lungs may react alone or simultaneously; their involvement is first evidenced by chest tightness, then by overt shortness of breath and wheezing, but rarely by acute pulmonary edema. The gastrointestinal tract may produce nausea, vomiting, bloating, cramps or persistent abdominal pain and tenderness, and finally diarrhea (often a late occurrence). Shock may result from these respiratory changes or from direct cardiovascular effects, leading to arrhythmias, hypotension, hypovolemia, syncope, or total cardiovascular collapse.

Exercise-induced anaphylaxis has been recently described.[30–32] It appears to involve concomitantly a specific food ingested prior to exercise and then activity itself. Neither will produce anaphylaxis alone in some cases; in others, exercise alone appears to be the stimulus.

SUMMARY

Allergy is a dynamic process. Alterations in sensitivities and their expressions may occur throughout life, in response to changes in the body's metabolism and physiologic processes as well as to stress. In addition, chronic exposure to potential allergens may lead to the development of new allergic sensitizations. Heredity plays a basic role. If one parent has allergies, approximately 35 per cent of the children will develop symptoms; if both parents are allergic, 75 to 80 per cent of children will be affected.

The diagnosis in a particular patient is aided by awareness that allergy may readily mimic many other medical problems. The fact that symptoms occur intermittently and may vary from one exposure to another provides a clue to an allergic cause. Further, there is usually a total body response as well as the response of a specific target organ.

Finally, a very optimistic note: the allergic reaction is usually reversible, with few or no residual pathologic effects once the allergens are identified and properly eliminated or treated.

REFERENCES

1. Cowen DE: Clinical symptomatology of the allergic response. JCE ORL Allergy 40:42, 1978.
2. Shambaugh G Jr: Serous otitis media: are tubes the answer? Am J Otol 5:63, 1983.
3. Lim D, Bluestone C, Klein J, Nelson JD: Recent Advances in Otitis Media with Effusion. Philadelphia, BC Decker, 1984, pp 5–44.

4. Kraemer MJ, Richardson MA, et al: Risk factors for persistent middle ear effusion. JAMA 249:1023, 1983.
5. Bernstein JM: The possible role of food "sensitivity" in the otitis-prone child. Manuscript presented at American Academy Otolaryngology–Head and Neck Surgery Symposium, Chicago, September 1987.
6. Veldman JE, McCabe BF, Huizing EH, Mygind N (eds): Immunobiology, Autoimmunity, Transplantation in Otorhinolaryngology. Amsterdam-Berkley, Kugler Publications, 1985.
7. Powers WH: Evaluation of the dizzy patient; metabolic and allergic aspects. JCE ORL Allergy 40:45, 1978.
8. Marks MB: Stigmata of Respiratory Tract Allergies. Kalamazoo, MI, The Upjohn Company, 1977.
9. Khosla VM, Khosla SV: Oral manifestations of allergy. *In* Frazier CA (ed): Dentistry and the Allergic Patient. Springfield, IL, Charles C Thomas, 1973, pp 131–171.
10. Allansmith MR: The Eye Immunology. St. Louis, CV Mosby, 1982.
11. English GM: Nasal Polyposis in Otolaryngology. Philadelphia, Harper & Row, 1985, Chapter 19.
12. Egger J, Wilson J, Carter CM, et al: Is migraine a food allergy? A double-blind controlled trial of oligo-antigenic diet treatment. Lancet 2:865, 1983.
13. Mansfield LE, Vaugh RT, Walter SF, et al: Food allergy and adult migraine: blind and medication confirmation of an allergy etiology Ann Allergy 55:120, 1985.
14. Krause HF: Upper airway obstruction as a cause of dental and facial deformities. Primary ENT 3:2, 1987.
15. Smith JF: Salivary gland manifestation of allergy. *In* Frazier CA (ed): Dentistry and the Allergic Patient. Springfield, IL, Charles C Thomas, 1973, pp 172–190.
16. Holinger LD: Chronic cough in infants and children. Laryngoscope 96:316, 1986.
17. Davidson FW: Acute laryngeal obstruction in children. Penn Med, October: 42–46, 1984.
18. Wolff AA, Levi R: Histamine and cardiac arrhythmias. Circ Res 58:1, 1986.
19. Graver LM, Robertson DA, Levi R, et al: IgE mediated hypersensitivity in human heart tissue: histamine release and functional changes. J Allergy Clin Immunol 77 709, 1986.
20. Machado FRD, Assem ESK, Ezeamuzie CI: Cardiac anaphylaxis: the role of different mediators. Part I. Histamine. Allergol Immunopathol 13:259, 1985.
21. Machado FRD, Assem ESK, Ezeamuzie CI: Cardiac anaphylaxis: the role of different mediators. Part II. The role of prostaglandins, thromboxanes, and leukotrienes in cardiac anaphylaxis. Allergol Immunopathol 13:335, 1985.
22. Georgitis JW, Reisman RE, Clayton WF, et al: Local intranasal immunotherapy for grass allergic rhinitis. J Allergy Clin Immunol 71:71, 1983.
23. Platts-Mills TAE: Oral immunotherapy: a way forward (editorial). J Allergy Clin Immunol 80:129, 1987.
24. Gerrard JW: Food Allergy: New Perspectives. Springfield, IL, Charles C Thomas, 1980.
25. Bernstein IL, Englander BE, Gallagher JS, et al: Localized and systemic hypersensitivity reactions to human seminal fluid. Ann Intern Med 94:459, 1981.
26. Kniker WR: Importance of food intolerance and etiology of atopic eczema. Allergy Observer 1:2, 1984.
27. Feingold BF: Introduction to Clinical Allergy. Springfield, IL, Charles C Thomas, 1973.
28. Shatz GS: Anaphylaxis. *In* Korenblat PE, Wedner HJ (eds): Allergy Theory and Practice. Orlando, Grune & Stratton, 1984 pp 147–158.
29. Schneider SB: Anaphylactoid reactions. *In* Korenblat PE, Wedner HJ (eds): Allergy Theory and Practice. Orlando, Grune & Stratton, 1984, pp 159–169.
30. Buchbinder EM, Block KJ, Moss J, et al: Food-dependent exercise-induced anaphylaxis. JAMA 250:2973, 1983.
31. Longley S, Panush RS: Familial exercise-induced anaphylaxis. Ann Allergy 58:257, 1987.
32. Scheffer AL, Tong AKF, Murphy GF, et al: Exercise-induced anaphylaxis: a serious form of physical allergy associated with mast cell degranulation. J Allergy Clin Immunol 75:479, 1985.

Additional Recommended References

Bernstein MM: The role of IgE mediated hypersensitivity in otitis media with effusion, a 1987 update. Am J Rhinol 1:67, 1987.

Hughes GB, Barna BP, Kinney SE, et al: Predictive value of laboratory tests in "autoimmune" inner ear disease; preliminary report. Laryngoscopy 96:502, 1986.

Irwin RS, Pratter MR, Holland PS, et al: Postnasal drip causes cough and is associated with reversible upper airway obstruction. Chest 85:346, 1984.

Middleton E, Reed CE, Ellis ER: Allergy: Principles and Practice. 2nd ed. St. Louis, CV Mosby, 1983.

Mygind N: Nasal Allergy. 2nd ed. Oxford, Blackwell Scientific Publications, 1979.

Sacha RF, Tremblay NF, Jacobs RL: Chronic cough, sinusitis and hyperreactive airways in children: an often overlooked association. Ann Allergy 54:195, 1985.

CHAPTER 9

Asthma Concepts

Shirley Murphy, M.D.

Conventional clinical wisdom is, "All that wheezes is not asthma." Although several pulmonary disorders, including foreign body aspiration or cystic fibrosis, may present with wheezing, most lung conditions that cause wheezing are asthma. However, pulmonary symptoms other than wheezing may also be caused by asthma. Asthma is clinically recognized by a classic symptom trio of wheezing, dyspnea, and cough. Asthma can present with only isolated dyspnea or cough that may then progress to classic wheezing. Few physicians have difficulty establishing the diagnosis of asthma in the adolescent child who presents with multiple bouts of wheezing. However, the adult who complains of fatigue with exercise or a chronic cough may also have asthma and will benefit from asthma pharmacotherapy.

This chapter reviews the pathophysiology and diagnosis of asthma with particular reference to how asthma relates to the otorhinolaryngologist's practice.

DEFINITION OF ASTHMA

The American Thoracic Society defines asthma as "a disease characterized by an increased responsiveness of the trachea and the bronchi to various stimuli which is manifested by widespread narrowing of the airways that changes in severity either spontaneously or as a result of therapy."[1] The hallmark of asthma is unusually responsive airways referred to as hyperreactive airways. When an asthmatic is exposed to or challenged with such nonspecific agents as cold air, smoke, or exercise, the airways constrict. This nonspecific reactivity does not usually occur in normal individuals.[2]

The mast cell is important in the development of airway reactivity and the pathogenesis of asthma. It is estimated that 32 billion mast cells guard the entryways into the body. In the lung, mast cells line the airways beneath the basement membrane, often near blood vessels, mucous glands, and nerve endings, and are also free in the bronchial lumen. Both immunologic and nonimmunologic stimulation can activate these cells, leading to the release of chemical substances called mediators, which cause mucosal edema, increased mucus secretion, bronchospasm, and inflammation of the airways[3] (Fig. 9–1).

Figure 9–2 outlines the mast cell mediators and their specific actions in asthma. In allergic individuals, inhalation of specific allergens results in mast cell degranulation with released mediators loosening tight epithelial junctions, allowing entrance of allergens to deeper mast cells. The once intact airway is then vulnerable to many stimuli and becomes unstable or hyperreactive.[3] An analogy relating the lung to the intact skin provides another way of understanding bronchial hyperreactivity (Fig. 9–3). The intact skin is not normally responsive to nonspecific irritants such as soap or alcohol, but once abraded becomes very sensitive to these minor irritants. The asthmatic airways, once only reactive to a

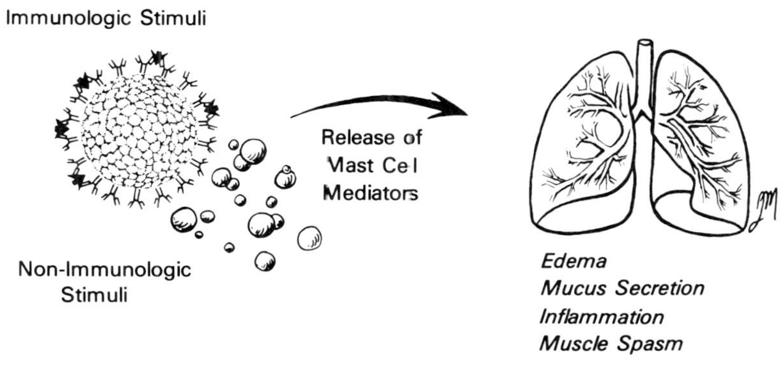

FIGURE 9–1. Development of hyperreactive airways.

specific allergen such as ragweed, now contract when exposed to nonspecific stimuli such as smoke, cold air, and other irritants.

Nonspecific airway reactivity can be quantitatively measured by challenges with exercise, cold air, methacholine, or histamine. A methacholine challenge is performed by first obtaining baseline spirometry measurements. The subject then inhales increasing doses of methacholine, a synthetic analog of acetylcholine, the neurotransmitter of the parasympathetic nervous system. After each increase in dosage, the patient undergoes repeat pulmonary function measurements. A positive test occurs when the forced expiratory volume in one second (or FEV_1) drops by 20 per cent. This is then referred to as the PD_{20} (or the provocative dose that decreased the FEV_1 by 20 per cent).

Allergic individuals who do not have nonspecific airway hyperreactivity demonstrated by methacholine challenge most likely do not have asthma. Normal individuals, however, can have transient increases in bronchial hyperreactivity following viral upper respiratory tract infections. Subjects with allergic rhinitis are intermediate in their levels of nonspecific reactivity when compared with normal and asthmatic subjects.[4]

The airway extends from the nose to the terminal bronchioles, and this results in a variety of asthma clinical presentations important to the otorhinolaryngologist.

CLINICAL PRESENTATIONS OF ASTHMA

Cough

Cough is part of the traditional symptom triad recognized as asthma and is often the predominant symptom of the asthma triad of wheezing, dyspnea, and cough. However, until recently it was not recognized that cough could be the *sole* presenting symptom of asthma.

In 1979, Corrao and coworkers reported six patients who presented with the sole symptom

Histamine	→	increased capillary permeability	→	mucosal edema
Neutrophil chemotactic factors	→	recruit neutrophils into lung	→	inflammation
Eosinophil chemotactic factors	→	recruit eosinophils into lung	→	inflammation
Prostaglandins (PGD_2)	→	smooth muscle constriction	→	bronchospasm
Leukotriene C_4 & D_4	→	smooth muscle constriction	→	bronchospasm
	↘	stimulation of submucosal glands & goblet cells	→	increased mucus secretion

FIGURE 9–2. Mast cell mediators important in pathophysiology of asthma.

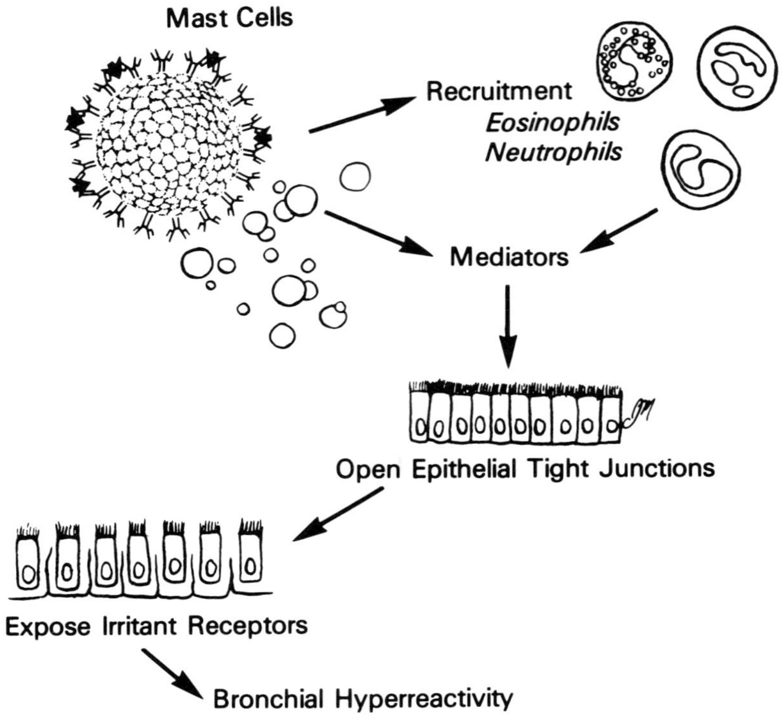

FIGURE 9–3. Development of bronchial hyperreactivity.

of chronic cough that had persisted for one to 48 months.[5] They had no sputum production, no wheezing or dyspnea, no history of atopic disease, and normal baseline pulmonary function measurements. A methacholine challenge was performed on the patients as well as on age-matched normal controls. After five inhalations of 25 mg/ml of methacholine, each subject in the cough group had a 20 per cent drop in FEV_1, whereas the control group remained at baseline values. Thus, this positive methacholine challenge was evidence of underlying reactive airways disease or asthma. The cough patients underwent a therapeutic trial of either theophylline or terbutaline. The cough disappeared in all patients within 48 hours. After six months of therapy, the bronchodilators were stopped and the cough returned. Reinstitution of therapy again stopped the cough. In an 18-month follow-up period, two out of six of the patients had gone on to develop frank wheezing.

Chronic cough has been shown also to be a presenting symptom of asthma in children by Drs. Cloutier and Loughlin.[6] They studied 15 patients, 6 to 16 years of age, who had a persistent nonproductive cough ranging from 10 weeks to 11 years. All 15 patients had normal baseline spirometry; however, after an exercise challenge, the pulmonary function parameters dropped significantly in all 15 patients. With a trial of bronchodilator therapy, all 15 patients became asymptomatic. When therapy was stopped, 11 of the 15 patients had a return of cough and two had the onset of wheezing.

Bronchoscopy is often performed in patients who present with cough; however, Poe and coworkers showed that this may be unnecessary.[7] They reviewed records of 109 patients who presented with isolated chronic cough, of whom 51 underwent bronchoscopy. The cause of the cough was discovered in only one patient using this method. However, in the 87 patients who underwent spirometry and/or methacholine challenge, the diagnosis was determined in 39 per cent of the patients.

The clinical approach to the patient with isolated cough should include a careful history eliciting atopy, seasonal or exertional exacerbations, and a complete physical examination. Sinus films may be helpful. If simple spirometry performed before and after a bronchodilator is normal, a challenge with methacholine, histamine, or exercise should be considered to document airway hyperreactivity. A therapeutic trial with either theophylline, cromolyn, or a beta$_2$-agonist may prove to be diagnostic in the patient presenting with cough variant asthma.

Recurrent Croup

Laryngotracheobronchitis or croup is recognized clinically by inspiratory stridor, hoarse voice, and barking cough and is of viral causation.

Recurrent or spasmodic croup begins suddenly with an acute nocturnal episode of inspiratory stridor lasting several hours and resolving spontaneously or with inhalation of a sympathomimetic. Spasmodic croup may be recurrent, and until recently, its cause was unknown.

In 1981, Zach and coworkers reassessed 110 patients who had been hospitalized for croup nine years earlier.[8] Patients were evaluated by questionnaire, physical examination, allergy skin testing, and pulmonary function tests including histamine challenge. Of these patients, 53 had only isolated croup limited to one to two attacks. However, 57 had recurrent croup ranging from four to 60 attacks in the nine years following their original admission.

Patients with recurrent croup could be distinguished from those with a single episode of viral croup by several parameters. A positive history of allergies occurred in 26 of 57 recurrent croup patients as contrasted with 7 of 53 with single episode croup ($p < 0.01$).

In another report, the same investigators evaluated 17 children with recurrent croup with a mean age of 9.6 years.[9] The episodes were noted to occur from 9:00 PM to 4:00 AM, with mean episode of six hours (1- to 36-hour range). Ten of 17 patients had allergies, and five of 17 had reported wheezing episodes. Fourteen (82 per cent) of 17 had a positive histamine challenge, and during the challenge four patients developed the actual onset of stridor.

A 1981 editorial on treatment of recurrent croup suggested that since sympathomimetics (e.g., inhaled racemic epinephrine) have been used for the effective management of acute croup, their use should be expanded to prevent bouts of recurrent croup.[10] The authors suggested prophylactic cromolyn and/or allergen avoidance might be useful in preventing recurrent croup.

Recurrent Pneumonias

The child with multiple episodes of recurrent radiographic areas of pulmonary infiltration or atelectasis presents an interesting diagnostic challenge. In 1982, Eigen and associates reported a record review of 81 children who had been referred for the evaluation of recurrent or persistent pneumonias.[11] Twenty of the 81 patients were found to have an underlying cause for these pneumonias. Of the 61 who had no obvious cause for these episodes, 48 per cent had a history of allergies, 41 per cent had a history of wheezing, and 18 per cent had documented wheezing during their initial episode of pneumonia. Methacholine challenge tests documented that 92 per cent of those children tested had bronchial hyperreactivity or asthma. The authors concluded that asthma is a common cause of persistent or recurrent pneumonias in children, which may be the initial symptom of asthma even in the absence of wheezing.

Sinusitis

Chronic sinus disease and its relationship to asthma is an important concern for the otorhinolaryngologist. Rachelefsky and coworkers[12] reviewed the records of 48 children in their practice whose asthma could not be controlled after three months of vigorous bronchodilator therapy. These patients had a radiographic evaluation of their maxillary sinuses, which revealed that 21 per cent of the children had greater than 6 mm of mucosal thickening, 25 per cent had one opacified sinus, 38 per cent had bilateral opacification, and 17 per cent had air-fluid levels present. All children were then treated with antimicrobial agents for two to five weeks. Of the 48 patients, 39 (80 per cent) responded both clinically and radiologically, and of these, 38 were able to discontinue taking bronchodilators after resolution of their sinusitis. The possible presence of sinus disease should be considered in patients with asthma that is refractory or difficult to control.

Exercise-Induced Asthma

The symptoms of exercise-induced asthma (EIA) range from severe wheezing and chest tightness with incapacitating dyspnea to mild chest tightness and cough. Some patients do not experience overt symptoms but have only a postexercise decrease in forced expiratory volume in one second (FEV_1).[13] It is important to recognize exercise-induced asthma, since the symptoms may frighten and discourage patients from gaining the fitness benefits of exercise.

The prevalence of exercise-induced asthma among asthmatic patients has been reported to be from 80 to 90 per cent,[14] but it is probable that all asthmatic patients will develop bronchospasm if the exercise is strenuous enough. Also, 40 per cent of people with allergic rhinitis have also been demonstrated to have exercise-induced asthma.[15]

The type and severity of exercise is important in the development of EIA, since there is a linear correlation between increasingly strenuous exercise and the severity of the exercise-induced asthma. Running causes more severe symptoms than does bicycling, swimming, or walking. Exercise lasting less than two minutes does not usually cause exercise-induced asthma, but that which lasts six minutes appears to cause the maximum exercise-induced bronchospasm. In longer exercise, it is sometimes possible for the person to "run through" the bronchoconstriction. The colder and drier the air, the greater the exercise-induced asthma. EIA may also worsen in the spring and the fall when the concentration of airborne allergens is high, or in the presence of air pollutants such as ozone and sulfur dioxide.

The pathophysiologic mechanism of exercise-induced asthma is controversial. As one exercises, there is an increased demand for oxygen to be delivered to the tissues. This results in increased ventilation, and an increased volume of air is presented to the airways to be warmed and humidified. This results in increased respiratory heat and water loss, which cools the airways and leads to hyperosmolarity in the airway mucosa. These events may translate into bronchospasm by alterations in autonomic neural activity, by release of chemical mediators from mast cells, or through the direct constricting effect of cooling on airway smooth muscle.[16] Regardless of the mechanisms that produce EIA, the resulting physiologic changes are identical to those occurring in spontaneous asthma.

When exercise-induced asthma is suspected, it can be confirmed with a trial of therapy with inhaled cromolyn sodium or inhaled $beta_2$-agonists while monitoring the therapeutic response. A "free running test" has been suggested for the diagnosis of EIA in children.[14] The patient is asked to run at near maximum capacity for five minutes, with FEV_1 or peak flow being measured pre- and postexercise. A decrease of 15 per cent or more in the peak expiratory flow or FEV_1 from the preexercise baseline is diagnostic.

The ideal treatment of exercise-induced asthma is prophylaxis so that the individual athlete can exercise at maximum capacity without medication side effects. Exercise-induced asthma induced by any activity can be prevented by the inhalation of 20 mg of cromolyn sodium via a Spinhaler or two puffs of an albuterol inhaler immediately before exercise. Studies have demonstrated that in severe asthmatics or with exceptionally strenuous exercise, both drugs may be more effective than either used alone.[17] Cromolyn is very effective in preventing or reducing bronchospastic responses to exercise or hyperventilation with cold, dry air and has the added advantage of blocking bronchospasm induced by allergens, sulfur dioxide, and ozone. It has no effect on the cardiovascular system and will also block both the immediate and late bronchoconstrictive response to exercise.

To avoid their cardiovascular side effects, inhaled beta-agonists should be $beta_2$-specific. Oral beta-adrenergic agents have the disadvantage of cardiovascular side effects and need to be taken an hour or more before exercise to achieve maximum effect. Theophylline is less effective, and exercise-induced asthma can often be produced despite therapeutic levels of theophylline.[18] Theophylline may be associated with side effects that interfere with maximum athletic performance, such as diuresis, headache, and tachycardia. Inhaled corticosteroids do not block EIA, and therefore are not of benefit in this condition.

It is important to recognize and treat EIA, allowing patients to exercise to their maximum potential.

REFERENCES

1. Definition and classification of pulmonary emphysema. CIBA Foundation Guest Symposium. Thorax 14:286, 1959.

2. Bleecker ER: Airways reactivity and asthma. J Allergy Clin Immunol 75:21, 1985.
3. Kaliner M: Mast cell mediators and asthma. Chest 87:25, 1985.
4. Cockcroft DW, Ruffin RE, Dolovich J, Hargreave FE: Allergen-induced increase in nonallergic bronchial reactivity. Clin Allergy 7:503, 1977.
5. Corrao WM, Braman SS, Irwin RS: Chronic cough as the sole presenting manifestation of bronchial asthma. N Engl J Med 300:633, 1979.
6. Cloutier MM, Loughlin GM: Chronic cough in children: a manifestation of airway hyperreactivity. Pediatrics 67:6, 1981.
7. Poe RH, Israel RH, Utell MJ, Hall WJ: Chronic cough: bronchoscopy or pulmonary function testing. Am Rev Respir Dis 121:979, 1980.
8. Zach MS, Erben A, Olinsky A: Croup, recurrent croup, allergy, and airways hyperreactivity. Arch Dis Child 56:336, 1981.
9. Zach MS, Schnall RP, Landau LI: Upper and lower airway hyperreactivity in recurrent croup. Am Rev Respir Dis 121:979, 1980.
10. Recurrent croup and allergy. Lancet 21:1150, 1981.
11. Eigen H, Laughlin JJ, Homrighausen J: Recurrent pneumonia in children and its relationship to bronchial hyperreactivity. Pediatrics 70:698, 1982.
12. Rachelefsky GS, Katz RM, Siegel SC: Chronic sinus disease with associated reactive airway disease in children. Pediatrics 73:526, 1984.
13. Speir WA, Chaudhary BA, Karlson KH: Exercise-induced asthma: meeting the challenge. J Respir Dis 4:10, 1983.
14. Shapiro GG, Bierman CU: Exercise-induced asthma. J Asthma 20:383, 1983.
15. Kawabori J, Pierson WE, Loveday L, et al: Incidence of exercise-induced asthma in children. J Allergy Clin Immunol 58:447, 1976.
16. Eggleston PA: Exercise-induced asthma. Clin Rev Allergy 1:19, 1983.
17. Latimer KM, O'Byrne PM, Morris MM, et al: Bronchoconstriction stimulated by airway cooling; better protection with combined inhalation of terbutaline sulphate and cromolyn sodium than with either alone. Am Rev Respir Dis 128:440, 1983.
18. Bleecker ER: Exercise-induced asthma: physiologic and clinical considerations. Clin Chest Med 5:L109, 1984.

CHAPTER 10

Inhalant Allergy

Hueston C. King, M.D., F.A.C.S., F.A.C.A.

Inhalant allergy is the best recognized and most fully understood form of allergy today. It is also known as "atopy" and has been recognized for over 150 years.

The symptom complex of sneezing, nasal congestion, conjunctivitis, and itching of the skin was first described by John Bostock of Liverpool and London in 1819 at a time when most disease was identified in a descriptive manner rather than on an etiologic basis. He was reviewing his own symptoms, which occurred from about the middle of June to the end of July, and which he originally attributed to the effect of sunbeams on the grass. He called the condition "summer catarrh."[1] In 1828, after years of observation, he associated the disease with an effluvium of fresh-cut hay and renamed the condition "hay fever."[2]

A variety of investigators commented upon the condition thereafter, but it remained for Morrill Wyman of Cambridge, Massachusetts, to clearly identify pollen as the causative agent in the disease in his classic description of hay fever, published in 1872.[3] The following year, Charles Blackley of Manchester, England, demonstrated the effect of applying grass pollen to the excoriated skin of a sensitive patient.[4] The result was a raised wheal surrounded by erythema that itched intensely. The demonstration of this phenomenon opened the way for traditional allergy skin testing still used widely today: the scratch, prick, and puncture.

Treatment of aeroallergen sensitivity did not come into being until 1911, when Leonard Noon of St. Mary's Hospital, London, began treating his patients with injections of pollen extract on the assumption that "antitoxins" would be formed to neutralize supposed "toxins" released by the pollens.[5] Most of his previous work had been associated with tetanus immunization, and his approach to allergy care, although incorrect, was logical. It also worked. His methods of standardization and comparison of extracts are of more than historical interest, as many of his problems continue to plague investigators today, making comparisons of treatment methods difficult.

To create a standardization of extract strength, Noon arbitrarily selected a "unit" of pollen toxin as the amount that could be extracted for the thousandth part of a milligram of Phleum pollen. All other quantities could then be expressed against this in terms of whole numbers. The strength of a pollen extract then was given in terms of the number of "units" in a cubic centimeter of extract.

Comparison of different extracts was made by instilling a drop of pollen extract into the conjunctiva of a known hay fever patient. The strength of the extract required to produce a minimal reaction would then represent the patient's "resistance"; i.e., if a dilution of four "units" was required to institute a reaction, the patient's resistance was rated as "4." These responses could then be used in selecting vaccine for injection therapy. Thus, from the outset of immunotherapy, when only clinical observation and arbitrary standards were available, quantification has been a primary goal.

By today's available standards, Noon's quantification methods were gross. Still his patients improved. Treated patients tolerated later pollen exposures significantly better than did their untreated counterparts. A treatment method had been developed on an empirical basis and had been shown to be effective.

RECOGNIZING THE PROBLEM

Today, the inhalants remain the most familiar offenders for the allergy sufferer. "Inhalants" are identified by their route of entry into the body—not their basic biologic makeup. These enter via the respiratory tree, making their initial contact with the mucosal lining of the nose, mouth, throat, and tracheobronchial tree. Since the entire lining of this part of the body is richly supplied with IgE, it is not surprising that essentially all inhalant allergy is IgE-mediated, producing immediate type I Gell and Coombs reactions. This rapid onset of action following exposure and limited duration when the exposure is removed are of considerable value in identifying the offenders. The vast majority of these consist of pollens, molds, dust, and various epidermals. The time of onset, the usual limitation of symptoms to the respiratory system, the symptoms themselves, and the physical findings all aid the clinician in diagnosing inhalant allergy.

APPEARANCE OF SYMPTOMS

Age

It is rare to find an infant severely affected by inhalant allergy. Prior to the age of 3 years, the IgE necessary to activate inhalant allergy is quite limited, and the investigation of active symptoms is likely to produce limited success under the age of 5 years. Thereafter, the IgE level increases in the inhalant-sensitive patient, peaking in the 20s. The symptoms tend to follow the IgE level. There is normally a slow drop from this peak to middle age, sometimes followed by a minor peak in the 60s. This pattern may vary in different individuals and may be affected by exposure, health, and various forms of stress.

The development of specific IgE quantitation has confirmed that many older patients do indeed have significant inhalant allergy despite the fact that their reduced skin reactivity may make skin testing appear negative.

Seasonal

Most of the continental United States experiences strong seasonal swings that have a marked effect on the inhalant allergy sufferer. Pollens are the most strongly seasonal allergens and their pattern is the most predictable. From year to year, the onset of pollination may be affected by unusual temperatures, rainfall, or other environmental factors; and the ecologic changes brought about by urban and rural development cannot be overlooked. Pollinating plants introduced into an area for agriculture or ornamentation will make their contribution. The tendencies of allergenic pollens to be airborne, sometimes over hundreds of miles, may simultaneously complicate the problem and smooth out the regional variations. To the beginning allergist this apparently overwhelming number of potential offenders may make identification and treatment appear prohibitive. Such, however, is rarely the case.

Pollens, to produce allergic problems, must meet Thommen's postulates:

1. The plant must be seed-bearing. Only seed-bearing plants produce pollen.
2. The pollen must be allergenic.
3. The pollen must be wind-borne for distribution.
4. The pollen must be produced in large quantities.
5. The pollen must be buoyant to be distributed over a wide range (15 to 50 micra in diameter).
6. The plant producing the pollen must be widely and abundantly distributed, or close to human habitation.

Patients habitually blame their symptoms on profusely flowering, bright-colored plants. The vast majority of these are insect-pollinated and not offenders. While the possibility of an unusual, specific offender cannot be overlooked, the use of regional pollen guides for an area, plus pollen counts, if available, will usually provide more accurate information. Throughout most of the temperate United States, three pollinating seasons are of importance: trees in the spring, February to May; grasses in the summer, April to frost, including active seasons; and weeds in the fall, July to frost. Regional pollen guides will be supplied upon request by many of the major allergy supply houses.[6–8] One laboratory has offered a guide based upon the user's zip code.[9] These vary somewhat in detail, but as the public's interest in allergy and therefore the demand for therapy has increased, they have become steadily more complete and accurate. A major book appeared in 1983[10] outlining pollen distribution in detail. Many major cities also carry out regular pollen counts, through either the Department of Agriculture or the Department of Pollution Control. Telephone calls will usually determine whether such reports are available. If so, they offer a valuable supplement to the regional guides. Not all pollens need be controlled to give relief to the average sufferer. A selection of the major offenders will generally prove adequate, and the number may be increased later if needed.

Molds are close to pollens in allergenic importance, although their seasonal pattern is far less predictable. Molds flourish in damp areas, increasing greatly in the rainy season. Since this seasonal change is less predictable than the four major seasons, so is the prevalence of mold problems. In accordance with the level of humidity, mold problems are greatest in the low-lying, subtropical parts of the United States. All areas east of the Mississippi River, however, are subject to long periods of high humidity and hence much mold. The problem decreases in the Rocky Mountain area and the Pacific coast; however, it never disappears. In dry climates, dampness accumulates around plumbing and in basement areas, fostering mold growth. The allergist must be aware of this and must be prepared, in such areas, to expect mold-sensitive patients to be bothered at different times and under different circumstances than those on the Atlantic coast. In the West, molds tend to be an indoor problem, peaking when homes are closed for long periods. In the East, mold problems peak when homes are open or when the patient spends much time outdoors.

Dust allergy is a study in itself. Dust is not dirt tracked into the house and allowed to dry; house dust is a unique allergen that has frustrated investigators for decades. It has repeatedly been dubbed the "universal allergen." If allergists were to be given a choice of one allergen to be used for treatment, house dust would be selected. Prior to the almost universal use of air conditioning, a predictable curve for dust allergy symptoms over the temperate United States was well established. As would be expected, dust symptoms peaked at the time that both homes and public buildings were closed for long periods of time because of winter cold. At present, there is much less seasonal variation in house dust problems in some areas, since offices, stores, airline terminals, and most public buildings are always air conditioned. Homes may still show the older pattern.

House dust is a heterogeneous mix containing 28 known or suspected allergens.[11] Probably the most potent of these is the house dust mite. Two species of mite are recognized as problems: *Dermatophagoides pteronyssinus* and *D. farinae*. These microscopic creatures are present in vast quantities in house dust in most areas, although rare in altitudes above 3000 feet. The mite feces produce most of the allergenic activity. Although mites are by no means the only significant allergens in house dust, dependence on immunologic identification and treatment of mite allergy may eventually replace traditional evaluation for house dust as a whole, since it appears that the less specific house dust vaccine may leave the market.

Epidermals, the hair and dander of animals, represent one of the most virulent group of allergens. Many allergists refuse to treat epidermal problems, demanding that the patient avoid the offender. Although it cannot be denied that treating epidermal allergy may be less effective than treatment for other inhalant allergens, if the offender is the family pet, the usual response to a demand for elimination is getting rid of the family allergist. The problem exists, it is common, and frequently it requires a degree of compromise.

Exposure is the key to identifying epidermal allergens. For the urban or suburban patient, most epidermals will peak during the months in which the house is closed. Cats and other "furry" animals represent the majority of offenders. The dander is light and permeates carpets, drapes, and upholstery. With an indoor animal, the "closed house" season produces a pressure cooker effect; the dander concentrates and is not allowed to blow away. Dog dander is heavier, and although it is a strong allergen, it is relatively easily removed. When a dog is taken out of a house and a thorough vacuuming is performed, a sensitive patient may move in after a few days with relatively minor problems. When a cat leaves a house, a three-month period should be expected before the sensitivity level is reduced significantly. For the rural patient, control of epidermal allergens may be essential to preserving his livelihood. The farmer or rancher must be carefully quizzed as to which animals he is exposed to day in and day out and appropriate sensitivity studies performed. While he must be advised of the potency of epidermal allergens and the difficulty in establishing good control, vigorous treatment may be expected to improve his situation and usually to make it tolerable. Seasonal effect on the farmer is minimal because the epidermal allergens to which he is exposed so permeate his environment.

Hidden epidermals present an infrequent but occasionally severe problem. Most wool carpets today have been replaced by synthetics. Wool blankets and clothing have decreased in popularity. When the patient fails to respond as expected, however, these should be investigated. Horsehair and cattle hair are still used in upholstery, and goat hair may be present in significant quantities in carpet padding. The seasonal pattern of such allergens follows that of house dust. They may not merit routine investigation, but should be examined in resistant cases.

An additional word of caution is merited here. Not all such exposures occur in the victim's home. The cat-sensitive child, seated next to a classmate who habitually sleeps with and plays with a cat, may react strongly to the cat hair and dander on the classmate's clothes. The same applies to exposure in a neighbor's house. All such exposures require investigation. This is the reason that the history is still the cornerstone of allergy diagnosis.

Diurnal

Although less clear-cut than seasonal exposure, fluctuation of symptoms on a diurnal basis may provide valuable information as to the type of inhalant allergen that is producing problems. Pollens reach their airborne peak as the sun's rays dissipate the early morning cool, and are much reduced by the filtration of central air conditioning and heating. The patient who complains of a sudden rush of symptoms on leaving the house in the morning may be expected to exhibit a strong pollen sensitivity. Mold spores, on the other hand, are extremely light and are carried on the higher wind currents during the warmth of the day. With the setting of the sun and the onset of the evening cool, the mold spores drop to levels nearer to the ground and may be more easily inhaled. The patient whose symptoms peak with sunset may be expected to be mold sensitive. Dust, of course, is present throughout the day and is primarily an indoor problem. For reasons still not clear, however, dust symptoms usually peak after the patient has retired. The allergy victim complaining of severe nasal congestion within minutes of going to bed will usually be found to be dust sensitive.

Exposure

Many problems related to specific allergy exposures have already been discussed. A complete and detailed history will bring out essentially all common exposures on the part of any patient. It is unfortunate, however, that many histories are taken in a stereotyped manner that leaves some of the most severe exposures unidentified. A Texas allergist often commented: "The history is everything. I take at least a four-hour history on every patient. I see 40 patients a day."[12] The implication, of course, is that taking a history is an ongoing process, never truly completed. Much information is gained through day to day contact with the allergy nurse. Specific exposures must be recognized. The advent of a new pet in the house may be important. A move to a new house or a change of job may add new allergenic problems. Prolonged travel increases dust exposures, since airlines and commercial buildings are poorly ventilated and usually overly air conditioned. No simple rule may be applied here, since by its very nature, allergenic exposure is an individual condition. Such exposure must be recognized, however, and assiduously investigated if the sensitive patient is to be given means of satisfactory relief.

SYMPTOMS OF INHALANT ALLERGY

Inhalant allergy, as has been noted, is essentially all IgE-mediated Gell and Coombs type I, immediate in onset and clearing quite rapidly upon removal of the offending substance. The symptoms are largely confined to the respiratory system and nearby mucous membranes. Best known are those of pollinosis or "hay fever," consisting of conjunctivitis, profuse rhinorrhea, repeated sneezing, and nasal congestion. More common but less obvious to others present are those of perennial allergic rhinitis. Here, the conjunctivitis is less apparent and the main complaint is nasal obstruction and postnasal drip. Sneezing may be intermittent but presents less of a problem.

A dry, irritated, and frequently sore throat may result from mouth breathing as well as direct irritation from the allergens. The chronic, irritated throat of dust allergy is well known. Its very chronicity differentiates it from infection. Deeper in the throat, a sensation of mucus constantly present, plus repeated clearings of the throat and a varying degree of hoarseness indicate involvement of the larynx. A cough, either productive or dry, and occasional wheezing lead to a suspicion of allergic tracheobronchitis with or without asthmatic bronchitis. Suspicions are confirmed by the symptom pattern, nasal smears or scrapings, negative sputum cultures, and a known allergic background. Certain symptoms, although not diagnostic, are characteristic of certain allergic problems.

Most cases of conjunctivitis are due to pollen sensitivity. Mold rarely produces this. Dust often causes a distinct itching of the inner canthus of the eye without mucous membrane involvement. A deep, wet cough leads the investigator to suspect mold sensitivity. The allergic patient, however, tends to be sensitive to a large number of inhalant allergens, and an overlap of symptoms is the rule rather than the exception. It must be remembered that allergy is a genetic defect in the immune mechanism, and in the presence of such a defect, repeated sensitization may be expected. The only guide to the presence of inhalants as the offenders lies in the tendency of the symptoms to remain in the respiratory system. Since such patients may also be food sensitive, the diagnosis may still be difficult.

PHYSICAL FINDINGS

The physical examination by the otolaryngologist is normally limited to the ears, nose, and throat, supplemented by radiographs of the lungs and sinuses. The nasal mucosa in pollen allergy tends to be congested, pale, bluish, and covered by copious watery mucus.

In the dust-sensitive patient, and sometimes in those sensitive to epidermals, the mucosa is dry and red, resembling that seen in a head cold. The pharynx tends to show increased vascularity and scattered lymphoid islands. The larynx may be somewhat edematous but rarely shows any indication of inflammation. Without other disease, the lungs will normally be clear. The sinuses may be cloudy owing to edematous mucosa, but this will generally be uniform and rarely will any fluid levels be present. As with most aspects of inhalant allergy, the physical findings will rarely be clear-cut, and the absence of infection is of more value than the presence of other findings. Many inhalant allergic patients will show nearly normal physical findings during less severe stages of their disease.

Inhalant allergy is the most common and best recognized form of allergic disease. Whereas its very widespread nature makes for a considerable range of variability, it presents an overall consistent pattern and is usually easily recognized.

REFERENCES

1. Bostock J: Case of a periodical affection of the eyes and chest. Med Chir Trans 10:161, 1819.
2. Bostock J: Of the catarrhus aestivus, or summer catarrh. Med Chir Trans 14:437, 1828.
3. Wyman M: Autumnal Catarrh. Cambridge, Hurd & Houghton, 1872.
4. Blackley CH: Experimental Researches on the Causes and Nature of Catarrhus Aestivus (Hay Fever or Hay Asthma). 1st ed. London, Balliere, Tindall & Cox, 1873.
5. Noon L: Prophylactic inoculation against hay fever. Lancet 1:1572, 1911.
6. Pollen Guide. Meridian Biomedical, 821 Wagon Trail, Austin, TX.
7. Pollen Aeroallergens of the United States. Center Laboratories, 35 Channel Drive, Port Washington, NY.
8. Antigen Labs, P.O. Box 125, 30–34 South Main Street, Liberty, MS.
9. Hollister-Stier Division of Miles Laboratories, P.O. Box 3145, Spokane, WA.
10. Lewis WH, Vinay P, Zenger V: Airborne and Allergenic Pollens of North America. Baltimore, Johns Hopkins University Press, 1983.
11. "House dust." National Institute of Allergy and Infectious Diseases. Publication No. 83–400.
12. Oscar Hamilton, M.D.: personal communication.

Suggested Additional Readings

Rinkel HJ: The management of clinical allergy. Parts I, II, III. Arch Otolaryngol 77:56, 1963.

Williams RI: Skin titration: testing and treatment. Otolaryngol Clin North Am 4:508, 1971.

Willoughby JW: Serial dilution titration skin tests in inhalant allergy—a clinical quantitative assessment of biologic skin reactivity to allergenic extracts. Otolaryngol Clin North Am 7:579, 1974.

Cowen DE: Serial dilution titration: technique and application. ORL Allergy Digest 41:37, 1979.

Cowen DE: Serial dilution titration: technique and application. *In* King HC (ed): Otolaryngologic Allergy. 1981, pp 179–207.

King HC: Endpoint titration and immunotherapy. Otolaryngol Clin North Am 18:703, 1985.

King WP: The role of the skin endpoint titration method in allergy. *In* Goldman JI: The Principles and Practice of Rhinology. New York, John Wiley & Sons, 1987, pp 283–292.

Ward WA: Skin endpoint immunotherapy. *In* Krause HF: Otolaryngic Allergy. Philadelphia, WB Saunders, 1989.

CHAPTER 11

Molds: Good News—Bad News

Walter A. Ward, Jr., M.D.

A perplexing disease struck the inhabitants of the small French village of Pont-Saint-Esprit in 1951. Victims were certain that evil spirits had entered their bodies; several victims died. Attending physicians were baffled by the mysterious malady, until they identified it as a form of ergotism, commonly known as "Saint Anthony's fire," caused by eating bread that had been made from contaminated flour. Ergotism had been common in northern Europe during the Middle Ages, especially in regions with a high consumption of rye bread. Modern methods of grain cleaning and milling practically eliminated ergotism, a disease caused by the fungus ergot. To be more precise, ergot is a sclerotium, a special part of a fungus that develops on grass, particularly rye. The fungal spores are carried by the wind to flowers of rye grass; there, the spores germinate, infect, and destroy the ovaries of the rye plant, replacing them with masses of microscopic threads joined together into a hard fungal structure shaped like the rye kernel but much larger and darker. This is ergot, and it contains numerous poisonous, organic compounds called alkaloids. A mature head of rye may carry several ergots in addition to the noninfected kernels. In the process of harvesting, much of the ergot falls to the ground, but that which remains is mixed with the grain. If the ergot is not removed before milling, ergotized flour may be used in baking, causing "Saint Anthony's fire," for which no cure is known.[1]

The threat of ergot is broader, however. That which falls to the ground may produce further problems. Cattle that graze in the rye field after harvest may consume enough ergot to cause the abortion of fetuses or even their own death. Then, when the rye blooms in the spring, ergot remaining on the ground will produce tiny, black, mushroom-like bodies that expel quantities of spores, starting the cycle of infections all over.

One of the many chemicals in ergot is lysergic acid, the active principle of the psychedelic drug lysergic acid diethylamide (LSD). Thus, a single fungus containing ergot may reduce crop yields, sicken and even kill humans, cause abortion or death in cattle, and be used as a source of LSD. However, on a positive note, ergot also provides drugs useful in inducing labor in pregnant women and controlling hemorrhage after birth, drugs for which no good substitutes have yet been found.

So, in any consideration of molds there is good news and bad news. The good news dates back to the first loaf of leavened bread ever baked and the first vat of grape juice that was fermented into wine to the many antibiotics that have revolutionized the practice of modern medicine.

The bad news is that molds probably contribute to more dollars lost in destructive value to humans and their property than all other organisms put together from the Dutch elm and chestnut diseases that have destroyed entire forests, to the smut that destroys grains, to the rusts and molds that have contributed to the rusting, mildewing, molding, and rotting of metal, paper, cloth, leather, and farm products. However, despite the extensive use of molds for productive purposes in modern times, many of these molds produce allergy problems in sensitive individuals. It is this bad news that shall be the focus here.

CLASSIFICATION

The terms "fungus" and "mold" are frequently used interchangeably. However, the term fungus is more inclusive, as it includes yeasts, smuts, and rusts, all of which are fungi but are not molds. The most conspicuous of fungi is the mushroom, which lends its Latin name, *fungus* (pl., *fungi*), to the whole family of these plants. The study of fungi is known as mycology, which is derived from the Greek word for mushroom, *mykes*. Fungi other than mushrooms are sometimes collectively called molds. However, the term is best restricted to fungi of the type represented by bread mold. It is the imperfect fungi, the true molds, that are most often the cause of allergic manifestations, especially asthma. Thus, the term "mold allergy" is most frequently used to refer to this problem.

Molds are characterized by the fact that they are scavengers, requiring organic material that is synthesized by other organisms to survive. They require a very high concentration of oxygen, need considerable moisture, and thrive in temperatures of about 68° to 86° F (20° to 30°C). However, some molds exist at temperatures just above freezing, as evidenced by those found in the spoilage of foods in the refrigerator.

Approximately 50,000 species of fungi have been described, and it is estimated that as many as 100,000 to 250,000 species of fungi may occur throughout the world. Although more prevalent in warm, moist climates, fungi are also found in deserts as well as the Alaskan tundra. More important, because of the light weight of the spores, as the air expands in the heat of the day, spores may be carried to elevations where they become caught in wind currents and are transported hundreds of miles, thus affecting susceptible individuals in remote areas far distant from their place of origin. With so many different species of fungi, it is vital that the physician focus on the molds that are of greatest clinical importance.

Prince and his associates have conducted and published mold surveys of most regions of the United States.[2–5] It is important to be familiar with the geographic distribution of molds. Much has been written about outdoor molds and indoor molds. A study of these reports would indicate that basically the same molds are present in both locations, and except in unusual situations, there is no significant difference between indoor and outdoor molds, although in a given region of the country the relative importance of a given mold may shift in an indoor list versus an outdoor list. However, the same molds are usually present in both.

Prince divides fungi into three classifications: (1) universal dominants; (2) geographical dominants; and (3) local dominants.[6]

Universal dominants, found in significant number throughout the entire world and known to cause disease, include Alternaria, Hormodendrum (Cladosporium), Aspergillus, Penicillium, Pullularia, Phoma, Trichoderma, Fusarium, Helminthosporium, Curvularia, Epicoccum, and yeasts (Cryptococcus and Rhodotorula). The geographical dominants include Rhizopus, Mucor, Stemphylium, Botrytis, Paecilomyces, Monilia (*M. sitophilia*), and Spondylocladium.

Prince's final classification is the local dominants. These are clinically significant only in local situations under certain conditions. Although it is important to remember that these are allergenic and may present considerable problem for the susceptible individual who is exposed to them, they are not considered major offenders because of their restricted occurrence. Local dominants include Verticillium, Cephalosporium, Sporobolomyces, Absidia, Myrrothecium, and Chaetomium.

Since the pioneer work by Storm van Leeuwen of Holland in the third decade of this century, there has been increasing evidence of the importance of allergy to various inhaled mold spores in the causation of asthma, hay fever, and other allergic illnesses. Van Leeuwen reported a patient whose asthma recurred after her return home from a prolonged, symptom-free visit to the Alps. A careful mycological investigation of her home revealed that her kapok mattress was the host for a pure culture of *Aspergillus fumigatus*.[7] In 1934, Prince published the first treatise on his many molds and their relationships to diseases.[2] Similar studies followed by Feinburg and Randolph in Chicago, and others.[8–11] Statistics were reported that demonstrated the magnitude of the role molds play in causing allergic diseases. These figures emphasize the importance of learning as much as possible about these organisms.

SYMPTOMS OF MOLD ALLERGY

Patients with mold allergy will present with clinical symptoms that are similar if not identical to those caused by other inhalants. These may include sneezing upon exposure to the antigen accompanied by nasal obstruction, rhinorrhea, and frequently eustachian tube block and headaches associated with sinus obstruction, all due to histamine release within the nasal and sinus mucous membranes. Itching of the skin and eyes, pharyngitis accompanied by hoarseness, and itching throat are frequently seen. An itching throat is also associated with food allergies. These may well be those that have mold associated with their production, such as bread, wine, and cheese.

There are also a number of symptoms peculiar to mold allergy. A wet, gurgly cough that may or may not be productive, occurring especially at night, is significant. Burning and itching of the eyes in the absence of the redness seen in patients with inhalant and dust allergies is of great significance. In addition, environmental flares that occur under certain circumstances may be extremely important. The patient who enters a damp basement to do the laundry and has a flare-up, or the patient who reports congestion when mowing grass, is usually the victim of a mold allergy. Contrary to popular belief, most flare-ups resulting from mowing the grass in the usual lawn are not the result of a grass sensitivity, since most grasses must be 10 to 14 inches high before they can pollinate. Similarly, flare-ups that occur when raking leaves are due primarily to mold allergy from the decaying leaves, although dust may also be a factor. The patients whose symptoms flare in the evening rather than during the day may well have mold allergy, since the mold spores expand and are carried high in the atmosphere during the heat of the day, but descend at night when temperatures drop. A flare after a wind storm may be caused by dust, pollen, or mold (or a combination thereof), but the flare that occurs following a thunderstorm is normally due to mold because the heavy rain settles the dust and washes out the heavier pollen. Likewise, patients whose symptoms clear immediately after the first heavy snowfall of the winter are likely victims of mold allergy, since molds are carried out of the air in a very heavy snowfall.

It is important to give particular attention to the role of the seasons in mold allergy. In the South, for example, the symptoms of mold allergy are often seen year-round. In the North, molds are generally dormant in the cold winter months, so that symptoms are usually confined to the period between March and November, peaking from May to September, causing many physicians to mistakenly diagnose pollen allergy. Although these may be factors, if consideration is not also given to the importance of molds, treatment will not achieve optimal results.

The importance of an adequate history in evaluating the mold-allergic patient cannot be overemphasized. As previously noted, symptoms are very important, but an environmental history must also be carefully and thoroughly evaluated. This should include not only the patient's home, but also the surrounding neighborhood, the location and nature of employment, and hobbies of the patient that might bring exposure to molds.

Although a physical examination frequently reveals those findings suggestive of allergy, the overall physical examination may not offer specific indications to implicate molds. At this point, skin testing is appropriate. The author prefers serial dilution titration techniques, which are covered in Chapter 18.

ALLERGENIC EXTRACTS

Two criteria are used in identifying molds as allergens: (1) proven exposure—large quantities of the specific mold spore have been demonstrated repeatedly in air breathed by the patient with asthma and/or hay fever; (2) positive skin test—extracts of the particular mold spore produce a positive, immediate cutaneous or intradermal reaction in the patient with asthma and/or hay fever. Delayed reactions do occur with mold allergy. They are discussed in the chapter on pathogenic fungi.

The Food and Drug Administration assembled the Panel on Review of Allergenic Extracts to review the safety, efficacy, and labeling of allergenic extract products and related licensed biologic products. The findings and recommendations were reported in the Federal Register (January 23, 1985, vol. 50, #15). On the basis of the Panel's findings and recommendations, the FDA proposed classifying mold extract as follows: Category I: safe, effective, and not misbranded; Category II: unsafe, ineffective, or misbranded; Category IIIA: to remain licensed pending reclassification into either Category I or Category II; and Category IIIB: license to be revoked pending completion of studies permitting determinations of effectiveness and safety.[12]

Extracts of most of the mold spores meeting these criteria have been licensed for use in diagnostic skin testing and immunotherapy. However, only a small fraction of these have proved to be allergenic on the basis of the two criteria outlined previously combined with the following additional essential criteria necessary for including in Category I for mold immunotherapy: (1) clinical correlation—the patient with symptoms who is known to have environmental exposure and positive skin and/or laboratory tests must also show improvement both symptomatically and immunologically with immunotherapy; (2) safety—safety of the extract must be established.

Stock Cultures

Stock cultures of molds are obtained as isolates from soil and air samples or from culture collections such as the American Type Culture Collection. Two basic methods are used for obtaining allergenic extracts from the mature growth cultures.

Regular Process. The mature growth in production cultures is separated from the medium and dried at the end of the incubation period (generally two to three weeks). The dried mold is ground to a powder and stored in sealed containers at 20° to 24° C until ready for use in preparing extract. The dried mold is extracted with extracting fluid, sterilized by filtration, and then processed like other allergenic extracts.

MMP Process. This type of mold extract is prepared under franchise from the Association of Allergists for Mycological Investigation. The association's graduate mycologist maintains the stock cultures and provides them to the manufacturer. At the end of a five-week incubation period, the growth and broth are separated and the broth is concentrated, dialyzed, and dehydrated by freeze-drying. This dry material contains the nondialyzable mold metabolites including the allergens. It is stored in sealed containers at 1° to 5° C until needed in preparing liquid extract. The liquid extract is prepared by reconstitution of the dry material in either 50 per cent glycerin and 0.9 per cent NaCl solution, or in a buffered saline preservative solution (since the patient may be glycerin-sensitive, the buffered saline solution may be preferable). The extract is then sterilized by filtration. The stock concentrate is then tested for sterility and general safety, and the extract is stored at 1° to 5° C.[13]

Skin Test Diagnosis

Serial dilution titration testing of the clinically sensitive patient who develops asthma and/or hay fever after the inhalation of specific mold spores will usually produce positive skin tests to the mold extracts. However, patients will not have equal skin reactivity. Although most will react to low doses of the mold extract, a few will react only to high doses.[14–21]

Many atopic patients who are clinically symptom-free after exposure to the specific spores but have asthma and/or hay fever symptoms induced by exposure to other allergens will show a positive skin reaction to the specific extract.[17, 18, 20, 22] Typically, such clinically insensitive patients are "less skin reactive" than their clinically sensitive counterparts, so that higher doses are typically required to elicit the reaction. However, a few clinically insensitive patients will react to low doses of the extract just as some clinically sensitive patients react only to high doses. Thus, it is important that a positive skin reaction to a certain concentration of the specific mold extract should not be the sole diagnostic basis for initiating immunotherapy, but rather should be combined with the total picture demonstrated by the patient's history and physical examination.

There is considerable evidence of both cross-reacting and distinct antigens in various genera and species of the Dematiaceae, especially Alternaria, Helminthosporium, Curvularia, Spondylocladium, Stemphylium, Hormodendrum, and Pullularia. This has been demonstrated by skin testing,[23] neutralization of passive transfer,[24] antigen binding,[25, 26] and gel diffusion techniques.[27] The genera-specific antigens may be the only important ones in a particular case and should thus all be available for both diagnostic studies and immunotherapy.[23] There are reports of patients who are sensitive to only one species of dematiaceous mold. Other studies indicate that both the strain of *Alternaria tenius* (syn., *A. alternaria*) and the conditions of culture may influence the specificity of the extract.[28] Well-defined, potent mold cultures demand careful attention to both mold strain and cultural conditions.[13]

The aspergilli also show evidence of cross-reacting and distinct antigens.[18] Because of the specific antigens of these species, the physician needs extracts of multiple species of aspergilli. As with the Dematiaceae, the assurance of well-defined, potent mold extracts of aspergilli demands intensive study of the effects of both strain and cultural conditions on specificity.

Six mold spores have been shown to be effective aids for the diagnosis of hay fever and/or asthma induced by the inhalation of specific mold spores. These are Alternaria, Cladosporium (Hormodendrum), Helminthosporium, Aspergillus, Penicillium, and Mucor. The FDA Panel on Review of Allergenic Extracts recommended that these be placed in Category I for skin test diagnosis.[29]

There is less definitive but suggestive evidence indicating that five other extracts may also be effective for skin test diagnosis. These are Botrytis, *Candida albicans, Cephalothecium roseum, Monilia sitophilia,* and Pullularia. The Panel recommended that these be placed in Category IIIA for skin test diagnosis.

MANAGEMENT

Hyde has reviewed and revised Thommen's postulates about pollen allergy to apply to mold allergy. Hyde's postulates are:

1. The pollen or other spore type must contain an excitant of hay fever or asthma.
2. The spores must be produced in sufficiently large quantities.
3. The spores must be sufficiently buoyant to become airborne.
4. The plant species must be widely and abundantly distributed.
5. In order that any type of spore shall be regarded as the causative agent in a particular case of hay fever or asthma, it must be shown that the patient experienced symptoms at a time or times when the spores concerned were present in large quantities in the air.[30, 31]

As in the management of other allergic conditions, the avoidance or elimination of the causative fungi should be given primary consideration. In the case of most ingestant fungi and in certain environmental and occupational types, avoidance of the offending allergen is relatively easily accomplished. Since the mold-supporting peculiarities of the patient's own environment may influence his particular allergic responses, environmental mold surveys together with a detailed patient history will be invaluable in the successful management of the mold-sensitive patient.

Precautions in the elimination or avoidance of the source of the allergen should be followed, much the same as for house dust (Tables 11–1 and 11–2). Pillows and mattresses are important sources of fungi and should be enclosed in dustproof covers, or sponge rubber may be substituted. In areas with excessive humidity,

Table 11–1. CHARACTERISTICS OF THE MORE IMPORTANT MOLD AND FUNGUS SPORES

Alternaria	An atmospheric mold, dirty gray or brown, found in dead, dying, or decaying vegetation; causes a known disease of the potato and beans; may be a factor in house dust sensitivity
Aspergillus	Most commonly found in old, damp, musty houses, in kapok, or on dried fruits such as figs and dates, where it assumes a bluish color; also found in onions as the black mold
Hormodendrum	An atmospheric mold, brown like Alternaria, found in decaying vegetation (tomato and peaches) and responsible for the brown discoloration; also found in spoiled meat and tobacco
Mucor	Commonly found in old, musty houses, furniture, and furnishings; the grayish-white growth known as whiskers, which is observed upon the surface of meat, is formed by this mold; also found in decaying fruits
Monilia	May be found in the sputum; common in aging nutmeats, in bakery goods, in yeast, and as the brown rot in stone fruits
Penicillium	The cause of common bread molds; a factor in the ripening of Camembert and Roquefort cheeses; may be found in apples, pears, and citrus fruits as the blue mold rot

Table 11–2. COMMON SOURCES OF FUNGI

Alternaria	Parasite or saprophyte on plants and plant material
Aspergillus	Fowl (chicken), damp hay and grain, damp cloth, leather goods, spoiled foods (bacon, sausage, etc.), damp paper, decaying plant and vegetable material
Chaetomium	Damp paper, fabric, and straw
Epicoccum	Decaying vegetative material, plant leaves, and uncooked fruit
Fusarium	Parasitizes green plants (peas, beans, cotton, tomato, corn, sweet potato, rice)
Geotrichum	Cheese, pickles, decaying plants
Helminthosporium	Cereal grain, plants, grasses (i.e., wheat, oats, rye, etc.)
Hormodendrum (Cladosporium)	Leather, rubber, cloth, foods, and wood products
Monilia sitophilia	Bread and pastries
Mucor	Barns, barnyards (decaying vegetable or animal material)
Penicillium	Plant rot, cheese, fruits, bread, leather, fabrics
Phoma	Books (paper), paints containing lead, green plants
Paecilomyces (Spicaria)	Damp paper, decaying vegetable material
Pullularia	Plastics, paints, caulking compounds
Rhizopus	Breads, cured meats, root vegetables (i.e., potatoes)
Stemphylium	Paper, wood, canvas, cotton fabrics

The sources given for the individual fungus in no way cover all the areas where it can be found. All of the fungi listed have been isolated from soil samples, and the majority are also commonly isolated from air samples. Specific sources listed are those in which man has come in contact with the fungi in either of two manners: (1) a useful nature, such as cheese and wine production; (2) a detrimental relationship, such as destroying food plants or textiles and discoloring paints or plastics.

the growth of molds on shoes, leather goods, and clothing should be eliminated. Burning an electric light in a closet at all times will help protect the contents. Upstairs rooms or apartments are less susceptible to mold than are those on a lower level. In almost any climate, basement rooms may become damp and grow mold profusely if adequate precautions are not taken. Adequate ventilation as well as the use of an electric dehumidifier should help, but some situations are very difficult to control. Attention should be given to the insulation on air conditioning and refrigeration equipment to keep it as dry as possible, thus reducing mold growth. Similarly, cold-mist vaporizers must be carefully cleaned or they will merely aggravate rather than relieve the patient's symptoms.

The mold-sensitive patient must also take care to avoid contact with molds in certain environments such as wooded areas, swamps, open country, and farms, especially those with threshing or grain-handling operations. Haystacks, feed barns, and dead vegetation (grass, leaves) all support mold growth readily, especially before the first killing frost in the fall. Symptoms exacerbated by lawn mowing have been discussed previously. Libraries may provoke symptoms in the mold-sensitive patient, since book bindings are a primary source of environmental mold. Rather than depriving the mold-sensitive child of favorite stuffed animals, regularly placing them in a clothes dryer for 20 minutes of drying will kill most of the offending mold. Much of the success of treatment will depend upon careful detective work and trial and error to determine the sources of the offending molds.

Where the elimination or avoidance is not possible, or in cases in which inadequate relief is achieved, immunotherapy is indicated. It should be noted that in some instances house dust is a contributory factor, so it may be necessary to treat both dust and mold to achieve optimal results.

Acknowledgment

Special gratitude is expressed to Alison McConnell Spransy for her editorial assistance in preparing this chapter.

REFERENCES

1. Foust JW: Mold allergy. Personal correspondence with author, 1983.
2. Prince HE, Selle WA, Morrow MB: Molds in the etiology of asthma and hay fever: a preliminary report. Texas State J Med 30:340, 1934.
3. Prince HE, Morrow MB: Molds in the etiology of asthma and hay fever with special reference to the coastal areas of Texas. South Med J 30:754, 1937.
4. Prince HE, Morrow MB: Airborne molds in the etiology of respiratory allergic diseases. Tri-State Med J 11:2277, 1939.
5. Morrow MB, Lowe EP, Prince HE: Mold fungi in the etiology of respiratory allergic diseases. I. A survey of air-borne molds. J Allergy 13:215, 1942.
6. Prince HE: Non-pollen factors simulating seasonal respiratory allergy. South Med J 32:956, 1939.

7. van Leeuwen WS: Allergic Diseases. Philadelphia, 1925.
8. Feinburg SM: Mold allergy: its importance in asthma and hay fever. Wis Med J 34:254, 1935.
9. Feinburg SM: Seasonal hay fever and asthma due to molds. JAMA 107:1861, 1936.
10. Feinburg SM, Little HT: Studies on the relation of microorganisms to allergy. III. A year's survey of daily mold spore content of the air. J Allergy 7:149, 1936.
11. Rackemann FM, Randolph TG, Guba EF: The specificity of fungous allergy. J Allergy 9:447, 1938.
12. Department of Health and Human Services, FDA: Biological products; allergenic extracts; implementation of efficacy review. Fed Reg 50:3082, January 23, 1985.
13. Department of Health and Human Services, FDA: Biological products; allergenic extracts; implementation of efficacy review. Fed Reg 50:3193, January 23, 1985.
14. Chobot R, Dundy H, Schaffer N: Relationship of mold reactions to clinical symptoms. J Allergy 12:46, 1940.
15. Blumstein GI: Mold allergy. II. Clinical analysis. Ann Allergy 3:341, 1945.
16. Halpern SR, Holman J, Whittaker C: The correlation between skin and respiratory mucous membrane tests with molds in allergic rhinitis. Ann Allergy 19:1407, 1961.
17. Pennington ES: A study of clinical sensitivity to air-borne molds. J Allergy 12:388, 1941.
18. Pennington ES: A study of the incidence of air-borne molds and of skin sensitivity to molds. South Med J 33:931, 1940.
19. Brown GT: Hypersensitiveness to fungi. J Allergy 7:455, 1936.
20. Fontana VJ, Wittig H, Holt LE: Observations on the specificity of the skin test. The incidence of positive skin tests in allergic and nonallergic children. J Allergy 34:348, 1963.
21. Colen J, Van Arsdel PP, Pasnick LJ, Horn JD: Observations on the experimental reproduction of asthma with mold antigens. J Allergy 35:331, 1964.
22. Bronsky EA, Ellis EF: Inhalational bronchial challenge testing in asthmatic children. Pediatr Clin North Am 116:85, 1969.
23. Prince HE, Morrow MB: Skin reaction patterns to dematiaceous mold allergens. Ann Allergy 29:535, 1971.
24. Prince HE, Arbesman CE, Sellers ED, et al: Mold fungi in the etiology of respiratory allergic diseases. XII. Further studies with mold extracts. Ann Allergy 7:597, 1949.
25. Schumacher MJ, McClatchy JK, Farr RS, Minden P: Primary interaction between antibody and components of alternaria. I. Immunological and chemical characteristics of labeled antigens. J Allergy Clin Immunol 56:39, 1975.
26. Schumacher MJ, Farr RS, McClatchy JK, Minden P: Primary interaction between antibody and components of alternaria. II. Antibodies in sera from normal, allergic and immunoglobulin-deficient children. J Allergy Clin Immunol 56:54, 1975.
27. Bonilla-Soto O, Rose NR, Arbesman CE: Allergenic molds. J Allergy 32:246, 1961.
28. Schumacher MJ, Jeffery SE: Variability of *Alternaria alternata:* biochemical and immunological characteristics of culture filtrates from seven isolates. J Allergy Clin Immunol 58:263, 1976.
29. Department of Health and Human Services, FDA: Biological products; allergenic extracts; implementation of efficacy review. Fed Reg 50:3196, January 23, 1985.
30. Coca AF, Walzer M, Thommen AA: Asthma and hay fever in theory and practice. Baltimore, Charles C Thomas, 1931, pp 598, 600, 601, 603.
31. Hyde HA: Atmospheric pollen and spores in relation to allergy. I. Clin Allergy 2:153, 1972.

CHAPTER 12

Pathogenic Fungi Allergy

Walter A. Ward, Jr., M.D.

Three groups of pathogenic fungi that can cause allergic reactions as well as infection are Trichophyton, Oidiomycetes (Candida or Monilia), and Epidermophyton. These three groups are the etiologic agents of the dermatomycoses, primary fungal infections that generally present on the nails, the mucous membranes, and the skin of various areas of the body, where they take the form of tinea (Fig. 12–1). Tinea can be caused not only by the Trichophyton and Epidermophyton organisms, but also by the group of pathogenic fungi called Microsporium.

The diagnosis is usually simple when a dermatomycosis is suspected. Scrapings of scales from the active lesion, nail scrapings, or roots of loose hair can be placed on a glass slide to which 15 per cent potassium hydroxide (KOH) has been added and a coverslip applied. Examination under a medium-power microscope allows visualization of any mycelia or spores, by which the primary pathogenic fungal infection can be identified. When a mucosal fungal infection is suspected, diagnosis must often be based on cultures and biopsy. Other types of fungal infections include the dermatophytoses (athlete's foot), onychomycosis (Fig. 12–2), and candidiasis.

The purpose of the preceding paragraph was to introduce the usual presentation of these primary fungal infections so that their allergic presentation can be recognized. This allergic presentation is called a dermatophytid, or "id" reaction. "Id" reactions are characteristically erythematous, vesicular, bullous, or eczematoid

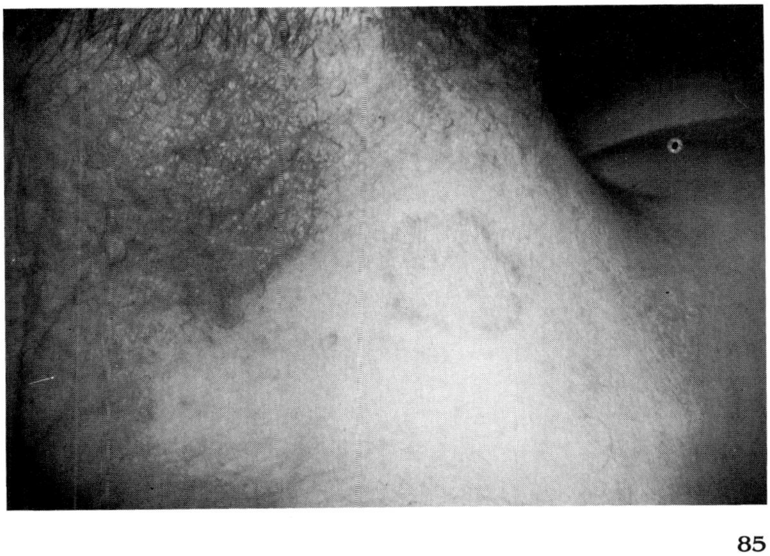

FIGURE 12–1. Tinea on the back of the neck.

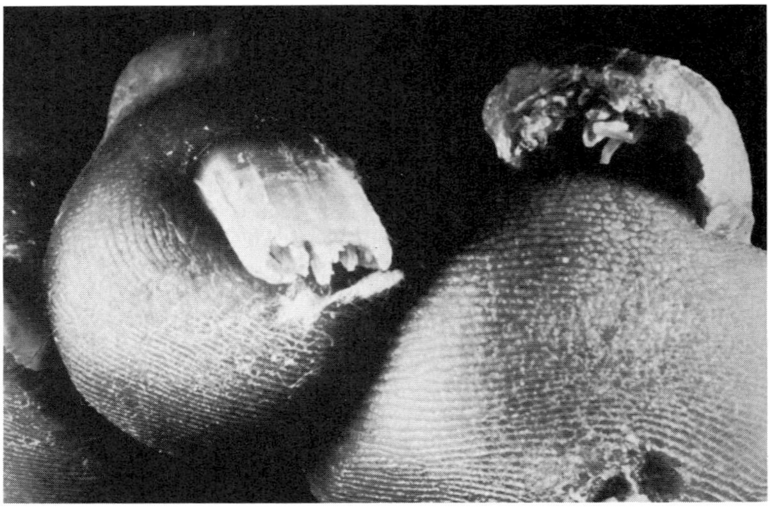

FIGURE 12–2. Onychomycosis, fungal infection of the toenails.

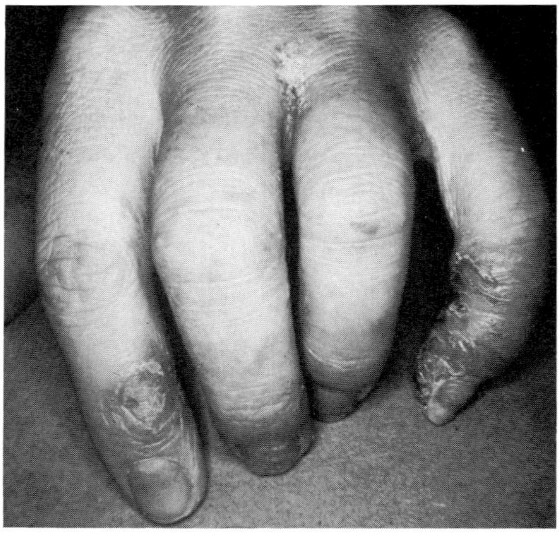

FIGURE 12–3. Id reaction of the hand.

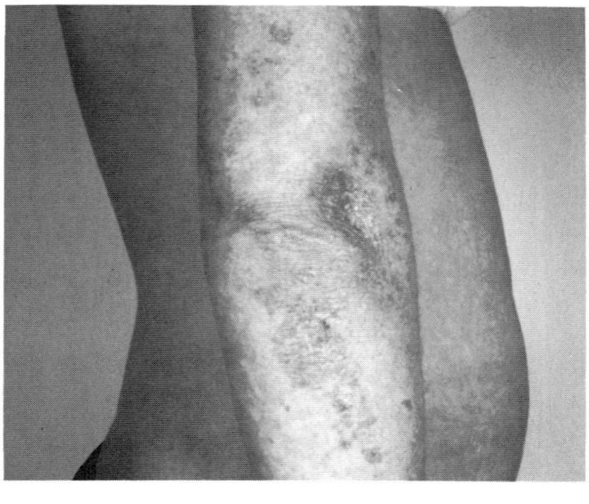

FIGURE 12–4. Id reaction on an arm.

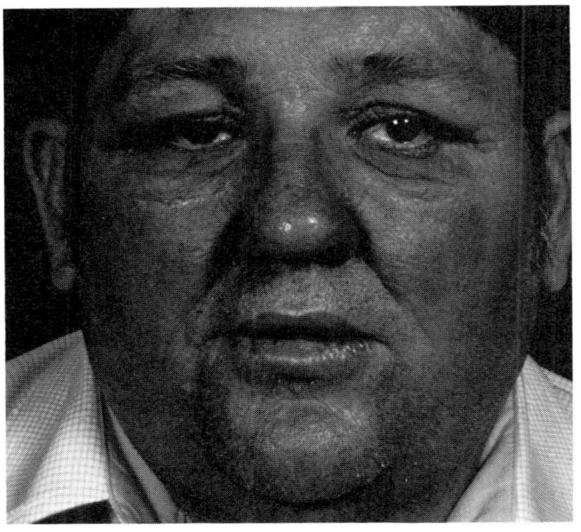

FIGURE 12–5. Facial id reaction.

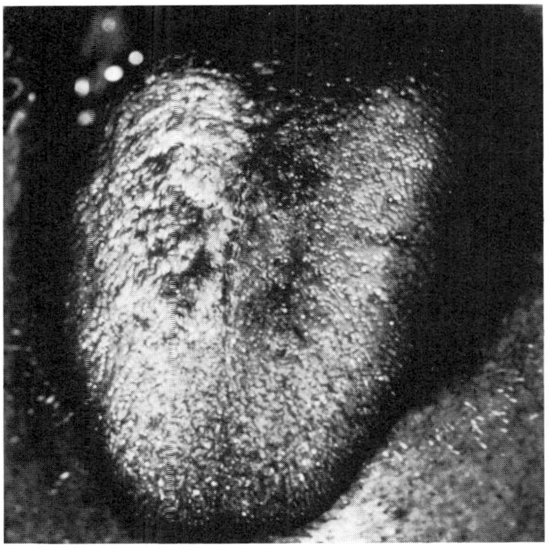

FIGURE 12–7. Black hairy tongue.

pruritic eruptions, the pruritus varying from mild to insufferable (Figs. 12–3 to 12–6). They are always the result of an allergy sensitization to the fungus protein from a primary fungal infection. The criteria for diagnosis of the "id" reaction are (1) the diagnosis of a primary fungal infection, either present on the body at the time of the "id" eruption or previously present by history; (2) the absence of demonstrable fungi at the secondary, or "id," site; and (3) a positive hypersensitivity skin reaction to the combined trichophytin, oidiomycetes, and epidermophytin antigens (TOE antigen) or to any one or more of the separate antigens for these three groups. By separating these antigens into separate skin tests, you decrease the risk of possibly sensitizing a previously nonreacting patient to any of the antigens in the combined TOE mixture.

While we speak of a cutaneous manifestation of the "id" reaction, we should not forget other signs and symptoms representative of this al-

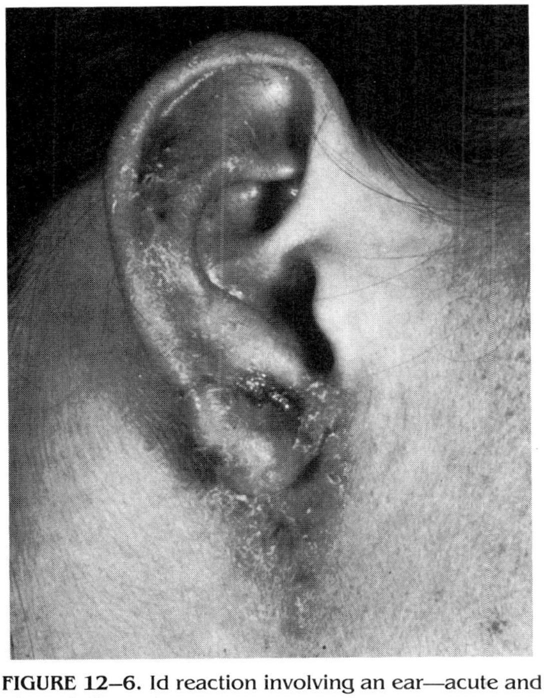

FIGURE 12–6. Id reaction involving an ear—acute and highly inflamed.

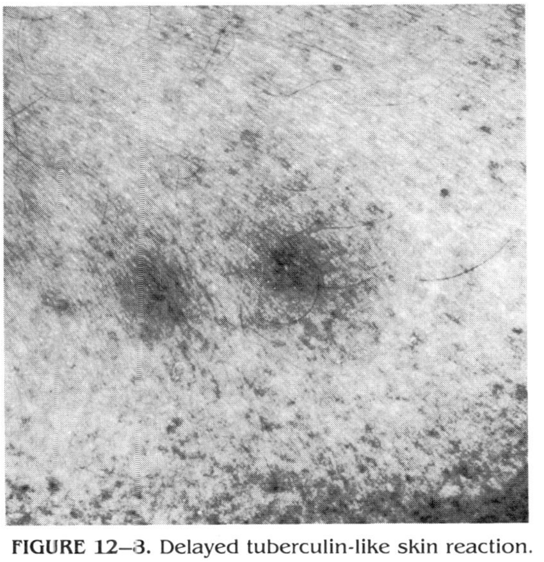

FIGURE 12–8. Delayed tuberculin-like skin reaction.

lergy: a hairy, often black, tongue (Fig. 12–7); halitosis; chronic heartburn or dyspepsia; excessive flatulence; pruritus ani; chronic vaginitis unresponsive to the usual treatment; headache; a cough unresponsive to the usual treatment; and otomycosis.

TESTING FOR "ID" REACTION

In skin testing for the allergic manifestation of these fungi, one must begin testing, as in all testing by the serial endpoint titration method, with a weak, nonreactive dilution. In 1959, Brown[1] recommended that testing be started with a #9 dilution, because he had found that of 109 positive reactors, all had reacted to a #5 or stronger dilution (e.g., #4, #3, #2), except for one who had reacted to a #9 dilution on original testing. In actuality it is safe to begin testing with a #6 dilution.

As in all serial endpoint titration (SET), you must obtain an endpoint for fungal atopy. The classic definition of the endpoint is the dilution that produces a 7 mm or larger wheal preceded by a nonreactive wheal on the preceding weaker dilution, and followed by a 2 mm larger wheal on the next stronger dilution. In the majority of instances when testing for fungal allergy, a perfect 4 mm wheal has been applied, the nonreactive wheal will measure 5 mm at the end of 10 to 15 minutes, and the first reactive wheal will measure 7 mm at the end of the same length of time. However, in contrast to the recommendations for SET testing with food and other inhalant allergens, the author does not recommend that you go any farther, that is, that you obtain the confirming, or 9 mm, wheal on the next stronger dilution for fungi, because you may cause an exacerbation of the patient's symptoms. If on your initial test dose of a #6 dilution you should obtain a reaction larger than 7 mm, it is imperative that you prepare dilutions weak enough to obtain the 7 mm wheal. If symptoms have been exacerbated, these symptoms, as a general rule, will abate when the true endpoint is obtained. It is wise to warn your patient when testing for fungal allergy that there may be a zone of erythema not seen during testing for pollens and that there is quite often a delayed tuberculin type reaction, which may take one week or more to subside (Fig. 12–8). If an "id" reaction is suspected and a negative skin response is obtained, the patient should return the next day for evaluation of any evidence of delayed skin reaction. When a delayed reaction is present, the author generally chooses the dilution that caused the minimal type of skin reactivity as the "probable" endpoint.

In conclusion, the skin endpoint titration method is ideally suited for the treatment of fungal allergy problems because it has a safety factor that allows testing and treatment without danger of precipitating severe symptoms. A mild increase in symptoms while testing for these fungal antigens will always confirm your preliminary diagnosis. This response was first noted by Brown in 1959,[1] and it continues to hold true.

REFERENCE

Brown DW Jr: The clinical use of T.O.E. in E.E.N.T. practice. Arch Otol 70:558, 1959.

CHAPTER 13

Stinging Insect Allergy

Hueston C. King, M.D., F.A.C.S., F.A.C.A.

In the past few years, stinging insect allergy has gained a position of importance unprecedented in the allergy field. This is in part due to an increasing recognition of the importance of stings in producing severe illness and death. It is well established that more people die from insect stings every year than from the bites of poisonous snakes.[1] There is reason to suspect that the actual mortality from insect stings may be considerably higher. Recent serologic evidence indicates that a significant number of sudden deaths, especially in rural areas, may actually be due to allergic reactions to insect stings, as significant levels of IgE antibodies have been found in the victim's blood.[2, 3]

Part of the interest is due to anticipation among researchers that stinging insect allergy may represent a microcosm that in years to come will predict the direction of all IgE-mediated allergy diagnosis and therapy. In view of the random development and frequently conflicting studies concerning most aspects of allergy care, a field with a limited format allowing detailed study, monitoring of laboratory parameters and documentation of results without other sensitivities clouding the issue is greatly to be desired. Whether stinging insect allergy will fill the bill has yet to be determined.

THE STINGING INSECTS

All stinging insects belong to the Hymenoptera family, lacy-winged insects with an abdominal stinger, a modified ovipositor. The members of the group will be considered individually.

Bees

By far the most virulent venom is produced by the honey bee, family Apidae. No honey bees are native to the United States. All have been imported from Europe for their product and have adapted well throughout the land. They are found in profusion throughout the country. Since the honey bee is a pollen gatherer, it is usually found on flowers and is attracted to bright colors and sweet smells. Stings occur only during the day and only when the bee is threatened, since administering a single sting kills the bee. In spite of this, the honey bee remains moderately aggressive when challenged. The venom of the honey bee has been the most extensively studied of the Hymenoptera. It is a complex substance containing kinin, acetylcholine, serotonin, histamine, phospholipase A, and hyaluronidase. Four major allergenic proteins have been identified: phospholipase A, hyaluronidase, apamin, and melittin. Of these, phospholipase A has exhibited the greatest allergenic activity.[4]

Other members of the bee family include the bumble bee and the sweat bee. An occasional anaphylactic reaction has been reported from stings by these bees, but these have been too infrequent to evoke enough concern to have had a venom supply developed for treatment.

Vespid Wasps

The vespid wasps, superfamily Vespoidea, include the common wasp, the yellow hornet, the white-faced hornet, and the yellow jacket. While there is much overlap in the geographic distribution of these insects, they are most prevalent in the northeast area of the United States and all along the Atlantic coast. In the south central United States these wasps, especially the yellow jacket, are relatively rare. The vespid wasps are much more aggressive than the bees, and the yellow jacket has a well-deserved reputation for its bad temper. Like the bees, these wasps are social insects and build nests of paperlike material that are hung beneath branches, eaves of houses, or any projecting surface. Some nest in holes in the ground. With the coming of cold weather the entire colony is destroyed except for the new queens, which go into hibernation to start new colonies in the spring.

Because of their narrow waists, wasps can consume only liquids. Their diet consists of nectar and the juice of ripe or rotting fruit; hence, they are commonly found around orchards and garbage pails. The wasp returns to the nest at night, and essentially all stings occur during the day.

Wasps, hornets, and yellow jackets come in a variety of shades and patterns of black, brown, tan, and yellow. Identification of the living insect is possible by close observation, but few nonentomologists will take the time or effort required to make such identification. This is especially true if the potential victim has a known sensitivity to insect stings. This can produce a serious problem in therapy, since accurate identification of the offending insect is a prerequisite to initiating venom therapy. This is discussed at greater length in Chapter 28.

The venom of all the vespid wasps is similar but not identical. Some substances appear throughout the group whereas others do not, making cross-reactivity only partial. Both wasp venom and hornet venom contain histamine, serotonin, and phospholipase A and B. Wasp venom also contains dopamine and hyaluronidase, which hornet venom does not. Hornet venom contains acetylcholine, which wasp venom does not, and both contain a variety of insect-specific kinins. Not all the ingredients of the venoms of stinging insects have yet been fully identified. It is of interest that dialysis does not diminish the toxic action of vespid venoms, indicating that the critical agents are high molecular weight substances, whereas the toxic principles of bee venom are dialyzable.[5]

Treatment of vespid-sensitive patients has been performed with reasonable success with a mixed vespid venom. This is a compromise on cost, since all venom treatment is expensive. When attaining the desired level of 100 μg of venom for each vespid included in the venom treatment mix, however, a 20 per cent failure rate has been reported. Treatment of vespid-sensitive patients with 200 μg of yellow jacket venom alone is under consideration as being possibly superior, but no definite recommendations for this have as yet been made (Fig. 13–1).

Polistes Wasps

The Polistes wasp is a reddish-brown wasp with a slender, spindle-shaped abdomen. It is prevalent through the south central United States, where the vespid wasp is rare. Certain Polistes species are indigenous to the Pacific coast. Unlike the vespid wasp, the Polistes wasp seeks the shelter of houses and attics in the winter, and it may become a nuisance when it emerges from hibernation in the spring. Fortunately, it is not aggressive, and stings are relatively rare. Its habits otherwise resemble those of the vespid wasp.

The venoms of all the Polistes wasps cross-

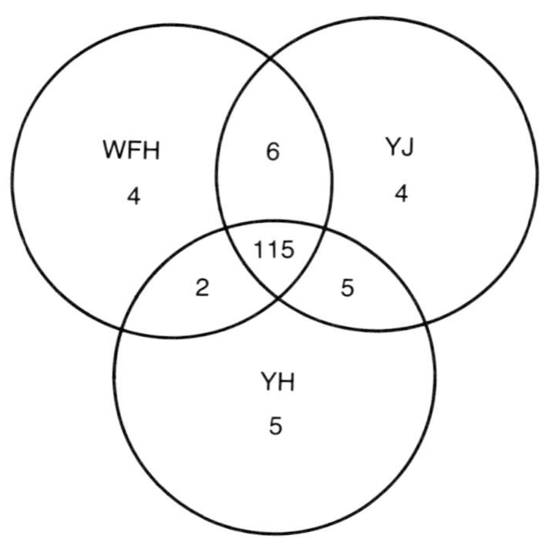

FIGURE 13–1. Distribution of positive skin tests within the vespid genus. WFH, white-faced hornet; YJ, yellow jacket; YH, yellow hornet. (From Ramirez DA, et al: Diagnosis of hymenoptera hypersensitivity. Ann Allergy 47:303, 1981. Used by permission.)

react well. They contain two minor and one major kinin. At least one species is known to contain hyaluronidase. Polistes venom does not cross-react with any other stinging insect venom.[6, 7]

Imported Fire Ant

Two species of imported fire ants are present in the United States, *Solenopsis richteri* and *Solenopsis invicta.* There are five species of native fire ants but none are dangerous. The imported fire ants appear to have arrived originally in Mobile, Alabama, probably in fruit shipments from South America. From there, *Solenopsis invicta* has spread rapidly throughout the southeastern United States. These insects now represent the greatest cause of manpower loss over this area and are spreading more widely every year. It is estimated that their progress will be stopped only by 10° low winter temperature line.[8] *Solenopsis richteri* has adapted poorly and remains near the Mobile area.

The fire ant is unique among the Hymenoptera in being both a biting and a stinging insect. When aroused, the ant seizes the victim with its mandibles, inflicting a painful bite. Without releasing its hold, it stings and pivots, stinging repeatedly until dislodged. The easily identified fire ant mark is a central bite surrounded by a crescent of sting marks. Field workers may be swarmed over by these insects, sustaining multiple stings and becoming completely disabled for prolonged periods. The ants nest in open fields, and it is there, when a nest is encountered, that the stings occur. Although deaths from fire ant stings are rare, morbidity is common and severe. The fire ant venom is unique in the animal kingdom. It is composed of more than 95 per cent simple disubstituted piperidine alkaloids. The venom is necrotoxic, hemolytic, insecticidal (except for the ant), and bactericidal and causes activation of the complement pathway. To date, no fire ant venom is commercially available, and treatment must be given with whole body extract.

THE STING

Whereas there has been some debate on the subject, most investigators consider insect sting anaphylaxis an IgE-mediated phenomenon.[9] The anaphylactic reaction is different from the pure toxic reaction to the sting. Literally hundreds of stings would be required to kill an adult from toxin alone, and most deaths are reported from one or two stings. No relationship has been shown between the patient subject to large local reactions from stings and those undergoing anaphylaxis. In addition, the tendency to insect sting anaphylaxis is no higher in the atopic population than in the nonatopic group. An allergic background, then, is of little value in anticipating the patient likely to be at risk from stings. Only a previous record of anaphylactic-type systemic reactions from previous insect stings is of value.

The systemic allergic reaction to the sting is prompt in onset, occurring within minutes and sometimes within seconds. The first indication of trouble may be a hacking cough and a sensation of constriction in the throat. This is usually followed by generalized urticaria, sneezing, respiratory distress, a fall in blood pressure, rapid pulse, and various degrees of angioedema. The victim suffers from acute anxiety and a sense of impending doom. Death may occur, and when it does it is anoxic in nature. Various degrees of systemic reaction may occur, and have been classified for convenience into four levels of severity:[10]

Slight General Reaction. Generalized urticaria, malaise, and anxiety.

General Reaction. Any of the above plus two or more of the following: generalized edema, chest constriction, wheezing, abdominal pain, nausea and/or vomiting, dizziness.

Severe General Reaction. Any of the above plus two or more of the following: dyspnea, dysphagia, hoarseness or thickened speech, weakness, confusion, severe anxiety.

Shock Syndrome. Any of the above plus two or more of the following: cyanosis, fall in blood pressure, collapse, incontinence, unconsciousness.

This older format has been refined into a new grading system, the Systemic Reaction Index (SRI), with a maximum score at 1.0.[11]

This breakdown may serve as a rough guide to the treating physician, but the possibility of severe morbidity or death should indicate the need for instituting therapy on an emergency basis if any signs of a systemic reaction appear.

An additional form of systemic reaction to insect stings is occasionally seen. This occurs 10 to 14 days after the sting, and resembles a serum sickness with symptoms such as low-grade fever, malaise, lymphadenopathy, and polyarthritis. These may be vague and frequently not associated by the patient with the sting. The true allergic reaction is the immediate one, but the delayed form may result in sensitization. The exact relationship is not yet clear.

Stinging insect allergy represents a special and unique aspect of the field. Much new knowledge has emerged in the past few years and more is appearing almost daily. It may be anticipated that the field will change radically over the next few years, and may very possibly offer unique insights into the mechanism and treatment of other allergic problems.

It should be noted that this discussion is limited to stinging insect allergy. These insects use their stings as weapons. Biting insects such as mosquitoes, flies, and sandflies do not sting but possess a toxic saliva. Although in some cases this may produce an allergic reaction, it is not life-threatening. Biting insects may be repelled by a variety of substances marketed commercially for the purpose of disguising or making unappetizing the odor of humans. These cannot be counted on to repel stinging insects. Stinging insects attack when threatened and are not attracted to humans usually.

REFERENCES

1. Parrish HM: Analysis of 460 fatalities from venomous animals in the United States. Am J Med Sci 245:129, 1963.
2. Hoffman DR, Wood CL, Hudson P: Demonstration of IgE and IgG antibodies against venoms in blood of victims of fatal sting anaphylaxis. J Allergy Clin Immunol 71:193, 1983.
3. Schwartz HJ: Report to American Academy of Allergy and Immunology. Chicago, 1984.
4. Haberman E: Bee and wasp venoms. Science 177:314, 1972.
5. King TP, et al: Protein allergens of white-faced hornet, yellow hornet and yellow jacket venoms. Biochemistry 17:5165, 1978.
6. Tu AT: Venoms: Chemistry and Molecular Biology. New York, John Wiley & Sons, 1977.
7. Findlay, SR, et al: Polistes wasp hypersensitivity: Diagnosis by venom-induced release of histamine in vitro. J Allergy Clin Immunol 60:230, 1977.
8. Schmid WH: Medical implications: Imported fire ants, *solenopsis invicta*. Cutis 19:794, 1977.
9. Reisman RE: Allergic reactions to insect stings. South Med J 71:208, 1978.
10. Frazier CA: Clinical Symposia, vol 20. CIBA Pharmaceutical Co, 1968.
11. Lockey RF: Director, American Academy of Allergy and Immunology Committee on Insects.

PART II

Diagnostic Procedures

CHAPTER 14

Office Evaluation of the Allergic Patient

Joseph P. Keenan, M.D., F.A.C.S.

Patients with signs and symptoms of allergic disease affecting the head and neck area frequently choose to be treated by an otolaryngic allergist. Due to embryologic development, the mucous membrane lining the upper respiratory tract is often the target organ for allergic disease in this area.[1] It may be the source of entry of the allergen into the body as well as the target organ in which the symptoms of allergic disease are produced. The interaction of the antigen-antibody complex, its fixation to the mast cell, and the subsequent release of histamine and other mediators generate the signs and symptoms of allergic disease. These signs and symptoms are manifested by many disease states that otolaryngologists are often the first to see and treat. Some of these are sinusitis, otitis, rhinitis, and laryngitis. The modern otolaryngologist must be well versed in both the diagnosis and management of these diseases if the "total patient" is to be treated effectively.

HISTORY

It is of paramount importance for the otolaryngologist to spend adequate time eliciting a detailed, comprehensive, and exceedingly complete allergy* and medical history to ensure a correct diagnosis and the proper course of therapy. This history should be comprehensive in that the entire state of health of the patient is evaluated. There must be careful questioning of the patient concerning overall health, any co-

*See Allergy Questionnaire.

existing systemic illnesses of which the patient is aware, and whether or not these illnesses are directly or indirectly related to the allergy problem.

The physician must also obtain a careful medication history. In this way, illnesses that the patient might fail to mention may be discovered. For example, the patient may fail to mention that he has hypertension but on further questioning about medications may reveal the use of antihypertensive medications, and the doctor will discover additional factors that might impact on the allergy diagnosis. Antihypertensive medications, such as some of the beta-blockers, may at times cause symptoms of nasal stuffiness, exacerbating an underlying allergic rhinitis. The physician should carefully elicit from the patient, or parent in the case of children, all known allergies—drug, inhalant, ingestant, and chemical—and closely question the patient about previous treatments undertaken with other physicians. A detailed surgical history should be obtained. From this, a wealth of information will be gained ranging from adverse reactions to anesthetics and postoperative analgesics to discovering surgical procedures that might or might not be related to the allergy for which the patient is currently seeking treatment. Patients with histories of surgical procedures on the upper respiratory tract, such as nasal polypectomies or sinus procedures repeated over a number of years, would be highly suspect for possible underlying allergic diatheses as the cause for the recurrent obstruction leading to the need for repeat surgeries.[2]

Because allergic disease has an increased incidence in some families, a careful family history should be obtained. Although reports vary as to the exact incidence, it is probable that if both parents have allergic disease, allergy will be manifest in 80 to 85 per cent of the offspring, indicating a definite familial predisposition to the allergic disease. One should also be aware that certain diseases might not be recognized initially as due to allergy, such as sinusitis or headache related to congestion and edema of the mucous membranes surrounding the sinus ostia. This edema and chronic inflammation of the mucous membranes might have nasal allergy as its underlying cause. The physician should be cognizant that certain symptom complexes (i.e., nasal polyps with chronic sinusitis) certainly should make one suspicious of a personal or family history of allergy.

It is well known that environmental exposure can markedly aggravate symptoms related to allergy. A patient whose primary occupation is in a fairly sheltered environment, such as an assembler of computers working in a semisterile environment, obviously has different stresses placed upon the immune system than does a house painter who is working outside and being exposed to pollens and molds as well as the chemical outgassing from paint with a petrochemical base. These two patients are going to have radically different degrees of stress placed upon their immune systems. A person with the same degree of allergic predisposition in these two different environments will exhibit significantly different degrees of symptoms. In other words, the patient working in a fairly sheltered environment is going to have some masking of allergic symptoms because of the lack of challenge and stress placed on the system. The house painter, on the other hand, is most likely going to exhibit more symptoms, even assuming the same underlying familial/genetic predisposition, because the total allergic load placed on the immune system is markedly greater.

Home and Work Environment

In obtaining the history in the potentially allergic patient, there are several areas that should be included. Ascertaining the presence or absence as well as the type of pets in the home and work environment is important, since certain animals are much more allergenic than others, such as dogs and cats, whereas some, such as fish or reptiles, are fairly low in allergenicity. The patient must also be asked detailed questions about hobbies and other out-of-work exposure. Certain pesticides, fumigants, and fertilizers might also tremendously aggravate the underlying allergic condition of a person who has gardening as a hobby. Also, furniture refinishing and artistic endeavors may lead to chemical or toxic exposures, especially in a poorly ventilated environment.

The patient must be carefully questioned in regard to exacerbations of symptoms: When and where do they occur? If the individual is better during the workday and symptoms are aggravated after working in the garden on the week-end, then this would lead one to believe that certain chemicals to which the person is being exposed when gardening are the culprit in this case. On the other hand, if a patient whose occupation involves plastics reports worsening symptoms during the work week but notices some improvement in symptoms after being at home for two days, then it is the possible outgassing and fumes generated from these plastics that become suspect as the etiologic agent. The housewife or chef working near a gas stove for hours may complain of symptoms primarily related to that location.

Smoking can aggravate the symptoms of allergic rhinitis. Patients in general are strongly encouraged to stop smoking. Children whose parents smoke are at just as much risk as the parents themselves in terms of aggravation of allergic disease. The question of second-hand smoke is one that is just starting to be addressed by our society, and such smoke, too, can aggravate allergic disease, especially in relatively enclosed spaces such as restaurants, airplanes, and enclosed offices.

PHYSICAL EXAMINATION

General

It is incumbent upon the otolaryngic allergist treating a patient for allergic disease to carefully exclude any other contributing local or systemic illness. If indicated or warranted by age, by general state of health, or because of a pathologic process detected on the physical examination performed by the otolaryngologist, detailed physical examination by an internist should be strongly recommended prior to starting allergic testing and treatment.

Regional Examination

A careful examination of the head and neck area is of paramount importance. Different stigmata of allergic disease can be seen in the patient with allergic disease, and these should be actively sought for in all areas of the head, neck, and upper respiratory tract.

It is wise to have some method of dealing with this examination, and a systemic approach is the most productive if followed consistently. Start the examination of the head and neck with a careful examination of the area in toto. In examining the general features (e.g., the nature and quality of the hair), any scaling on the scalp, any abnormalities of skin turgor, or any obvious lesions or growths should be looked for and excluded.

Ears

A careful examination of the auricles should be carried out. Attention should then be turned to the external auditory canals. If there is any abnormal increase in desquamation of epithelium, a chronic eczemoid external otitis might be diagnosed. The tympanic membrane should be examined to ensure that the eardrums are healthy and do not show signs of repeat chronic ear infection or atelectasis, scarring, or retraction. The mobility of the eardrum should be checked to make sure there is no effusion present in the middle ear space, which could be a result of chronic eustachian tube dysfunction because of obstruction of the orifice in the nasopharynx due to edema of the mucous membrane secondary to allergy. As always, the otolaryngologist should be alert to the presence of a persistent unilateral secretory otitis media, often one of the common presenting signs of a nasopharyngeal neoplasm. It would be disastrous for the physician and patient alike for a nasopharyngeal angiofibroma or carcinoma to be misdiagnosed and treated as a case of allergic rhinitis.

Nose

The nose should then be carefully examined. The nasal apparatus is the organ system that serves as the portal of entry of the allergen as well as the target organ in which the allergic reaction develops in humans. First, the mucous membranes should be evaluated. Is there swelling of the nasal membranes? Does there exist a bluish color or boggy distention of the mucous membrane overlying the turbinates and nasal septum? These can be judged by both inspection as well as palpation with a cotton-tipped applicator. One should look for clear watery discharge, especially of an excess quantity. Is there marked hypertrophy of the mucous membrane covering the turbinates? Are there nasal polyps, or is septal deviation present? There are often combinations of these abnormalities present, and it is important to separate the relative contributions of each in the generation of the patient's complaint. One way to separate mechanical deformities such as a nasal septal deviation as a cause of nasal dyspnea from the mucous membrane swelling is the careful examination of the tissues before and after the application of a vasoconstrictive nasal spray. The result of this examination, before and after the spray, accompanied by the patient's report of improvement or lack thereof will help the physician distinguish swelling of the mucous membranes versus some cartilaginous or bony obstruction as being the primary source of the patient's discomfort. Rhinomanometry is a very helpful procedure in measuring nasal functional ability. Pressure flow studies pre- and posttreatment with a topical vasoconstrictor spray will help to objectify and document improvement in nasal pulmonary function that could be expected once the allergic rhinitis and resultant mucous membrane edema is satisfactorily managed.

Oral Cavity

Examination of the oral cavity should begin with an overall view of the relative health of the teeth and gums. At times, poor dental health is related to obligatory mouth breathing and the subsequent drying of the teeth and gums because of the inability of the patient to breathe through the nose. Advanced periodontal disease is aggravated by similar nasal obstruction. One should also be aware of any abnormal or fetid odor, which can have the same cause or may be due to chronic sinusitis. The oral pharynx as well as the nasopharynx should be carefully examined with a mirror both to detect "cobblestoning" of the posterior pharynx, which is seen in patients with allergic rhinitis, as well as to rule out any space-occupying neoplastic disease of the nasopharynx.

The hypopharynx and larynx should be carefully examined by indirect laryngoscopy with a mirror or with a flexible nasal pharyngoscope. Hoarseness can be caused by many different sources, such as neoplastic disease of the vocal cords of either a malignant or benign process, or can result from the accumulation of mucus on the vibratory surface of the true or false vocal cords. Often, an excess amount of this mucus causes symptoms directly related to its prodigious production in patients with an underlying allergic rhinitis. The separation of these causes is of utmost importance to both the patient and physician. During this examination, it should be noted whether there appears to be normal, moderate, or excess amounts of secretions and whether they are clear, mucoid, watery, or thick in the nasopharynx and hypopharynx, and if there is pooling of secretions in the vallecula or pyriform sinus. Frequently, the allergic patient will report feeling a "lump in the throat." Many times what this represents is the pooling of excess secretions in the hypopharynx and larynx (which will resolve when the allergy is brought under control) or edema due to a secondary inflammatory reaction.

Neck

Examination of the neck should be carefully and methodically carried out. One should first check for any localized lymphadenopathy. At times this would be a result of recent ear infection in younger children or of recent bacterial pharyngitis in adults. At times there is some localized regional lymphadenopathy, a result of infection years ago that has never totally resolved. A lump in the neck, especially in the jugular digastric area, may be a sign of nasopharyngeal disease, emphasizing the importance of the previous examination of the nasopharynx. One of the most common presenting signs of nasopharyngeal carcinoma is a mass in the neck in the jugular digastric area. One should also palpate for any hypertrophy of the neck muscles and the strap muscles. The increased frequency of swallowing that the allergic patient will perform in an effort to clear the mass-type sensation experienced in the throat will be evidenced by hypertrophy of some of these muscles. One should also examine the thyroid during swallowing to ensure there are no tumors, cysts, or masses in this area.

Chest

Careful auscultation, percussion, and examination of the chest should be carried out during respiration. In some patients, a mild degree of wheezing or other evidence of bronchospasm may accompany allergy. One should also listen

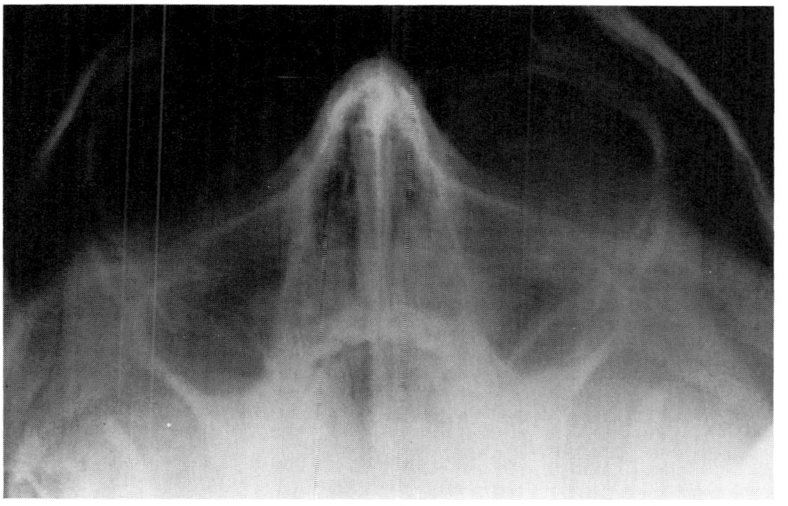

FIGURE 14–1. Clouding of maxillary sinus (Waters view). (Courtesy of Lincoln Russin, M.D.)

for any abnormalities of heart function such as murmurs, thrills, or gallops, which may suggest pulmonary congestion.

LABORATORY TESTS

Laboratory evaluation of the patient provides additional aids in the diagnosis of disease of allergic diathesis. A complete blood count (CBC) identifies any increase in leukocytes or any sign of recent infectious disease of bacterial or viral origin. In selected patients, depending on presenting symptoms, additional tests such as thyroid function studies, 5-hour oral glucose tolerance testing, and total eosinophil counts might be helpful. A screening IgE level may be obtained. This should not be viewed as an absolute indicator of allergic disease, for many times a patient with relatively severe rhinitis might have a normal total IgE level. It has been helpful in distinguishing those patients who are at increased risk of having major systemic reactions during the intradermal skin testing procedure, recognizing that the IgE level varies according to the age of the patient. At times, although not as a routine screening test, a general immunologic screen of the other immunoglobulins is indicated. In a pediatric patient with recurrent infections of the upper respiratory tract, this screen would help rule out any underlying major immunologic defects. In a relatively healthy middle-aged patient whose sole symptom is that of allergic rhinitis, it is probably not indicated. Other tests are sometimes indicated, especially in cases of unilateral facial swelling where angioneurotic edema is suspected. Tests such as C1, C2, and C1q esterase inhibitor help to distinguish those cases due to enzyme defect from those idiopathic in origin. Sometimes of a minor degree, angioneurotic edema as evidenced by swelling of the side of the face or tongue can be confused with a local reaction to a recent ingestion of a food to which the patient is allergic. The C1q inhibitor will be helpful in excluding at least a portion of these patients. Certainly it should be noted that a large portion of patients with angioneurotic edema are of the idiopathic type and, in this case, will have normal levels of the inhibitor enzyme.

Causes of regional lymphadenopathy in the neck, such as acute or chronic mononucleosis, should be investigated. Initially, the monospot test is indicated, but as many as 50 per cent may be negative, especially early, and the diagnosis must then be made by serial heterophil titers.

IgG levels, both pretesting and posttesting, are not widely used except in an experimental fashion at this time. However, it has been noted that there usually is a rise in IgG_4 antibody levels in those patients having a favorable clinical response to immunotherapy. In the future, it is possible that routine monitoring of the IgG levels will be used to gauge and document response to immunotherapy.

RADIOLOGIC STUDIES

Since many of the diseases related to allergic rhinitis involve organ systems that directly interact with the mucous membranes of the nasal cavity, ruling out disease in those associated structures is important. It generally is helpful in a person with long-standing allergic rhinitis to obtain sinus radiographs or tomograms or CT scan of the sinuses when the clinician deems them appropriate. Occasionally tomograms may be helpful, although they are replaced usually when CT scans are available. At times, clouding of the maxillary sinus (Fig. 14–1) or a fluid level (Fig. 14–2) will be seen. Polyp or mucocele formation may be noted in the sinuses because of long-standing nasal obstruction due to interference of the normal aeration and drainage of these sinuses through the maxillary ostia (Fig. 14–3). When the sinus films are obtained, it is also helpful to develop clear communication with the radiologist so that, as a routine, careful attention is given to the lateral radiograph to visualize the nasopharyngeal area well. This coupled with the careful mirror examination of the nasopharynx excludes neoplasm of this area. A computed tomography (CT) scan may be obtained; this is particularly imperative in those patients with marked symptoms related to the face and head, such as severe pain or pressure. A CT scan of the sinuses (Fig. 14–4) and/or the brain gives a very detailed and exact view of the health of these structures. Severe, persistent headaches may be caused by sinus blockage or by a brain tumor. In carefully selected patients, a CT scan is invaluable in the differential diagnosis of these cases. They are very helpful postoperatively to ascertain that the nasal antrostomies created at the time of the surgery are still patent, these areas being clearly seen on CT scan. Chest films are indicated if the patient has any signs or symptoms related to pulmonary disease. These are especially important in a person with a heavy smoking history to rule out such associated diseases as emphysema, bronchitis, or primary neoplasm.

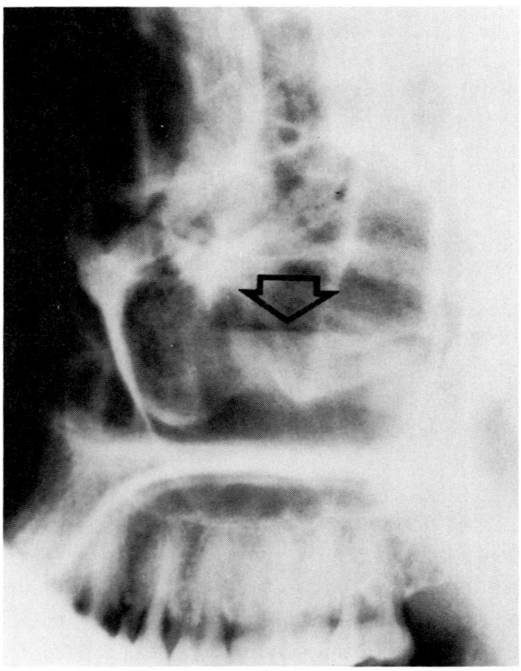

FIGURE 14–2. Air-fluid level in maxillary sinus (lateral view).

PULMONARY FUNCTION TESTING

An important part of the evaluation of the person with allergy of the upper respiratory tract may be pulmonary function testing. This is indicated at times even if frank compromise of pulmonary function is not present. Often after successful management by immunotherapy of an allergy that is affecting primarily the nose and sinuses, patients will report that they never breathed so well or they "are able to get more air." Some of this subjective improvement is most likely related to subclinical bronchospasm present in those patients with allergic rhinitis that has been relieved by the successful immunotherapy. It is wise to obtain the pulmonary function test as part of the initial allergy evaluation to establish a baseline level. Marked improvement of pulmonary function may well be demonstrated after successful immunotherapy related to mild reversible restrictive lung disease that is also improved by the immunotherapy. Response to this pulmonary testing helps to objectify and document the patient's response to therapy, positive or negative.

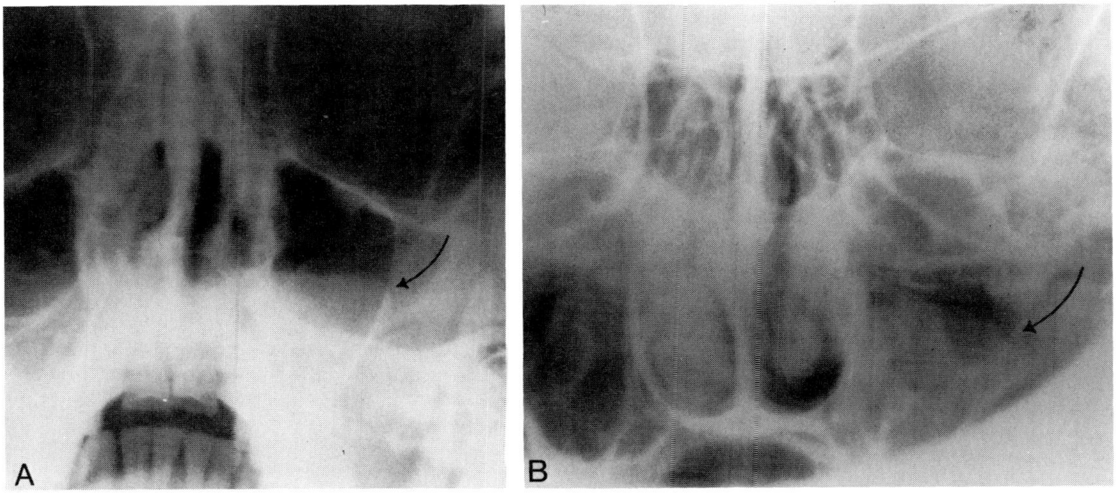

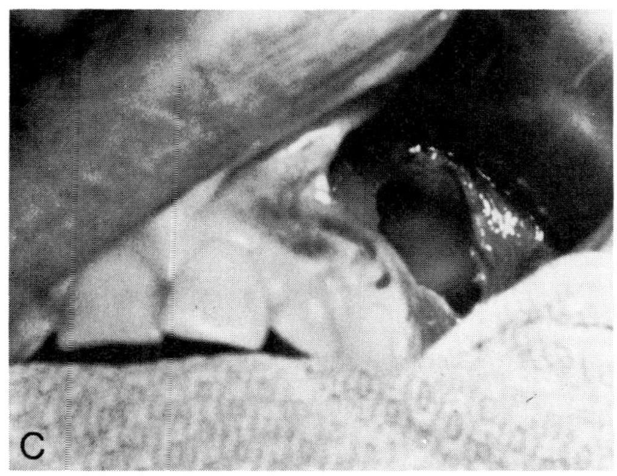

FIGURE 14–3. *A,* Polyp in maxillary sinus. *B,* Cyst in maxillary sinus. *C,* Cyst in sinus demonstrated via Caldwell-Luc surgical approach.

ALLERGY TESTING

Allergy testing quantitatively and qualitatively objectifies the patient's degree of allergic compromise. The testing can be broadly divided into two categories, that is, in vitro[3] and in vivo laboratory testing, which are discussed in subsequent chapters. Techniques of testing food allergy evaluation will also be discussed in detail. Skin endpoint titration is the most accurate in vivo method to document and objectively measure the degree of allergic reactivity. The major advantage of this technique is that both quantitative as well as qualitative parameters of the allergic disease are defined.

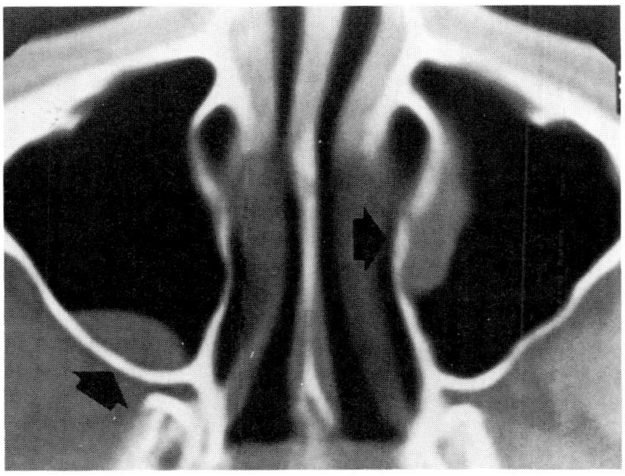

FIGURE 14–4. Computed tomography scan illustrating cysts (polyps) in each maxillary sinus.

SUMMARY

The otolaryngic allergist is the specialist of choice to evaluate and treat allergic disease. The target organ for inhalant allergens in humans is the upper respiratory tract, and diseases related to the ears, nose, and throat oftentimes have an allergic causation. As in all areas of medicine, the paramount importance of detailed history and physical examination is stressed. The importance of understanding the role of home and work environment in the aggravation of allergic disease as well as the role of familial predisposition is noted. Ancillary testing procedures, including roentgenographic, laboratory, and pulmonary, should be utilized when indicated. In vivo and in vitro tests may be used for testing; both have advantages and disadvantages, and it is incumbent upon the clinician to judge which modality will best serve the individual patient being treated at that time.

REFERENCES

1. Druce HM, Kaliner MA: Allergic rhinitis. JAMA 259:261, 1988.
2. Druce HM: Diagnosis and management of chronic sinusitis and its complications. Immunol/Allergy Clin North Am 7:117, 1987.
3. Nalebuff DJ, Fadal RG: RAST-based immunotherapy. Rhinology 22:11, 1984.

Allergy Questionnaire

Joseph P. Keenan, M.D., F.A.C.S.

Name ______________________ Age ________ Date ______________

Onset of symptoms ____

Major symptoms ____

____

____

1. Is your condition worse during any particular season, or is it a year-round problem? Season: ______________
2. Are you worse at any particular time of day? Time of day: ______________
3. Do you have any idea what is causing your symptoms? Cause: ______________

____

4. Do you take any medicine for your condition?	NO	YES
Does it help? When did you last take it? Rx: ______________		
5. Does the inside of your nose itch?	NO	YES
6. Do you have sneezing attacks? In morning?	NO	YES
7. Does your nose block often?	NO	YES
8. Do you get headaches when your nose blocks?	NO	YES
9. Do you have to blow your nose? Is it watery or thick mucus?	NO	YES
10. Are you bothered by postnasal drip?	NO	YES
11. Is your nasal blockage worse at any time of the day? When?	NO	YES
12. Have you ever been treated for sinus trouble or had polyps removed from nose or sinus?	NO	YES

THROAT

13. Does your throat or roof of the mouth ever feel itchy or tingly? When?	NO	YES
14. Do you usually have a sore throat in the morning that passes?	NO	YES
15. Do you clear your throat frequently?	NO	YES
16. Do you get ulcers or canker sores in the mouth?	NO	YES
17. Do you cough frequently? Upon arising?	NO	YES
18. Do you have asthma or have you ever had bronchitis? Frequency ______________ Last episode ______________	NO	YES

SKIN

19. Do you suffer with eczema or any chronic skin condition?	NO	YES
Describe: ______________		
20. Have you ever had hives? When? ______________ What caused it? ______________	NO	YES

21. Do you ever have swelling of the skin for no apparent reason—eyes, hands, ankles? NO YES
22. Are you bothered by itching skin when no rash is present? When? ______ NO YES
23. Does contact of your skin with certain substances cause a rash—fabrics, soaps, plants? NO YES

MISCELLANEOUS

24. Do you have frequent headaches? NO YES
    How often: ______
    Does medicine help: ______
    What kind: ______
25. Do you feel tired after a good night's sleep? NO YES
26. Do you have any muscle, back, or joint aches or pains on a chronic basis? Do you have growing pains? NO YES
27. Do your eyes, ears, or feet ever itch/athlete's foot? NO YES
28. Do you ever have ringing in your ears, dizzy spells, or loss of consciousness? NO YES

MEDICAL HISTORY

29. Did you have eczema as a child or excessive diaper rash? NO YES
30. Did you have colic or feeding problems as a baby? NO YES
31. Did you have croup as a child? NO YES
32. Have you ever had:
    - Measles
    - Tonsillitis
    - Pneumonia
    - Recurrent ear infections
    - Asthma
    - Hay fever
    - Migraine Dx by Dr.
    - Mononucleosis
33. Have you had any previous ENT surgery? NO YES
    Appendectomy? NO YES
34. Do you have high blood pressure or low blood pressure? BP ______
35. Is your mother living? NO YES Cause: ______
    Is your father living? NO YES Cause: ______
36. Any of the following in the family:

Cancer	Chronic skin conditions
Epilepsy	Frequent headaches
Diabetes	Hay fever
Severe mental illness requiring hospitalization	Bronchitis
	Hives
Sinus problems	Asthma

37. Do you drink alcohol? NO YES
    Frequency: ______
    Type: ______
38. Do you smoke? Frequency: ______

39. Do you use nosedrops or nasal sprays? Frequency: ______ Type: ______
40. Are you worse indoors or outdoors? INDOORS OUTDOORS

DUST

41. Are your symptoms worse when . . .
    You clean the house.
    The heat goes on in the fall.
    After you go to bed at night.

MOLD

42. Are your symptoms worse when . . .
    The weather is damp.
    You are around when grass is being mowed.
    You are in the basement of an old house.
    You are out in the early evening.
    Early fall or winter begins.

MISCELLANEOUS

43. Do you have any feather or down products that you use? NO YES
44. Does smoke bother you? NO YES
45. Do you have problems with cosmetics, perfumes, soaps, shampoos, or deodorants? NO YES
46. Do insect sprays, moth balls, household cleaners aggravate your symptoms? NO YES
47. Do you have any pets? NO YES Type: ______
48. Do you use wool blankets or have wool carpeting? NO YES
49. How old is your home? ______
50. What type of heating is in your home? ______
51. Do you use a wood-burning stove? NO YES
    Primary or secondary?
52. What type of stove do you use? ______ GAS ELECTRIC
53. Do you have air conditioning or fans? FANS AIR BOTH
54. How many houseplants do you have? ______
    Where in the house? ______
55. Do you have mostly carpeting or hardwood floors? CARPET HARDWOOD BOTH
56. How old is your bed mattress? ______
    Is it in a vinyl cover? NO YES
57. Do you do any work or hobby in the home that requires special equipment, chemicals, etc.? NO YES
58. Describe your work environment. ______
    ______

59. Do your symptoms seem better or worse when at work, on vacation, or away from home? WORK HOME VACATION CAN'T TELL
60. Are you presently on medications for any other medical problems? NO YES
    What are they? ______________________________
61. Are you on birth control pills? NO YES
62. Do you use any nonprescription drugs or supplements regularly? WHAT? NO YES
63. When was the last time you were on antibiotics? ______
    How long?______
64. Have you ever been tested or treated for allergy before? NO YES
    How long ago? ______
    Successfully? NO YES QUESTIONABLE
65. Are you allergic to any drugs or medications? What? NO YES
66. Have you ever had a bad reaction to an insect sting or bite that required you to go to the ER for treatment? NO YES

FOOD

67. Are there any foods that you avoid because you have an adverse reaction to them—GI upset, headache, etc.? NO YES
    ____
68. Are there any foods that you eat regularly that you respond to in a specific way: coffee—wake up, chocolate—headache, milk—bloating, etc.? NO YES
    ____
69. How many servings do you have on a daily basis (D)? Weekly basis (W)?
    e.g., Coffee ______ Wheat and Pasta ______

Editors' Addendum

Helen Fox Krause, M.D., F.A.C.S.
Jerry D. Shamblin, M.D., F.A.C.S.
Lee Foley, R.N.

FOR OUR PATIENTS

As a patient in our office, you have consulted us for evaluation of your ear, nose, or throat problem. There is an indication that your health problem is caused by or seriously affected by allergic disease. You may be considering an allergic evaluation (tests, etc.) in our office. We have prepared the following information for you so that you may be better informed before you decide to undertake the expense and time required for proper allergic evaluation.

WHAT ARE ALLERGIES?

Common allergic problems that are easily recognized are "hay fever" and asthma. Skin eruptions from food ingestion, e.g., hives from strawberries and eczema from chocolate, are also commonly recognized allergic problems. More recently, medical investigators have demonstrated that many common and puzzling ear, nose, and throat problems may be the result of chronic allergy.

Allergies are sensitivities that susceptible persons develop to normally harmless substances. The tendency to become susceptible to various things in our environment is usually inherited. Parents frequently deny any knowledge of allergy in the family history, but further questioning will usually reveal patterns of food intolerances, "sinus trouble," and other changes to suggest long-standing, although mild, allergic disease. If the susceptibility to allergy is inherited, then it is the amount of exposure to an offending substance (allergen) that will determine whether the individual will develop a severe illness as a result of his or her allergy, or will only be aware of mild changes. The greater the time and/or amount of exposure, the greater the chances that a susceptible person will develop an allergic problem that will require medical management.

Allergens are substances that are capable of producing allergy. When an allergen enters the body, substances called antibodies are produced. The interaction of the allergen and the antibody produces an irritation in the affected tissue. The swelling of the nasal lining during the hay fever season would be an example of this interaction.

Allergens may enter the body by ingestion, inhalation, injection, and external contact with the skin. It is then apparent that foods, dust, pollens, fumes, and almost anything in the environment may cause allergic diseases. In testing for allergy, emphasis is placed on the two most important groups: foods and inhalants (dust, pollens, and molds). Methods for detecting allergy to other substances are also available.

ALLERGY TESTS

There are several ways to test for allergies: the scratch test, punch or prick test, inhalation and ingestion tests, intradermal tests, and RAST (radioallergosorbent test) done on the patient's blood sample. In our office, we do titration testing using the intradermal method and the RAST method, because we feel they are the most scientific and the safest procedures available. We have multiple dilutions of our allergens that are used in testing. The intradermal test is made by injecting a minute amount of allergen just under the skin. The resulting wheal resembles a small mosquito bite, and after 10 minutes of observation, an increase in size generally indicates a positive reaction to that dilution. The number of tests required will depend on a patient's detailed history and on the test reactions. RAST involves taking a sample of blood from the patient and using a sophisticated laboratory procedure for allergy determination. A few intradermal skin tests are then used to correlate the results and institute treatment. Several techniques are available to test for food allergies also. All treatments will be explained in detail if you are to undergo allergy testing.

By establishing the endpoint dilution, we are able to reach the level of optimum relief of allergic symptoms more rapidly. We are also able to recheck the endpoint dilution when we fail to obtain optimum relief in a reasonable period.

TREATMENT

Treatment of allergy is a cooperative venture with both patient and physician as participants. The goal of treatment is to produce an allergic balance so that the patient may be freed of existing allergic illness and avoid the development of new allergic problems. A basic part of management is teaching the patient to eliminate offending allergens whenever possible. Since certain allergens cannot be eliminated, the reaction of the patient to these substances is controlled by desensitization.

Desensitization is the technique of injecting small but increasing amounts of the allergen to control the allergic reaction so that the patient has little or no reaction when he or she is exposed to the offending substance. In our office, desensitization by injection is used for inhalant allergens.

In conjunction with desensitization, patients will be taught to avoid and eliminate allergens. The use of dust-free programs, mold control in the home, and control of animal danders are essential to achieve balance when these sensitivities exist. For patients with food allergies, lists of common contacts for specific foods are available. The use of a rotary diversified diet is often recommended to restrict the intake of offending foods and avoid the development of new food allergies.

The length of time a patient will require desensitization will depend on his or her particular allergic problem. If a patient has a severe ragweed allergy (hay fever), injections each year may be required. A patient with symptoms due to food allergy may be relieved when the offending food is eliminated, and further trouble may be avoided with a rotary diversified diet.

Allergy History Questionnaire

Helen Fox Krause, M.D., F.A.C.S.
Jerry D. Shamblin, M.D., F.A.C.S.
Lee Foley, R.N.

Name ______________________ Referred by Dr. ______________________ Date ________
Address ____
Telephone: Home ____________ Work ____________ Employer ________________
Birthdate ____________ Age ______ Marital status ______________________
Insurance information: Name of insured ___________________________________
Insurance company ______________________ Insurance numbers ____________

PLEASE STUDY EACH QUESTION CAREFULLY,
AND ANSWER IT AS BEST YOU CAN.

YES NO

____ ____ *Cough?* Constant? ____ Intermittent? ____ Daytime? ____ Nighttime? ____
____ ____ *Frequent colds?*
____ ____ *Temperature with colds?*
____ ____ *Sneezing?*
What might precipitate it or increase it? ____________________
Is it seasonal or related to location? ______________________
____ ____ *Sore throats?* Frequency? ____
From infections? YES ___ NO___ From drainage? YES___ NO___
____ ____ *Nose drainage?* From the front, or down the throat? Circle which one.
Drainage clear or colored? Thick? Thin? From right side? Left side?
____ ____ *Nose blockage?* Right side? Left side? Both sides?
____ ____ *Eye symptoms?* Burning, puffy, or watering? Circle which one.
Itching? YES ____ NO ____ Where? Inside corner? ____
Outside corner? ____ All over? ____
____ ____ *Headaches?* Which part of head? ________
What starts a headache? ______________________________
What makes it worse?________ Headache worse at any time of day? ___
Can you tell when a headache may be starting? ____ How? ________
____ ____ *Fatigue?* When? Certain times of the day?____ Before eating?________
After eating? ____ Certain days of the week? ____ When?________
Chronic (all the time)? ____________
____ ____ *Shortness of breath*? Do you know why? Explain__________________
____ ____ *Wheezing*? Now? ________ As a child?________ With exercise?______
Out in the cold?____________ With infections? ________________
Other things that cause your wheezing? ____________________
____ ____ *Asthma*? Now? ________ As a child? ________
____ ____ *Earaches?* Do your ears drain or run?________ If so, clear? Or cloudy
drainage? Itchy?____ Stuffy?____ Flaky?____ Ring?____ Buzz?____
Crackle? ____ Pop? ____ Other sounds? ____ Hearing loss?____
____ ____ *Vertigo* (Dizziness)? ____ When? ______________________
____ ____ *Loss of smell?* When? ______________________________
____ ____ *Loss of taste?* When? ______________________________

YES NO

_____ _____ *Laryngitis?*

_____ _____ *Eczema?* Now? _____ As a child? _____ Describe type and location. _______

_____ _____ *Hives?* When? _____________ Where? _____________ Specify. _________

Any known material that causes a rash? _____________________________

Soap _____ Ointments? _____ Paint? _____ Clothing? _____

Cosmetics? _____ Poison ivy? _____

_____ _____ *Fungus infections?* Athlete's foot? _____ Vaginitis? _____ Jock rash? _____

_____ _____ *Pets?* Kind? __________________ Kept inside or outside? ____________

Breed? __________________ How long have you had your pet?________

Symptoms worse when visiting friends who have pets? YES ____ NO ____

Animal contact that causes symptoms? ______________________________

_____ _____ *Do you smoke?* Cigarettes? _____ Cigars? _____ Pipe? _____

Chew tobacco? _____ Snuff? _____

_____ _____ If you do not smoke, does someone else's smoking bother you?

_____ _____ Do you perspire excessively?

_____ _____ Do you regard yourself as being nervous?

_____ _____ Problem with personality or behavioral changes? Certain times of the day? ________ Certain seasons? ________ With certain foods? ________

_____ _____ *Itchiness?* Nose? _____ Roof of mouth? _____ Ears? _____

Hands? _____ Feet? _____

_____ _____ Were you a premature baby?

_____ _____ As an infant, were you taken off formula or any foods? Specify. __________

_____ _____ Were you a colicky or fussy baby? Breast or bottle fed? Circle one.

_____ _____ Do you suspect any food of increasing your symptoms? Specify. __________

____

_____ _____ Do you have any specific cravings, or do you overindulge in certain foods? List. ____

_____ _____ Does any certain food give you indigestion, hives, or otherwise upset you? Specify. ____

____

_____ _____ Are you awakened during the night with any symptoms? Which symptoms?

_____ Headaches _____ Bloating _____ Dizziness _____ Thirst

_____ Stomach cramps _____ Heartburn _____ Dry cough

_____ Sore throat

_____ _____ Do you awaken in the morning with any symptoms?

_____ Joint pain/stiffness _____ Increased congestion

_____ Increased drainage _____ Nausea Others? _______________

DO YOUR SYMPTOMS INCREASE OR DECREASE WITH THE FOLLOWING CONDITIONS?

INCREASE	DECREASE	SAME	
____________	____________	____________	Cold weather
____________	____________	____________	Warm weather
____________	____________	____________	Air conditioning
____________	____________	____________	Windy days
____________	____________	____________	March to May
____________	____________	____________	May to July
____________	____________	____________	August to October
____________	____________	____________	November to March

INCREASE	DECREASE	SAME	
______	______	______	Damp weather
______	______	______	Housework (dusting, etc.)
______	______	______	High pollution levels
______	______	______	Change of seasons
______	______	______	When furnace goes on
______	______	______	Going to bed
______	______	______	After asleep for a short time
______	______	______	On arising
______	______	______	Later in day, 4 to 9 PM
______	______	______	Being in or mowing grass

HOME AND WORK ENVIRONMENT

Please specify by H for Home and W for Work
What is your occupation? ______________________________
Do you participate in any particular activities, hobbies, or recreation? Specify ______________
____
Are your symptoms increased at home; at work; or no change? Circle one.
Are you exposed to excessive amounts of dusts, fumes, chemicals, noise? ______________
Are there plants, dried flowers, fresh flowers at home or at work? ______________

Heating System (Home and Work)

Electric _____ Gas _____ Oil _____ Kerosene heater _____ Forced air _____
Hot water _____ Fireplace _____ Wood-burning stove _____ Coal-burning stove _____
Air conditioning _____ Air cleaner _____ Humidifier _____

Cooking

Gas _______ Electric _______

Laundry

Do you use softener sheets, liquid softener, or bleach in laundry? Circle.

Cosmetics

Do you use makeup? _____ Eye makeup _____ Perfume _____ After shave _____

Housing

Do you live in a house? _____ Two story _____ Split level _____ Ranch _____ Trailer ________
Do you live in an apartment? _____ Small building _____ Large building _____
Older building _____ Newer building _____
Have you had insulation blown into your house? _____

Furniture

_____ Upholstered
_____ Not upholstered

_____ Fabric
_____ Vinyl

_____ Others

Floor Coverings

_____ Carpeting & pads
_____ Carpets & pads
_____ Rugs & pads
_____ Throw rugs
_____ Linoleum

Wall Coverings

_____ Wallpaper
_____ Fabric
_____ Paneling
_____ Tapestries
_____ Pennants

Window Coverings

_____ Washable curtains/drapes
_____ Unwashable curtains/drapes
_____ Shades
_____ Blinds
_____ Others

Mattress

_____ Innerspring
_____ Foam rubber
_____ Waterbed
_____ Other (specify)

Beds and Bedding

_____ Number of beds (your room)
_____ Comforters
_____ Chenille bedspread
_____ Stuffed animals

Pillows

_____ Feather or down
_____ Foam rubber
_____ Kapok
_____ Dacron or polyester

Do your symptoms improve, get worse, or stay the same when on vacation? Circle one.
Where do you usually go on vacation? Mountains, seashore, other ____________________

FAMILY HISTORY

Have any of your blood relatives had any of the following illnesses? If so, underline and check the relationship.

	Father	Mother	Brother	Sister	Child
Bronchial asthma	_____	_____	_____	_____	_____
Emphysema	_____	_____	_____	_____	_____
Hay fever	_____	_____	_____	_____	_____
Sinus problems	_____	_____	_____	_____	_____
Hives	_____	_____	_____	_____	_____
Postnasal drainage	_____	_____	_____	_____	_____
Eczema	_____	_____	_____	_____	_____
Thyroid problems	_____	_____	_____	_____	_____
Food allergies	_____	_____	_____	_____	_____

How long have you had specific symptoms that brought you to our office?
_____ Years _____ Months _____ Weeks _____ Days
Have you had allergy testing before?
Dr. who performed the tests? ____________________ Address ____________________
Date last testing ______________ Type of testing: Scratch, Intradermal, RAST (Circle one)
Were these positive reactions? _____ To what? ____________________
Were you treated? _____ For what? ____________________
With injection? _____ Medication? _____ Other treatment? _________ How long? _________
Did you improve with treatment? ____________________
List all medications you are now taking: ____________________
Allergies to any medications (oral or injectable)? ____________________

Have you had any steroids (cortisone) in the past month? ______________________
Do you feel we have missed something that is pertinent to your symptoms? Please list. __________
____
____
____
____

Please check over your answers. If you are satisfied that you have answered to the fullest extent, send this back to the office so it can be evaluated. If you have not been seen by other doctors, please bring this questionnaire with you at the time of your initial visit.

Thank you

CHAPTER 15

Nasal Cytology in Clinical Allergy

Helen F. Krause, M.D., F.A.C.S.

In a routine physical examination, it may be difficult to differentiate clinical allergy, infection, or mechanical obstruction resulting from a deviated septum. However, studies of the cellular patterns of nasal secretions or tissues often provide helpful information. For example, increases or alterations in specific cell types are generally important. Repeated cytologic studies may be helpful when an infection has been treated but symptoms persist. Such cytologic examination may reveal the presence of an allergy that was previously hidden by infection.

The study of cells in respiratory secretions dates back to the mid-1800s. The cells first identified were the eosinophils and the mast cells, the latter being first described by Ehrlich in 1879; and in 1927 Eyermann noted their relationship to the complex becoming known as "allergy." In the 1920s and 1930s, further reports were made by Hansel and by Lindsay and Walsh, who described eosinophils and neutrophils. Additional progress was made when Papanicolaou developed a stain specific for epithelial cell studies in 1942. Extensive work by Dr. and Mrs. Bryan in the 1950s and 1960s detailed mast cells and goblet cells as well as viral effects on epithelial cells of the nose. Subsequent studies have also emphasized cytology with respect to malignant alterations. These and other techniques developed over the years allow identification of many cells in the respiratory epithelium of the nose, paranasal sinuses, trachea, and lungs, and even in salivary secretions and middle ear fluids.

In the practice of allergy, we are most concerned with nasal cytology. Various cell types are characteristic of healthy noses, others of disease states. Some cells are merely suggestive of pathologic processes; some are pathognomonic.

Normal respiratory mucosa contains a variety of cells resting on a basement membrane over a lamina propria (Fig. 15–1). Those in the nasal vestibule and anterior fossa are squamous epithelium with hair follicles. Cells become hair-free more posteriorly, and ultimately convert to a transitional type. The epithelium in the middle and posterior portions of the nose is classic respiratory pseudostratified, composed of a number of cells all attached to a thin basement membrane: basal and intermediate, both ciliated and nonciliated columnar, and goblet cells. Basal cells are the primitive source from which columnar and goblet cells develop after passing through an intermediate stage. The ratio between columnar and goblet cells in the normal nasal epithelium is 5:1. The surface of each columnar cell is covered with 300 to 400 minute cytoplasmic projections, microvilli, which help retain fluid on the epithelial surfaces and promote chemical exchange. Some columnar cells are ciliated, others are not. As goblet cells develop, they fill with mucinogen granules containing primarily acidic glycoproteins.

This ciliated epithelium is covered by a mucous layer overlying a less viscous periciliary fluid that bathes the microvilli. This fluid and a portion of the mucous blanket are secreted by a number of serous glands, the important seromucinous and intraepithelial glands that are scat-

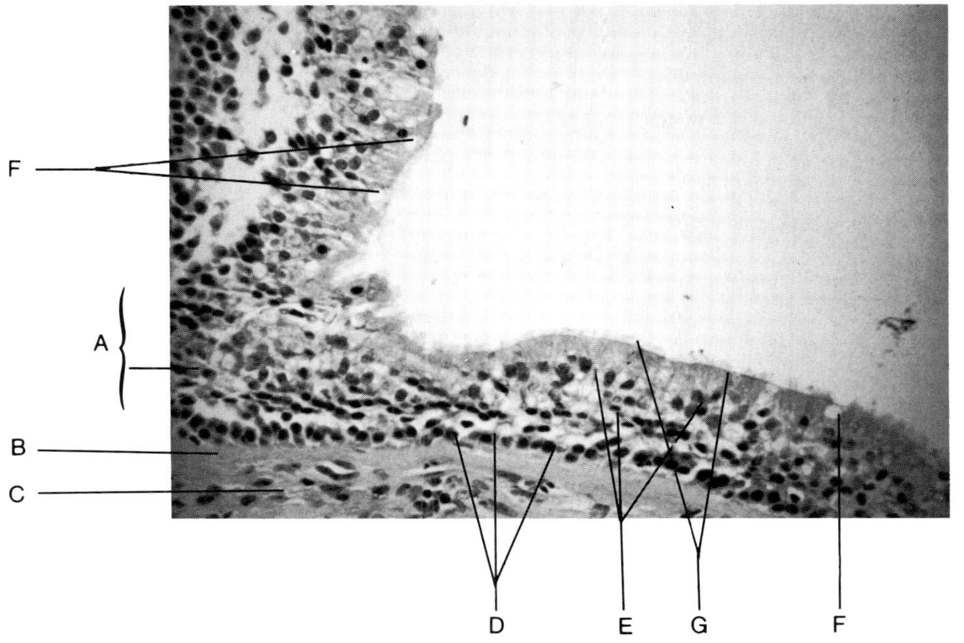

FIGURE 15–1. Normal respiratory mucosa. *A*, Pseudostratified columnar epithelium; *B*, basement membrane; *C*, lamina propria; *D*, basal cell; *E*, columnar cell; *F*, goblet cell; *G*, cilia.

tered in the mucosa. Bowman's glands, found only in the olfactory area, may or may not contribute to these layers.

Cilia are essential for the normal flow of the mucous blanket. Each ciliated columnar cell contains 50 to 100 projections on its surface. The individual cellular projection consists of an epithelial membrane enclosing a multistructured axonema—a complex including doublet microtubules, nexin links, spokes, dynein arms, and a central tubelike sheet in a specific pattern (Fig. 15–2). Genetic alteration of this pattern, especially loss of dynein arms, transposition of microtubules, and lack of radial spokes, is seen in the immotile-cilia syndrome described by Kartagener. Patients with this defect suffer from chronic rhinosinusitis, bronchiectasis, and often situs inversus. Chronic secretory otitis media is also frequently present, although there are normally few ciliated cells in the middle ear mucosa. In these patients, the mucociliary transport is severely impaired or absent. Electron microscopy is necessary for the diagnosis of such ciliary abnormalities.

Other cells seen in cytologic studies migrate to the epithelial surface from the lamina propria. In addition, granulocytes and lymphocytes derived from bone marrow stem cells eventually travel to the venous circulation in the nose. There, under the proper stimulus, they move out to the loose connective tissue of the lamina propria and continue by amebic activity through the epithelium.

Many areas of the nose have been sampled and studied. Some experts recommend that material be evaluated primarily from the middle turbinate and meatus and possibly from the roof

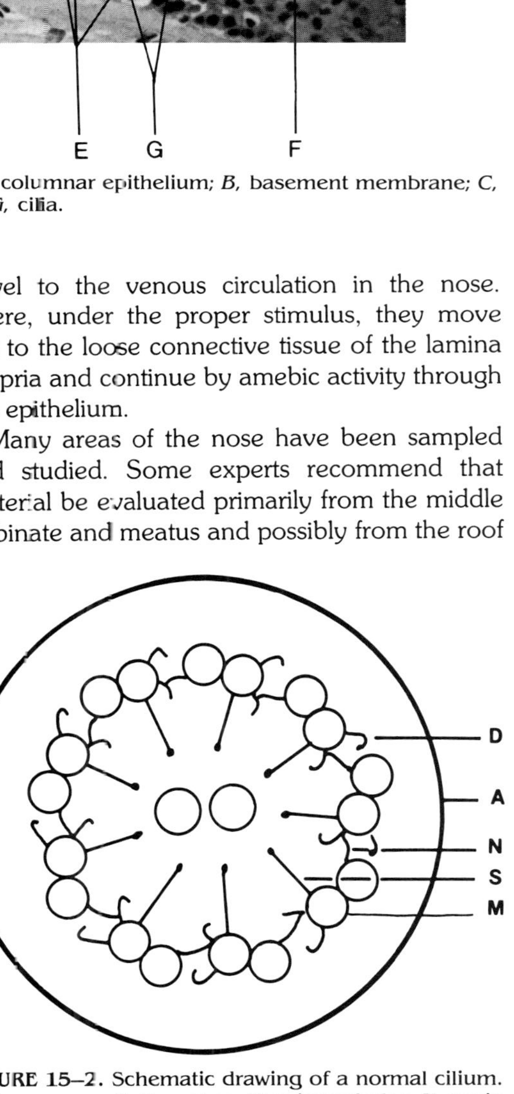

FIGURE 15–2. Schematic drawing of a normal cilium. *A*, Axonema wall; *S*, spokes; *M*, microtubules; *N*, nexin links; *D*, dynein arms.

of the fossa; others suggest the septum or middle turbinate. Today, however, the inferior turbinate is considered most representative (Fig. 15–3). Techniques for obtaining nasal secretions or tissues and the art of preparing slides for cytologic examination have engendered discussion for years, yet these valuable and simple procedures have not become routine in many offices—possibly because of a lack of understanding and training.

Secretions may be obtained by having the patient blow the nose into a plastic bag or waxed paper, by aspiration with a hand-held bulb, or with the use of a very small cotton swab, such as the "Calgiswab." The Bryans recommended the "wipe and roll" technique, with the swab being rubbed over the middle turbinate and posterior portions of the inferior turbinate two or three times. The swab is then gently rolled on a clean, dry glass slide that is dried quickly and stained. Advocates of the blow or swab techniques believe that these provide adequate demonstration of cellular elements. Others feel the blow technique identifies only cells that have been present for some time.

More recently, Alfredo Jalowayski, Ph.D., developed a small plastic spoon (Rhino-probe) for microscraping that produces intact and well-preserved cellular elements—a nontraumatic "mini biopsy." This can be done with a patient of any age comfortably and safely. The middle and inferior portions of the inferior turbinate are the recommended sampling sites (Fig. 15–3). The scrape technique, if done carefully, affords undistorted cells. Under direct vision, the mid-inferior portion of the inferior turbinate is gently scraped two or three times with the minispoon, avoiding the septum and anterior tip of the inferior turbinate (Fig. 15–3). A combination of this scraping and a roll of blown secretions on one slide has also been described.

A few cautions: The use of a vasoconstrictive spray may alter the cellular studies. Mast cells are very "twitchy" and easily destroyed. Samples for cytologic study should be taken before any manipulation is done.

A number of stains are available for nasal cytograms (Tables 15–1 and 15–2), each having its own advantages. Hansel stain is simple to use and remarkable in demonstration of eosinophils and neutrophils, but it is poor for basophils and epithelial elements. The Wright-Giemsa stain is excellent for granulocytes, goblet cells, epithelial cells, and bacteria. Papanicolaou, as mentioned, developed a stain specifically for epithelial elements. The Wright and hematoxylin-eosin (H & E) stains are more problematic in an office setting because they do not always yield consistent results.

STAIN TECHNIQUES

For the Hansel stain, the secretions are rolled onto a clear, dry glass slide with a cotton-tipped applicator or applied from the Rhino-probe. The specimen is fast-fixed with unscented hair spray or methyl alcohol, which rapidly dries the material onto the slide. The slide is then covered with the well-mixed Hansel stain containing two alcoholic components: 1:500 eosin and 1:200 methylene blue. After 30 to 45 seconds, distilled water is added and the slide is washed with alcohol to remove the excess color. The slide is then washed with water and dried.

Wright-Giemsa stain is advocated for use with any technique of specimen preparation. The slide is lightly spread with contents of the Rhino-

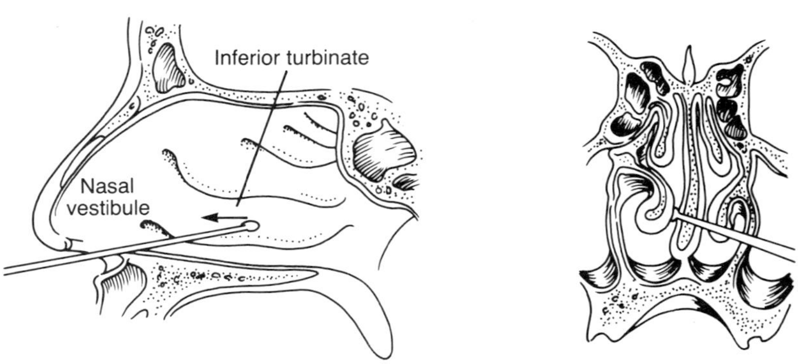

FIGURE 15–3. Nasal cavity site for scraping technique. (Courtesy of Synbiotics Corporation.)

Table 15–1. HANSEL STAIN TECHNIQUE

Prepare slide with secretions or scraping sample and fix
Flood with Hansel stain for 30 seconds
Add distilled water, pour off
Flood with methyl alcohol to remove excess color
Wash with water
Air dry or use warm blower

probe or lightly rolled with the cotton-tipped applicator, preventing thick layers of cells. Specially grooved glass slides are available to aid in spreading the cells; standard flat or partially frosted slides may also be used. If both blown or aspirated secretions and the scraping specimen are placed on opposite ends of the same slide, the two sources can be advantageously compared.

Slides must be fixed immediately with 95 per cent methyl alcohol or with unscented hair spray. Excess alcohol is absorbed by touching a paper towel to the edge of the prepared slide. Preparations may be stained on a rack or by use of dip bottles—Coplin jars (Fig. 15–4). If a rack is used, 1.0 ml of the Wright-Giemsa stain is added by pipette or syringe and left on for 10 seconds. The slide is gently agitated manually

Table 15–2. WRIGHT-GIEMSA STAIN TECHNIQUE

Prepare slide with secretions or scraping sample and fix
Flood with 1.0 ml of Wright-Giemsa stain for 10 seconds, gently agitating slide
Flood with 2.0 ml of special buffer solution and again agitate for 15 seconds
Flood with hematology rinse for 4 to 5 seconds
Dry in air or with warm blower

or by blowing on it. The buffer solution provided with the Wright-Giemsa stain is then added (2.0 ml), and the slide is again agitated. A violet, iridescent-metallic scum will form on the surface, indicating the reaction has been effective. The slide is then washed in a hematology rinse until clear of stain. Excess water is removed by touching the edge of the slide with a paper towel, and the back of the slide is wiped dry. Slides may be air-dried or more quickly dried for reading with a warm air blower. Permanent preparations can be made by dipping the slide in xylene for 5 to 10 seconds, then covering with a slide-mounting medium and a coverslip.

The dip method using Coplin jars is very simple. The three solutions—the Wright-Giemsa stain, the buffer, and the hematology rinse—are placed in the jars. With the aid of a slide holder or hemostat, the slides are dipped in the stain for 10 seconds, drained, then dipped in the buffer for 15 seconds. Again, the slide is drained and dipped into the rinse repeatedly for 4 seconds. The excess is removed and the back of the slide wiped.

Special chemical and fluorescent stains are available to identify various normal and pathogenic constituents in nasal secretions and tissues. Electron microscopy, although useful in studying special characteristics of cells, cilia, basement membrane, and lamina propria, is not practical in a clinical office. The microscope used in reading cytology slides may be monocular or binocular. (Many physicians find one of the old medical-school vintage quite acceptable.) Slides

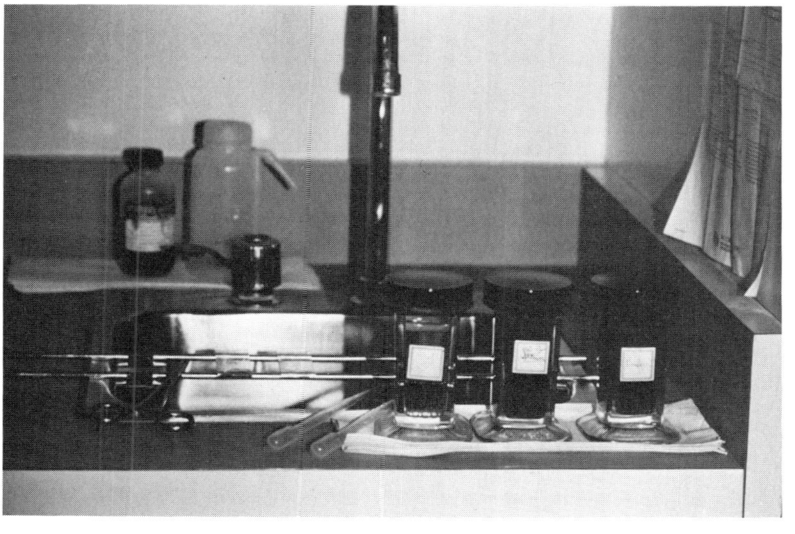

FIGURE 15–4. Laboratory equipment for cytologic staining.

should be viewed under low power scanning initially and selected fields reviewed under high power and oil immersion for better detail. A counter is very helpful. Grading the slides is discussed later in this chapter.

CYTOLOGIC CHARACTERISTICS

The cells found most abundantly in nasal cytologic examination are epithelial cells, which often appear as a background to more dramatically staining cells. Columnar cells may be seen as individuals or as clumps of connected cells. In normal respiratory epithelium (Fig. 15–1), all cells are in contact with the basement membrane but not all reach to the surface. They are not in contact with the lamina propria lying beneath the basement membrane. In tissue section, the smaller basal cells, which do not reach the surface, have dense cytoplasm and large, dark nuclei. The columnar cell cytoplasm is lighter than that of the basal cell. It appears bluish with finely dispersed chromatin and a large, nearly clear nucleus (Fig. 15–5). The microvilli cannot be identified, but the cilia may be seen on many cells.

Goblet cells (Fig. 15–6) are specialized types of apocrine glands containing mucinogen granules that appear frothy or foamy when stained. The nucleus is situated toward the base. The cell surface is covered with microvilli that are invisible in the usual preparation and has a small opening through which the granules are discharged. Goblet cell distribution in the nasal mucosa is very irregular. They are often seen along with eosinophils and mast cells. Exacerbation of allergy symptoms is usually reflected in increased numbers of goblet cells. Their numbers also increase in acute infection, slowly falling after the infection has cleared. In chronic inflammation (e.g., allergic rhinitis, rhinosinusitis), the numbers often remain elevated.

In preparations of secretions, mucous masses are often seen with no identifiable cellular structure.

Other cells not seen or rarely seen in appreciable numbers in the normal nose migrate from the lamina propria to the surface when appropriate physiologic conditions exist. Eosinophils—described as cells of beauty and mystery—are the classic cells of allergy (Fig. 15–7). They originate from bone marrow stem cells, travel in the bloodsteam, and are frequently seen in the lamina propria; only rarely do they appear in epithelium and secretions of the noses of normal individuals. They have a slightly dark cytoplasm filled with pink-red granules containing a high content of the enzymes peroxidase and aryl-sulfatase involved in arachidonic acid metabolism. The nucleus is bilobed and not obscured by the cytoplasmic granules. Inhalant allergy is suggested if 20 per cent or more of the granulocytes (eosinophils, mast cells, neutrophils, basophils) are of the eosinophil type. Frequently an increase in eosinophils is accom-

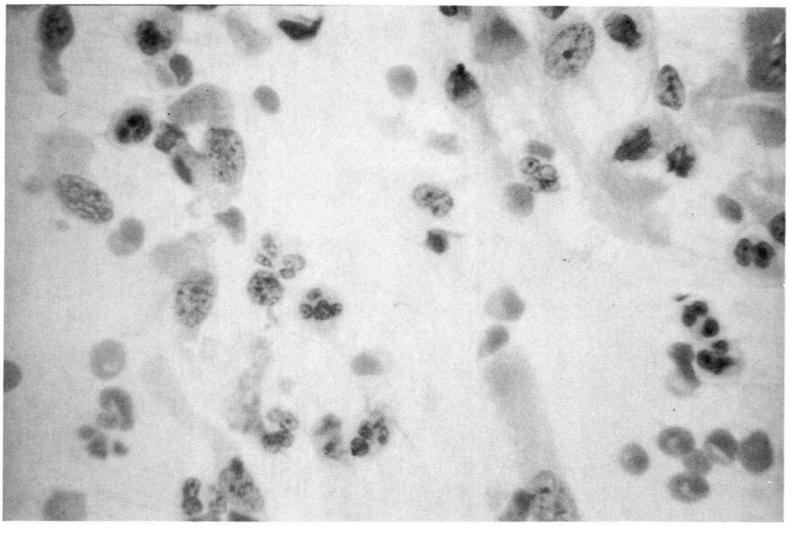

FIGURE 15–5. Epithelial cells, characterized by pale blue cytoplasm with a large, nearly clear nucleus; some have cilia.

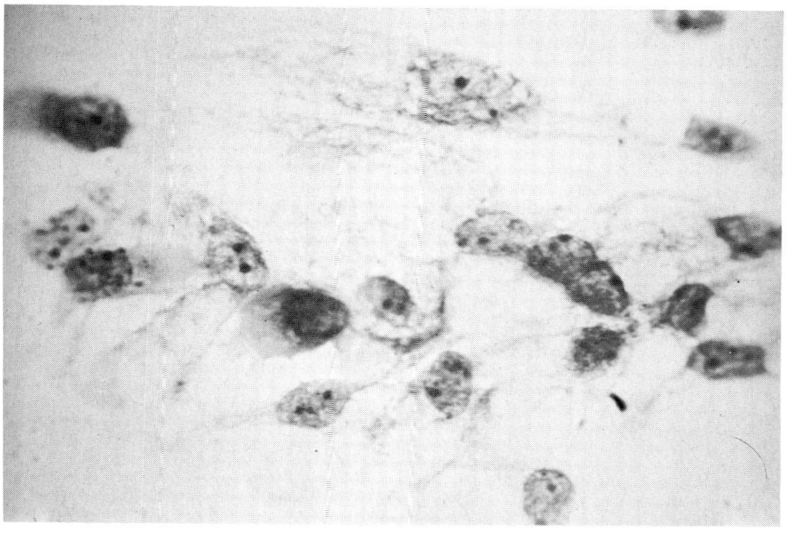

FIGURE 15–6. Goblet cells. Their frothy secretions push nuclei to base of cells.

panied by an increase in goblet cells. Large numbers of eosinophils are seen in some patients identified as having nonallergic eosinophilic rhinitis. Perhaps incitants of a chemical or irritative nature will one day be identified as the etiologic agent of the syndrome.

Mast cells (Fig. 15–8) are found in nearly all connective tissue in the body, particularly the skin, lymphoid tissue, bone marrow, and both respiratory and gastrointestinal mucosa. Variable in size and shape but larger than basophils, they probably originate from connective tissue cells around the blood vessels in the lamina propria of the respiratory mucosa. In normal people they rarely reach the epithelial layer and secretions. They are recognized by the large basophilic (reddish-purple) granules that nearly obliterate the oval central nucleus.

With degranulation, secretory granules spill outside the mast cell membrane. These granules and the cytoplasmic inclusions contain the mediators of allergic responses. Especially important are the preformed chemicals, eluted and granular (histamine, ECF–A, heparin, and other vasoactive amines) as well as the secondarily derived mediators. It was reported as early as 1933 that food allergy seems to stimulate more mast cells to appear in the nasal secretions. A rare nasal disease of undetermined cause, nasal mastocytosis, is characterized by the presence

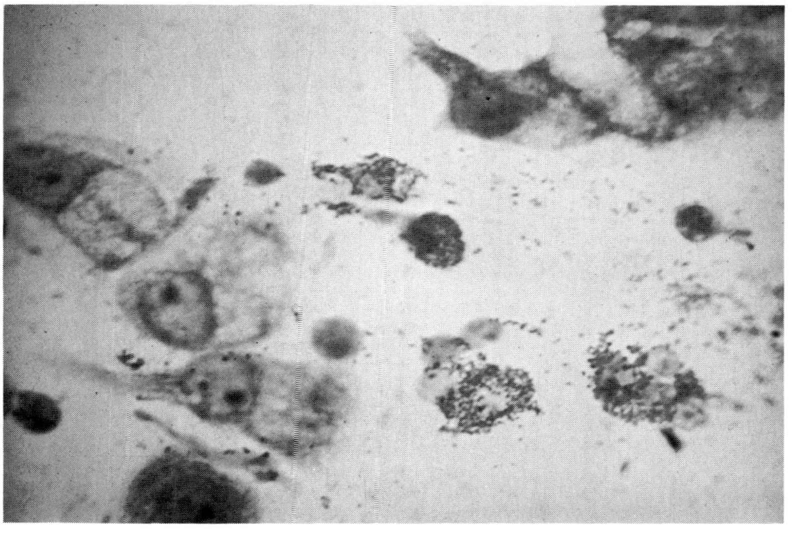

FIGURE 15–7. Eosinophils, including intact cells and disintegrating cells with spilling of pink-red granules. Goblet cells are nearby.

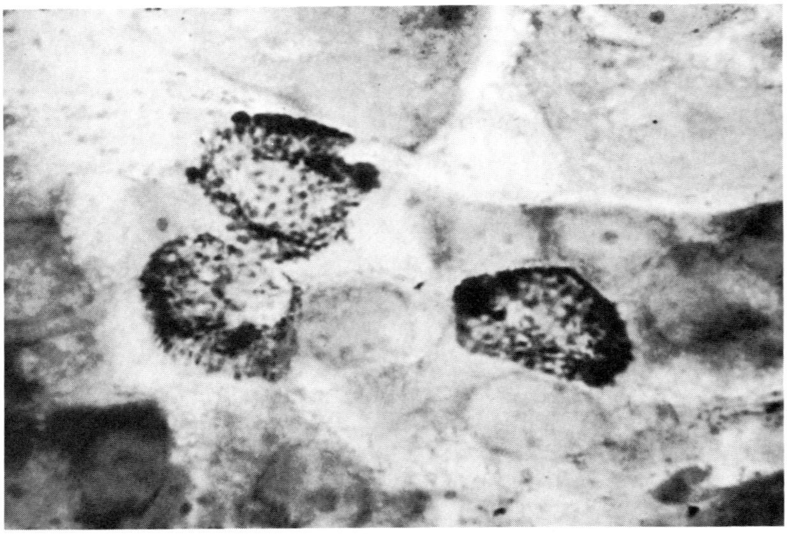

FIGURE 15–8. Mast cell cytoplasm is filled with reddish-purple granules nearly obliterating the oval central nucleus.

of mast cells in great quantities. Mast cells are seen more often in tissue studies than in smears.

Basophils may occasionally be present and must be distinguished from the larger mast cell, which is often called the "tissue basophil." The circulating basophil has a more distinct cell membrane, and the granules usually are also more distinctive (Fig. 15–9).

Polymorphonuclear leukocytes (neutrophils) and eosinophils are often seen together in nasal secretions (Fig. 15–10). Increased numbers of polymorphonuclear leukocytes suggest infection and are often seen with bacteria. Their major functions are migration and phagocytosis. Granules and lysosomes containing multiple enzymes that destroy bacteria and antibody-antigen complexes may be released and cause tissue injury if they are not inhibited. These cells have multilobulated nuclei and a pale, pink cytoplasm. They migrate into the epithelium and secretions from the venules in the lamina propria, and some are always present even in a normal, healthy nose. Bacteria seen with these leukocytes may be extracellular or (very often) intracellular. In acute infection, bacteria are most often gram-positive and intracellular (Fig. 15–

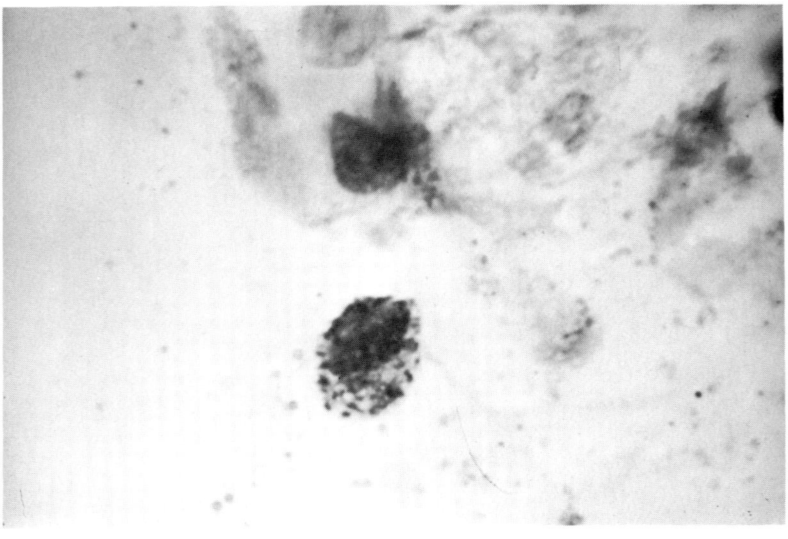

FIGURE 15–9. Basophil, having a distinct cell membrane with sharp purple granules.

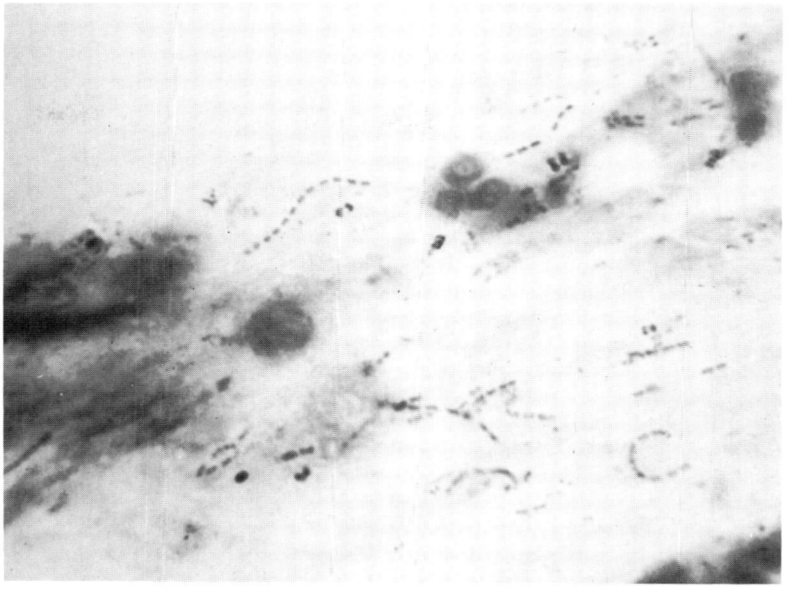

FIGURE 15–10. Polymorphonuclear leukocytes with multilobulated nuclei, occurring with both intracellular and extracellular bacteria.

10). Chronic infection is usually associated with multiple or mixed types of bacteria, more often extracellular (Fig. 15–11).

Lymphocytes with large central nuclei are seen scattered in the nasal mucosa in various numbers, most often when antigens are present (Fig. 15–12). Various other cells may be present, such as polymorphonuclear leukocytes, eosinophils, and epithelial cells. Plasma cells are large, ovoid cells with a single, small, spherical, eccentric nucleus. The light blue basophilic cytoplasm of B lymphocytes contains RNA from which the immunoglobulins originate.

Other cellular elements, such as macrophages (the phagocytes), are rarely present in nasal secretions, more often appearing in the mucosa. The activity of these scavenger cells consists of pinocytosis (engulfing substances in solution) and phagocytosis (engulfing particulate matter). They appear in areas of loose connective tissue in an irregular configuration of pseudopods and projections that, even in a fixed slide, gives the

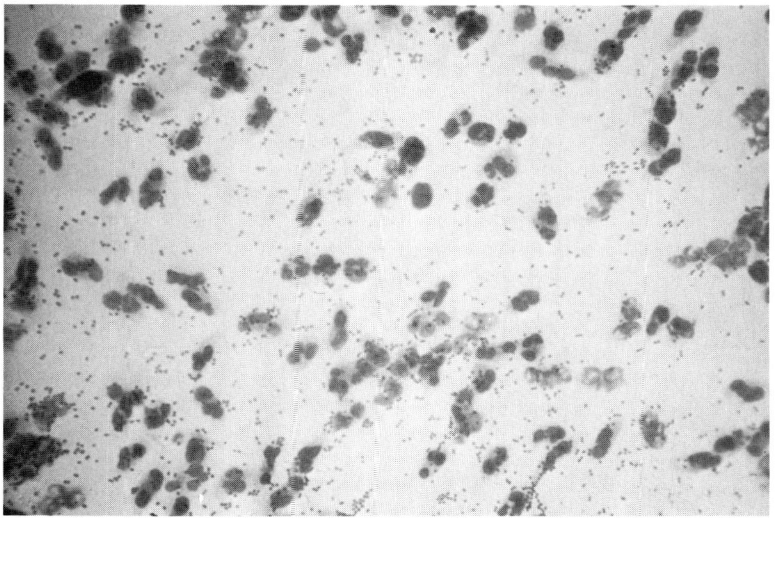

FIGURE 15–11. Polymorphonuclear leukocytes with extracellular bacteria.

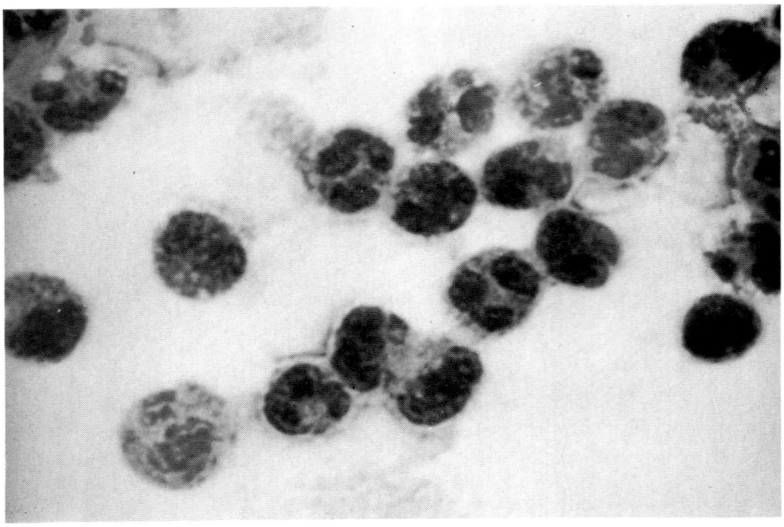

FIGURE 15–12. Lymphocytes with large, dark central nuclei. The ovoid plasma cells are larger and have smaller nuclei.

appearance of movement (Fig. 15–13). They also function in the immune system by marking antigens and processing and storing them for delivery to the mast cells and for interaction with specific lymphocytes.

Viral infections cause interesting degenerative changes in nasal epithelial cells that Papanicolaou labeled ciliocytophoria. The nucleus begins to degenerate very early in the infection and shows chromatin clumping. The cytoplasm alters its shape, becoming irregular, and a halo may appear around the pyknotic nucleus within the first four to five days of the onset of infection (Fig. 15–14). Finally, the cell appears to disintegrate, leaving nuclear fragments and ciliated tufts associated with small amounts of cytoplasm. These damaged cells are most easily seen during the first few days of the acute infection but are difficult to find if the infection persists. They are usually associated with many polymorphonuclear leukocytes.

There may be combinations of infection and allergy that cause symptoms similar to infection alone. Eosinophils, mast cells, and goblet cells most often accompany allergy. Polymorphonuclear leukocytes, bacteria, and epithelial cell degeneration may be present in the face of infections. On occasion, the acute infection may suppress the allergic effect.

Rarely, parasites, fungal mycelia, or mold

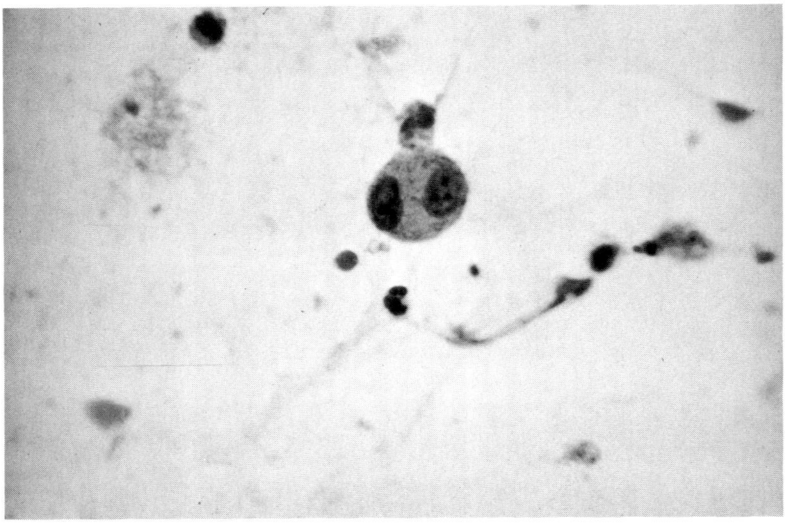

FIGURE 15–13. Macrophage extending a pseudopod.

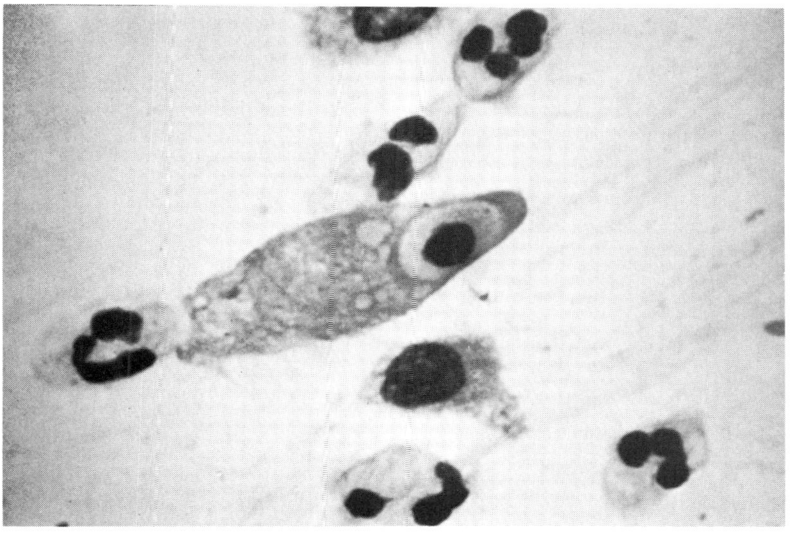

FIGURE 15–14. Epithelial cell demonstrating ciliocytophoria. Note halo around a pyknotic nucleus.

spores are seen on a slide. Cultures are necessary to make the final diagnosis.

Cytogram grading systems (Table 15–3) have been recommended, but cell populations may vary depending on the thickness of the preparation and the fields selected for review. Although some physicians and laboratories describe results of nasal cytology in terms of percentages of cells per field, an overall review by the technician or physician is often more valuable in assessing the suggested diagnosis. In general, eosinophils are increased in allergic rhinitis, in aspirin-sensitivity syndrome, and in nonallergic eosinophilic rhinitis. In a purely allergic response, we see primarily goblet cells with or without eosinophils and mast cells. Eosinophils are particularly seen in inhalant allergies, mast cells in food allergy. Numbers of mast cells and basophils rise in inhalant allergy, whereas goblet cells increase in bacterial and viral infections.

Table 15–3. GRADING OF NASAL CYTOGRAMS

Eosinophils (cells and clumps)	
0	None
1	Few scattered cells or small clumps
2	Moderate numbers and larger clumps
3	Many cells and large clumps
4	The field covered with cells
Basophils (number of cells/field)	
0	None
1	1
2	3
3	5
4	More than 5
Goblet cells (% goblet:epithelial cells)	
0	None
1	25
2	50
3	50–75
4	75–100

SUMMARY

Recognition of the usefulness of nasal cytology has increased in recent years, especially as it has become academically more important. Clues to treatment failure may be found; for example, previously well-controlled patients who escape from treatment effectiveness may show diagnostic changes in the nasal smear, often related to food allergy. Nasal cytology is an additional aid in the diagnosis and treatment of allergic patients. For them, it may bring into full bloom the sometimes obscure bud of diagnosis.

Photomicrographs provided through the courtesy of Volker Breitfeld, M.D., North Hills Passavant Hospital, Pittsburgh, PA; and Synbiotics Corporation, San Diego, CA.

REFERENCES

Anderson HA. Practical nasal cytology: key to the problem nose. JCE ORL Allergy, January:53, 1979.

Bickmore JT, Funkhouser JW: The clinical use of nasal cytography in upper respiratory allergy. Trans Am Soc Ophthalmol Otolaryngol Allergy 13:43, 1972.

Bickmore JT: Nasal cytology in allergy and infection. ORL Allergy 40:39, 1978.
Bickmore JT: Nasal cytology in allergy and infection. *In* King H (ed): Otolaryngologic Allergy. Miami, Symposia Specialists, 1981, pp 229–249.
Bryan MA: Nasal cytograms in the diagnosis of an allergy. Trans Am Soc Ophthalmol Otolarygol Allergy 8:24, 1967.
Bryan MA, Bryan WTK: Cytologic and cytochemical aspects of ciliated epithelium in the differentiation of nasal inflammatory disease. Acta Cytol 12:515, 1969.
Bryan WTK, Bryan M: Cytologic diagnosis in otolaryngology. Trans Am Acad Ophthalmol Otolaryngol 63:597, 1959.
Bryan WTK, Bryan M: Significance of mast cells in nasal secretions. Trans Am Soc Ophthalmol Otolaryngol 63:613, 1959.
Connell JT: Morphological changes in eosinophils in allergic diseases. J Allergy Clin Immunol 41:1, 1968.
Eyermann GH: Nasal manifestations of allergy. Ann Otol Rhinol Laryngol 36:808, 1927.
Hansel FK: Cytological diagnosis in respiratory allergy and infection. Ann Allergy 24:564, 1966.
Hilding AC: The common cold. Arch Otolaryngol 12:133, 1930.
Jahnke V: Electron microscopy in rhinology. Rhinology 23:173, 1985.
Jahnke V, Theopold HM: Elektronenmikroskopische Befunde bei allergischen Reaktionen der Nasenschleimhaut. Laryngol Rhinol Otol 62:603, 1983.
Lindsay JR, Walsh TE: Nasal secretions: the value of cytotoxic examination to the rhinologist. Arch Otolaryngol 17:783, 1933.
Mygind N: Nasal Allergy. Oxford, Blackwell Scientific Publications, 1979.
Mygind N: Essential Allergy. Oxford, Blackwell Scientific Publications, 1986.
Papanicolaou GW: A new procedure for staining vaginal smears. Science 95:438, 1942.
Papanicolaou GW: Degenerative changes in ciliated cells exfoliated from the bronchial epithelium. NY State J Med 50:2647, 1956.
Proctor DF, Anderson TB: The Nose. Amsterdam, Elsevier Biomedical Press, 1982.
Shioda H, Shiva MT: The significance of mast cells in nasal smears from patients with food allergy. J Allergy Clin Immunol 37:321, 1966.
Theopold HM, Jahnke V, Schinko I: Zur Feinstruktur der Zilien bei Kartagener Syndrom. Laryngol Rhinol Otol 63:33, 1984.

CHAPTER 16

Antigen Selection for Testing and Therapy

Hueston C. King, M.D., F.A.C.S., F.A.C.A.

For the beginning allergist, an essential hurdle is the selection of the proper antigens to be used in treatment. It can be intimidating to listen to the patient who declares he or she is "allergic to everything." Antigens are not available for "everything" nor, fortunately, are they needed. It can be equally frustrating, however, to have so limited a supply of antigens as to be unable to cope with realistic problems and fail to achieve relief. A realistic approach to the problem can be made by providing a good selection of antigens for a specific area that may be expanded as the need arises.

INHALANTS

Most treatment begins with aeroallergens, and these should form the nucleus of the treatment table. Pollens, dust, mold, and a group entitled "epidermals and miscellaneous" must be selected and purchased. A plan for individual selection will be considered one group at a time.

Pollens

These are the most regionally influenced antigens and the most affected by seasonal change. They are also the largest group of the aeroallergens. It may come as a surprise to know they are frequently not the most important elements in the patient's problem. In general, pollens of allergenic importance follow Thommen's postulates

1. The plant must be seed-bearing.
2. The pollen must be allergenic.
3. The pollen must be airborne.
4. The pollen must be produced in large quantities.
5. The pollen must be buoyant to be transferred over a large area (15 to 50 micra in diameter.
6. The plant producing the pollen must be widely and abundantly distributed, or close to human habitation.

As in most aspects of medicine, this is not entirely true. In areas of consistently high humidity, for example, major allergenic pollens may not be primarily wind-borne. Their exact portal of entry has not yet been determined. As a general rule, however, Thommen's postulates are valid, and the physician should resist the temptation to accept the patient's conviction that a highly visible and fragrant flowering plant is causing his or her problems. Most plants of this type are insect-pollinated and are not offenders.

In general, pollinating plants follow a predictable seasonal pattern. Trees pollinate in the spring. Grasses pollinate in the summer, usually overlapping the pollination season of the trees by a month or two. Weeds pollinate in the fall. All of these seasonal patterns are subject to variation caused by late or early seasonal changes, rainfall, and manmade changes in the ecology. Additional confusion can result from a patient's sensitivity to mold, dust, or food, which may become apparent at the same time as the pollinating season of certain plants.

A patient's history is of great value in anticipating sensitivities, but it must be borne in mind that the history may produce confusion in a field as large as allergy. Confirmatory tests are always essential.

Many antigen supply houses offer regional pollen lists developed by professional botanists. These lists provide an excellent starting point for assembling a basic armamentarium for the treatment of pollen sensitivity. Bearing in mind the ability of pollens to be carried hundreds of miles by wind currents, the use of regional lists is a practical necessity. Private practitioners are rarely equipped to develop a reliable list on their own. The regional pollen guide should not, however, be accepted without question by the practitioner. Reasonable caution should be observed.

An attempt should be made to find out how and when the pollen lists were obtained. Some currently published pollen guides are over 30 years old and have lost much of their validity owing to manmade changes in the area. Some guides list an inordinately large number of pollens. These may have been assembled by collecting all the pollen extracts required by allergists in the area over the years of the company's existence. Some of the allergists of previous decades were not knowledgeable botanists, and some were willing to experiment with rather rare allergens at their patient's requests. Such sources of information are not reliable for today's practitioner. On-the-spot regional pollen counts and field surveys of allergenic plants are the only definitive source of information. These should be reasonably current. In many locations, these are available from the Department of Agriculture or the Pollution Control Board.

A comparison of regional pollen guides from different laboratories may offer much information of value. When the same antigen appears on all lists, it is a reasonable assumption that it is indeed of real importance. An antigen that appears on only one list, especially if the list is extremely long, may be questioned as to importance and its purchase delayed until more concrete evidence is obtained.

Finally, it cannot be overemphasized that the allergist, to maintain credibility, should have a working knowledge of the appearance of allergenic plants. This is not difficult to obtain. A few visits to local botanical gardens and the Department of Botany at local colleges, junior colleges, and even high schools can be very rewarding. The Department of Agriculture is only too happy to have physicians show an interest in its activities. The allergist who can point out ragweed in bloom is held in much greater respect by patients than is the one who believes ragweed originates in a small glass vial. The allergist can also identify an allergen that, because of excessive growth in an area, is causing unusual problems for some of his or her patients. A reasonable familiarity with the major allergenic offenders in the area places the physician in a position of expertise.

What about the occasional offender or the rare patient who is indeed sensitive to a flowering plant that is not usually a problem? It is a basic tenet of allergy that anyone may be sensitive to anything, depending only on prior sensitization. A simple rule is to purchase a testing vial (5 ml) of an antigen that the patient feels is causing problems. Testing the patient will justify the individual purchase. It may then be included in the armamentarium for future tests. If it shows a minimal level of sensitivity on a succession of patients, it need not be replaced when it is used up or its shelf life expires. If it indeed proves a significant allergen, it may be added to the regular list. Using a selected combination of antigens from regional pollen guides plus the practitioner's personal observation, supplemented by individual allergens purchased by request, should provide a good testing board for pollens.

Over the years, many mixes of similar allergens have been made available by various laboratories and have become popular as a means of saving time and costs. Grass mix, tree mix, weed mix, and others, regionally oriented, may be purchased. These provide a reasonable level of success, but as in all short cuts, results are limited. Far greater versatility may be obtained by individual allergen evaluation.

Molds

Alternaria is the most important mold in the United States. Of additional major allergenic importance are Aspergillus, Pullularia, Hormodendrum, Penicillium, and Cephalosporium.

Other molds may be of equal importance on a regional basis.

Selection of appropriate molds rarely poses a problem. Regional mold surveys are available from the same sources as pollen surveys and may indicate a local mold of significance that should be added to the treatment and testing sets. In 1964, Morrow, Meyer, and Price published a map showing national surveys for molds (Annals of Allergy, vol. 22). This survey is still generally valid and of considerable value.

Molds are a problem everywhere. On the Eastern coast of the United States they are prevalent in the ambient air. Even in the driest desert areas, they are found indoors around plumbing. They are essential in any treatment armamentarium. It is fortunate that there is little major mold variation from one area to another.

TOE is not appropriate for an inhalant chapter. These are dermatophytes. Although they cause allergic problems, pathogenic fungi are not inhalant allergens and are discussed in Chapters 12 and 27.

Dust, Mite, Epidermals, and Miscellaneous

The final group of antigens needed for the testing and the treatment table is the dust, mite, epidermal, and miscellaneous group. Although this group is small in size, treatment often offers the highest degree of relief for the allergy patient. Antigens from this group are present in every environment, the exposure tends to be perennially high, and the allergenic activity is markedly significant.

House dust has been described as the "universal allergen." If practicing allergists found their armamentarium restricted to a single antigen, without exception they would choose house dust. Dust, however, is actually a composite of a large number of antigens acting synergistically, a fact that nearly resulted in the removal of house dust from the list of antigens approved by the Food and Drug Administration. Knowledge of this makes it easier to understand the recommendation that more than a single house dust extract should be included on the testing and treatment tables. Since extracting methods and sources are constantly changing, recommendations for dust extracts would be inappropriate. The beginning allergist should consult with others in the field, and the local area, to see what particular extracts are showing the highest degree of sensitivity in the local population, and have at least two of those extracts on the table.

Epidermals and miscellaneous may be grouped together. These are allergens that should be considered in accordance with specific exposure, not used as part of a panel. Exposures are variable from one patient to another. Dog and cat hair and dander (epithelium) are common enough to be included on every table. In farm and ranch areas, horsehair and cattle hair should be included. Beyond this, a specific industry may indicate the routine inclusion of an appropriate antigen in the collection. Otherwise, a good rule is to apply the same recommendations given for unusual pollens: If a patient suspects a specific sensitivity (e.g., guinea pig, parakeet, rabbit), buy a 5 ml testing vial of the antigen and test that patient. Other patients may be tested with the remainder until it is determined whether or not the particular antigen warrants routine inclusion in the set.

The preceding will provide a good basic set for testing and treatment of inhalant allergies, large enough to give a good picture without appreciable waste, and the cost will not be excessive. Within a matter of months, the list may be refined to provide appropriate continuing care. Additions may be made later as indicated, but the developing allergist will usually be surprised at how few are necessary.

SUMMARY

A reasonable list of antigens has been described for inhalant therapy. The reasons for their selection, and for varying their selection, have also been discussed. The number of antigens needed for practical therapy is not prohibitive and may be expanded without difficulty as needed. By following these considerations, the beginning practitioner should be able to provide a satisfactory range of allergy care.

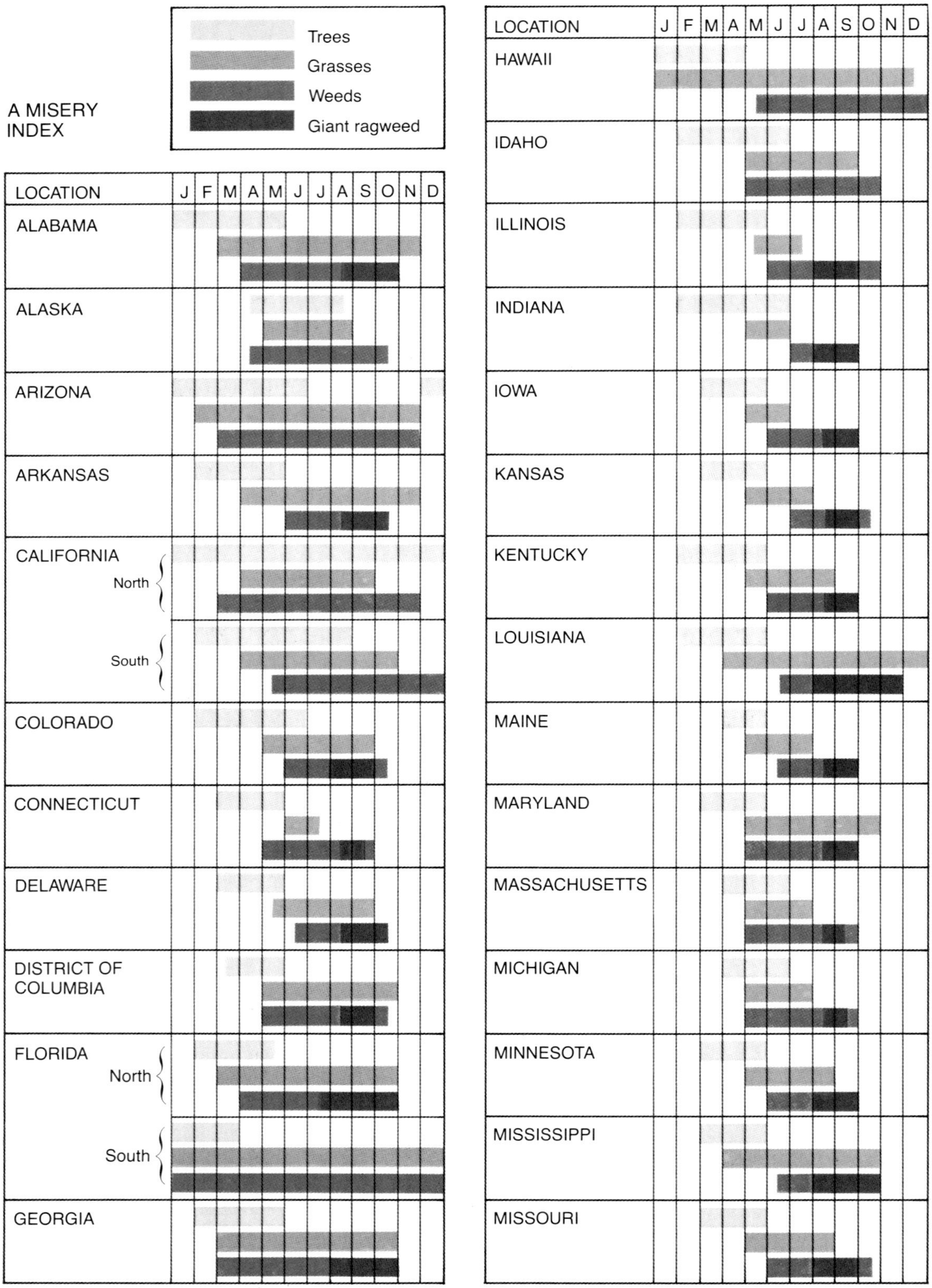
A MISERY INDEX
Trees
Grasses
Weeds
Giant ragweed
LOCATION
J F M A M J J A S O N D
ALABAMA
ALASKA
ARIZONA
ARKANSAS
CALIFORNIA
North
South
COLORADO
CONNECTICUT
DELAWARE
DISTRICT OF COLUMBIA
FLORIDA
North
South
GEORGIA
LOCATION
J F M A M J J A S O N D
HAWAII
IDAHO
ILLINOIS
INDIANA
IOWA
KANSAS
KENTUCKY
LOUISIANA
MAINE
MARYLAND
MASSACHUSETTS
MICHIGAN
MINNESOTA
MISSISSIPPI
MISSOURI

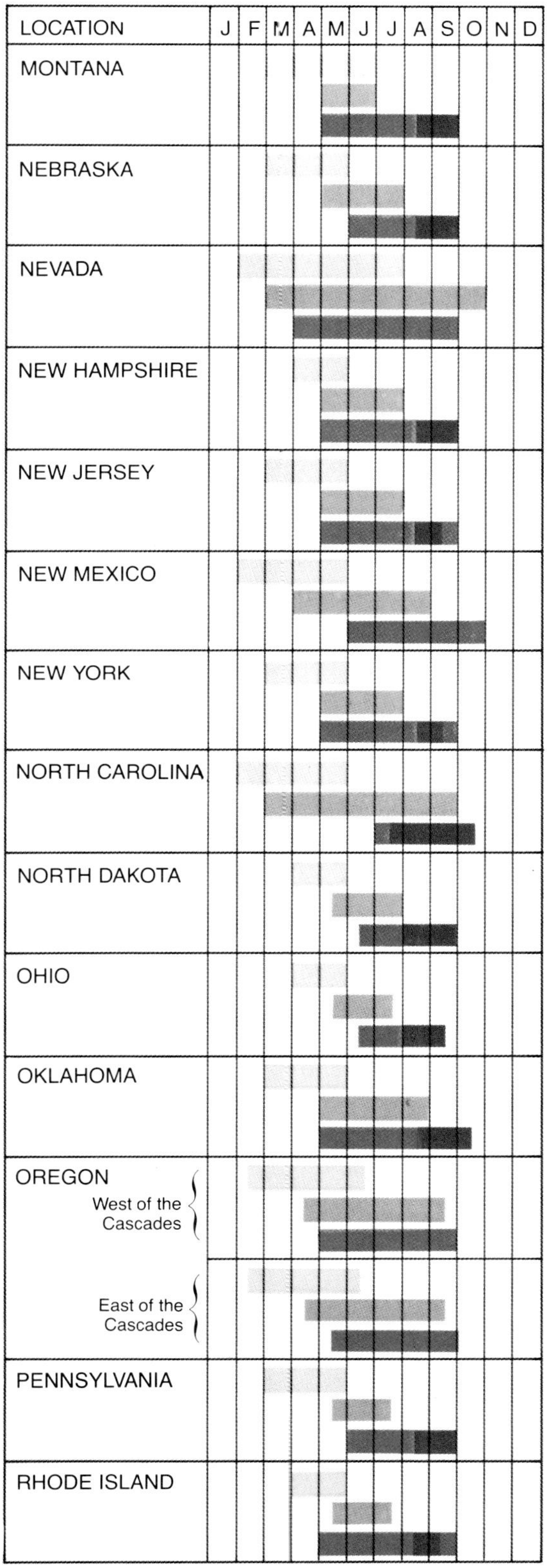

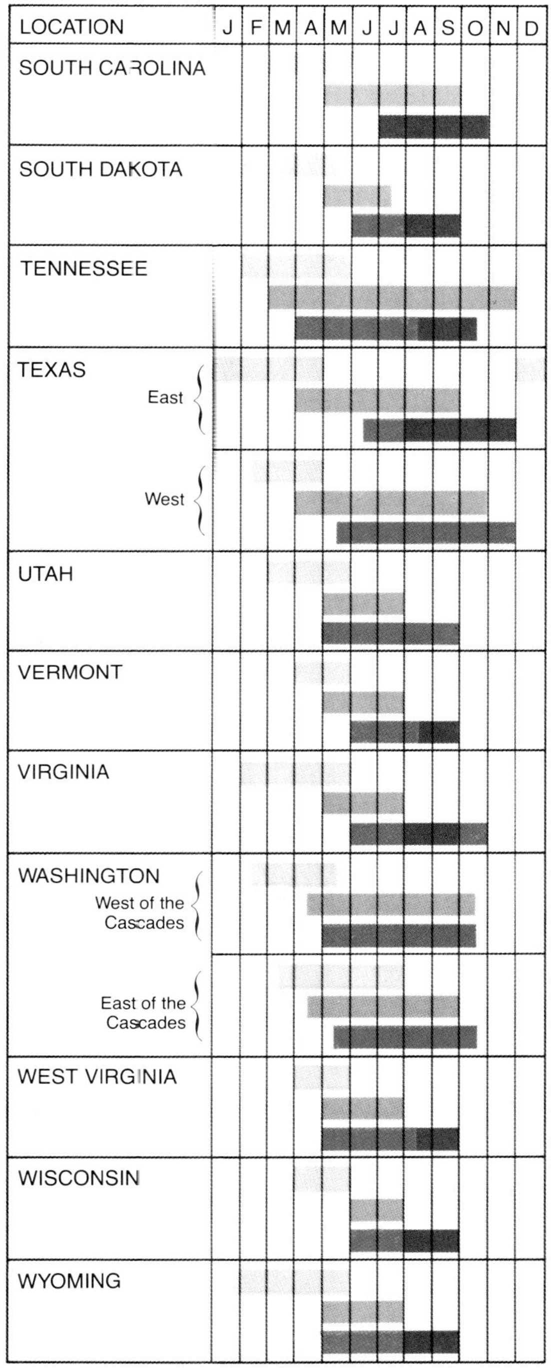

Pollen chart adapted from National Geographic, supported by a grant from Pharmacia Diagnostics Division of Electro-Nucleonics, Inc.

CHAPTER 17

Skin Endpoint Titration and the Modified RAST: Current Status

William P. King, M.D.

Recommended techniques for the diagnosis of inhalant IgE-mediated allergies are skin endpoint titration (SET) and the modified radioallergosorbent test (RAST).[1, 2] Both modalities have similar advantageous qualities: qualitative and quantitative diagnosis; that is, they indicate not only to what the patient is allergic, but also the degree of each specific allergy. In this manner, an individualized safe but potent immunotherapy starting dose for appropriate allergens is identified.

The American Academy of Otolaryngology–Head and Neck Surgery (AAO–HNS), the American Academy of Otolaryngic Allergy (AAOA), and the American Academy of Allergy and Immunology (AAAI) endorse escalation of immunotherapy dosage to either a symptom-relieving dose, that is, a dose that controls the patient's symptoms co-seasonally, or a maximally tolerated dose, whichever first occurs.[1–3]

The advantages of tests that quantitate specific allergen sensitivity are described by the AAOA as follows:

> The treatment starting dose indicated by either of the tests (SET or modified RAST) is usually more important than that empirically chosen after single dilution testing. Progressive increases result in the achievement of the final maintenance dose with notably fewer injections. This results in greater convenience and cost efficiency. There is also clinical advantage to be gained by the endorsed treatment modalities that follow these tests, since the potency of each contained allergen in a multi-allergen treatment vial differs according to the degree of sensitivity exhibited. Such a varied mixture allows a relatively equal advance in dosage for each contained allergen. This is in contrast to beginning treatment for all positive responding allergens with an equal strength mixture, as most often practiced after single dilution skin testing, where the final dose is limited by the most reactive contained allergen. Such therapy may result in clinically important but less reactive allergens failing to achieve the necessary dilution strength required to relieve symptoms.[4]

SKIN ENDPOINT TITRATION (SET)

First, let us review available skin testing techniques.

Patch Test. The patch test is used primarily for contact allergy diagnosis.

Scratch Tests. The scratch tests are highly criticized from all quarters because of lack of standardization of both technique and interpretation.[5–9]

Prick Tests. The usual single dilution prick test is more commonly used as a screen for severe sensitivities. Considering the fact that a prick test is equivalent to approximately a Rinkel #6 (1:312,500 wv) intracutaneous test wheal,[10] this test is very insensitive. A positive response, thus, indicates either a very high degree of sensitivity or a flash response. A prick test accomplished by the increasingly popular Multi-Test apparatus, however, is equivalent to intracutaneous testing with a 1:1000 wv to 1:1500 wv dilution[11] (between the 1:500 wv Rinkel #2 dilution and the 1:2500 wv Rinkel #3 dilution). Increased sensitivity allows this technique to be a more useful screening device.

Intracutaneous Test. Because of the more rapid assimilation of allergen, this test by nature is a much more sensitive test than any of the epicutaneous varieties. The primary shortcoming of intracutaneous testing is false-positive responses.[5, 6] It is imperative, therefore, that negative controls always be utilized to identify the degree of natural skin sensitivity and reactivity that exists in a given individual. The negative control solution must contain all of the ingredients in the same proportions contained in the active allergen mixture except the allergens themselves; specifically, it must contain the extracting glycerin, the preservative, and saline.

Single Dilution. This test variety is used more commonly by traditional allergists to test for the allergens that respond negatively on prior prick testing. Most often used is 1:1000 wv allergen dilution. The wide diversity of sensitivity between the prick test and this follow-up intracutaneous test actually disallows any meaningful quantitation of sensitivity.

Multiple Dilution. This technique of intracutaneous testing utilizes different dilutions of the same allergen to quantitate in bioassay fashion the degree of any existing sensitivity. This technique is commonly called skin endpoint titration.[12] Again, one must guard against misinterpretation of false-positive responses on application of stronger dilutions.

The precise makeup of the serial dilutions for skin endpoint titration (SET) varies with the SET technique employed. Norman, of Johns Hopkins, prefers 1:10 SET.[13] Dr. Turkeltaub of the Bureau of Biologics Section of the Federal Drug Administration utilizes 1:3 dilutions.[14] Norman states,

> Although a single concentration of a specific extract may be selected for testing and the reaction graded for positivity, much more information is obtained if a threshold dilution titration of skin tests is performed employing a ten-fold dilution series.[13]

Van Metre, also of Johns Hopkins, states,

> The absence of systemic and significant local reactions to 0.1 to 0.5 ml of endpoint dilution of ragweed pollen extract in this group of highly sensitive patients, suggests that immunotherapy by either the Rinkel (1:5) or current standard method (1:10) can be begun safely with 0.1 ml of the endpoint dilution and that there is no need to waste time and expense by beginning with a more dilute solution. Therefore, some form of titration may be useful prior to immunotherapy to determine the starting dilution.[15]

Turkeltaub notes,

> The best-fit linear regression line was calculated for the sum of erythema or wheal diameters obtained from four intradermal three-fold serial dilutions near the endpoint. . . . This quantitative skin-test assay is highly reproducible, yields potency data comparable to those of in vitro tests, can be applied to studies of extract stability and is suitable as a primary bio-assay of allergenic activity.[14]

An important discussion of the value of skin endpoint titration was held before the Health Care Delivery Committee of the Council of Medical Specialties Societies (CMSS) on July 28, 1981. At this meeting were representatives of the Medical College of Physicians, the American Academy of Allergy, the American Academy of Pediatrics, and the American Academy of Otolaryngology. The following statement pertaining to skin endpoint titration was issued at the conclusion of this meeting.

> Skin endpoint titration has been shown to be effective in quantifying patient sensitivity and for providing a rough guide to a safe starting dose for immunotherapy. It has not been shown to be an effective guide for determining the final therapeutic dose.[16]

On February 12, 1984, the leadership of the AAAI, the AAO–HNS, and the AAOA met and jointly reaffirmed this July 28, 1981, CMSS-composed statement on SET.[16]

Such agreement should be expected on review of the Position Statement of the AAAI in 1981.

> Studies indicated that some measurement of patient sensitivity, such as skin endpoint titration "by Rinkel or other standard methods," may be useful at the onset of immunotherapy to provide a guide to initial dose. Thereafter, costly repetitive endpoint titrations are usually unnecessary because regardless of what the titration indicates, the dose will be advanced either until the patient can tolerate no more or until a dose is reached that produces satisfactory results and has been shown in controlled studies to produce an effect superior to placebo.[3]

Skin endpoint titration testing is, therefore, a widely accepted modality.

Contention among allergy practitioners regarding the treatment technique suggested by Rinkel resulted in several critical papers. Indeed, Rinkel's writings are rather confusing regarding the proper manner of achieving a final maintenance dose. Although he repeatedly advocated advancing the dose based on clinical observations, he also stated that the selection of the top dose on the basis of a local reaction is only one third as accurate as the arbitrary administration of a top dose of 50X (0.50 ml of the endpoint dilution).[17, 18] Equipped with the modified RAST–provided knowledge that treatment need not be started with a dilution weaker than a Rinkel #6 dilution (1:312,500 wv),[19] it is readily understood why a limited 50X dose of a very dilute dilution may be of no therapeutic value, as verified by Van Metre[15] and Hirsch[20] in their separate studies. The Position Statements of the AAAI,[3] the AAO–HNS,[1] and the AAOA[2] disallow such predetermined dose limitation, regardless of the initial test modality utilized.

In view of all this agreement, one must be taken aback by published warnings to be wary of unproven diagnostic and treatment techniques, including "skin titration," without further explanation. Similarly, one must question the *how*'s and *wherefore*'s when third party payment institutions deny remuneration for "unproven" or "experimental" techniques such as "serial dilution titration," and even immunotherapy provided after such testing.

MODIFIED RAST

The radioallergosorbent test (RAST) was quickly developed after the discovery of IgE in 1967 by the Ishizakas and Johansson. Initial criticism for this in vitro method of allergy diagnosis and quantitation concerned lack of sensitivity despite excellent specificity, unavailability of many desired test allergens, and expense. All of these criticisms were justified, but were soon rectified.

With the appearance of the modified RAST, the most popular technique being that of Fadal and Nalebuff,[19] the lack of sensitivity problem was solved. As stated in the AAAI Position Statement,[3] skin testing is still more sensitive than is the RAST, actually to a fault when considering the propensity of intracutaneous skin testing for false-positive responses. Unmentioned is that the RAST is much more specific than is skin testing, disallowing unnecessary allergen, or even patient, treatment that may result after skin testing.

Scarcity of specific allergen discs is no longer a significant problem. Only rarely is skin test supplementation now necessary because of unavailability of some desired allergen.

With the introduction of a valid RAST screening technique by King[21] in 1982, and reaffirmation by Nalebuff[22] in 1984, the cost of RAST testing was significantly reduced.

As reaffirmed by Kniker, immunotherapy following the RAST, and to a somewhat lesser degree SET, "can be started safely at doses generally higher than those of the conventional approach, thereby saving months of delay and the expense of many ineffectual doses."[23] He notes that immunotherapy following the RAST, as after SET, allows the therapeutic advantage of the antigens' being "mixed in proportions relative to patient sensitivity, theoretically abrogating the likelihood of adverse reaction and permitting a steady advancement to the symptom relieving or maximally tolerated dose."[23]

Even prior to the now widely utilized RAST screen, Hamburger noted

> The high cost of the RAST is something that will correct itself in time with competition from several companies entering the field. Third party coverage problem, with local societies limiting the legitimate use of RAST, is a dangerous precedent. It should not be the case that a worthwhile test can be used only for people who can afford it.[24]

Similarly, Dockhorn stated,

> If prudence is utilized in selecting allergens for RAST testing, then the information obtained from these specific tests far outweighs the expense of these laboratory tests available. If this selective method is followed, then the information obtained from these specific tests far outweighs the expense of these laboratory tests.[25]

As far back as 1979, the National Institute of Allergy and Infectious Disease (NIAID) stated the following:

> Finally, one must confront the questions of desirability of quantifying IgE antibodies in patient sensitivity and the cost-benefit ratios of such studies. If an affordable, effective, and safe drug were to be made

available for treatment of rhinitis, monitoring immunologic changes during immunotherapy would be purely academic. In the absence of such a pharmacologic panacea, the time, effort, and expense of developing procedures to quantify the patient's sensitivity in IgE antibodies can be justified.[26]

At the July 1981 CMSS meeting, the following was approved by the attending organizations afore listed:

> Radioallergosorbent technique (RAST) is an in vitro test for the measurement of specific IgE antibody related to patient sensitivity and may be a useful adjunct in estimating the initial dose of immunotherapeutic extract. RAST has not been shown to be an effective guide to final therapeutic dose.[16]

Like the statement on skin endpoint titration, this proclamation was also reaffirmed in February 1984 by the AAAI, the AAO–HNS, and the AAOA.[16]

The AAAI Position Statement[27] wisely denotes concern about potential abuse of the RAST. Unfortunately, such potential does exist, as it does with any procedure. The ills of ignorance and lack of ethics are always with us, but do not fault the procedures.

Along with superior specificity, in the author's opinion, probably the greatest advantage of the RAST is convenience to the patient and to the physician. Whereas it is true that the test requires two days before an answer is at hand, as opposed to immediate skin test responses, there is seldom an acute need for such knowledge. Even this small objection is being overcome to a degree by some of the new second-generation enzyme tests, which require less than a day for completion.

SUMMARY

Quantitation is the key word—quantitation for medical efficiency and quantitation for cost efficiency.

The advantage of a quantitative test procedure is well illustrated by Lee, Kniker, and Campos in their mountain cedar co-seasonal allergy study.[28] A SET-tested group of patients was compared with a traditional group and a placebo group. While the traditional group's immunotherapy was started with a relatively brave 1:62,500 wv dilution, the 20 SET patients were begun at either a 1:2500 wv or 1:12,500 wv dilution. Injections were administered twice a week from December 24 to February 11. Over this period of time, the SET group received 11 times more allergen than the traditional group did. In addition, the SET subjects had substantially blunted total and specific IgE response in season; they produced lower specific IgE at season's end, and they had less shift of skin endpoint toward higher dilutions than normally occurs. These findings demonstrate that substantial immunologic effects are possible in the first month of aggressive co-seasonal immunotherapy when one is allowed to safely begin immunotherapy with a stronger dosage than is usually empirically selected.

Trevino[29] illustrated this same advantage in a different manner. He compared the resulting IgG-blocking antibodies after one year of immunotherapy in patients who were initially tested by either scratch testing, SET, or the modified RAST. The two groups tested by the last two quantitating techniques both produced significantly larger amount of blocking IgG antibody. Because the RAST typically allows a beginning dose even stronger than SET, the modified RAST group produced the greatest amount of IgG-blocking antibody.

Cost effectiveness in medicine has become a major issue, and rightfully so. The total cost of allergy care is a sum total of the cost of the initial testing procedures plus the cost of the therapy. Quantitative test procedures may be somewhat more expensive than nonquantitative techniques. The small expense is more than offset by the decrease in treatment costs that follows.

Therapy is composed of both immunotherapy and required symptomatic medications. Immunotherapy is subdivided into two phases: phase one, the time required for build-up to maintenance dose; and phase two, delivery of the maintenance dose at least two to three years. The total length of immunotherapy, thus, is largely a variant of the time required to complete phase one.

The reason a 1:62,500 wv empirical starting dose was referred to earlier as being relatively brave: empirical starting doses are more typically 1:500,000 wv, 1:1,000,000 wv, or even 1:1,000,000,000 wv dilutions.[22] With a dose escalation of 0.05 ml per injection until a total dose of 0.50 ml is reached, followed by progression to a concentration 10 times stronger, if treatment is started at the latter dilution, over 40 injections would be required before getting to the point at which a patient started at 1:62,500 wv, a SET #5 dilution, would begin. At one injection a week, this would require almost 10 months. Kniker estimates the average maintenance dose after traditional testing is reached in two to 12 months, whereas after quantitative endpoint titration or modified RAST testing the maintenance dose is achieved in several weeks.[23]

As a secondary result of more time-efficient symptom control, quantitative testing enhances cost effectiveness by both decreasing medication requirements and, owing to decreased morbidity, increasing patient productivity.

REFERENCES

1. American Academy of Otolaryngology–Head and Neck Surgery Policy, approved by Board of Directors, Washington, DC, 1982.
2. 1983 Position Statements of the American Academy of Otolaryngic Allergy. Washington, DC, American Academy of Otolaryngic Allergy, 1983.
3. American Academy of Allergy: Position Statements—Controversial techniques. J Allergy Clin Immunol 67:333, 1981.
4. Elaboration of Position Statements of the American Academy of Otolaryngic Allergy (AAOA). Washington, DC, American Academy of Otolaryngic Allergy, 1983.
5. Fadal RG, Nalebuff DJ: Tools of the allergist: old and new. Continuing Education, May 1979.
6. Kniker WT, Hales SW, Lee LK: Diagnostic methods to demonstrate IgE antibodies: skin testing techniques. Bull IV/Acad Med 57:524, 1981.
7. Imber WE: Allergic skin testing: a clinical investigation. J Allergy Clin Immunol 60:47, 1977.
8. Krause HA, Klaustermeyer WB: Immediate hypersensitivity skin testing: a comparison of scratch, prick and intradermal techniques. Immunol Allergy Pract 2:13, 1980.
9. Council of Scientific Affairs: In vivo diagnostic testing and immunotherapy for allergy: report 1, part 1, of the allergy panel. JAMA 258:1363, 1987.
10. Smith MP: Comparison of current techniques. *In* Becker GD (ed): Introduction to Otolaryngic Allergy. Washington, DC, American Academy of Otolaryngic Allergy, 1986, pp 12–13.
11. Murphree JT, Kniker WT: Correlation of immediate skin test responses to antigens introduced by Multi-Test and intracutaneous routes. Ann Allergy 43:274, 1979.
12. King WP: The role of the skin endpoint titration method in allergy. *In* Goldman J (ed): The Principle and Practice of Rhinology. New York, John Wiley & Sons, 1987, pp 283–292.
13. Norman PS: In vivo methods of study of allergy: skin and mucosa test techniques of interpretation. *In* Middleton E (ed): Allergy Principles and Practice. Vol 2. St. Louis, CV Mosby, 1983, p 297.
14. Turkeltaub PC, Rastogi SC, Baer H, et al: A standardized quantitative skin-test assay of allergen potency and stability: studies on the allergen dose-response cause and effect of wheal, erythema, and patient selection on assay results. J Allergy Clin Immunol 70:343, 1982.
15. Van Metre TE, Adkinson NF, Asmodio FJ, et al: A controlled study of the effectiveness of the Rinkel method of immunotherapy for ragweed pollen hay fever. J Allergy Clin Immunol 65:288, 1980.
16. AAOA News 2:1, 1984.
17. Rinkel HJ: The management of clinical allergy, part 2. Arch Otolaryngol 77:42, 1963.
18. Rinkel HJ: The management of clinical allergy, part 3. Arch Otolaryngol 77:205, 1963.
19. Nalebuff DJ, Fadal RG, Ali M: Local approach to immunotherapy. *In* Fadal RG, Nalebuff DJ (eds): RAST in Clinical Allergy. Miami, Symposia Specialists, 1981, pp 201–215.
20. Hirsch SR, Kalbfleisch JB, Golbert TM, et al: Rinkel injection therapy: a multicenter controlled study. J Allergy Clin Immunol 68:133, 1981.
21. King WP: Efficacy of a screening radioallergosorbent test. Arch Otolaryngol 108:781, 1982.
22. Nalebuff DJ: Use of RAST screening in clinical allergy: a cost effective approach to patient care. Ear Nose Throat J 64:15, 1984.
23. Kniker WT: Common sense. Continuing Education, May 1979.
24. Hamburger RN: A cautious view of the use of RAST in clinical allergy. Immunol Allergy Pract 5:10, 1981.
25. Dockhorn RJ: Using the RAST and PRIST with an overview of clinical significance. Ann Allergy 49:1, 1982.
26. NIAID Task Force Report. NIH publication No. 79–387, May 1979.
27. Position Statement: Skin testing and radioallergosorbent testing (RAST) for diagnosis of specific allergens responsible for IgE mediated disease, American Academy of Allergy and Immunology. J Allergy Clin Immunol 72:515, 1983.
28. Lee LK, Kniker WT, Campos T: Aggressive coseasonal immunotherapy in mountain cedar allergy. Arch Otolaryngol 108:787, 1982.
29. Trevino RJ: IgG levels after treatment with antigen based on the scratch testing, intradermal testing, modified RAST testing. Otolaryngol Head Neck Surg 95:307, 1986.

CHAPTER 18

Diagnostic Skin Testing: Skin Endpoint Titration

Walter A. Ward, Jr., M.D.

Skin endpoint titration is a technique for determining the endpoint of reaction to an inhalant allergen and the safe initial dosage for treatment of the detected allergies. The technique was developed in 1935, when French K. Hansel and his colleagues began using what they called "serial dilution testing" to establish guidelines for the co-seasonal treatment of hay fever.[1] They were immediately impressed by the striking symptomatic relief that followed the intracutaneous introduction of small amounts of the extract being tested. Soon, they adapted this small optimal dose to inhalant desensitization therapy, discarding the more traditional method of desensitization.

Herbert J. Rinkel was intrigued by Hansel's work, and after visiting Hansel to be taught the technique, he began in the early 1940s to use serial dilution titration routinely in his practice.[2–5] This text teaches the updated version of Rinkel's original technique,[6, 7] the preferred term for the technique being skin endpoint titration (SET). Currently, well over 3000 physicians throughout the world are using SET, having been guided by such pioneers as Cowen,[7, 8] W. P. King,[6] H. C. King,[9] Williams,[10, 11] and Willoughby.[12]

The advantages of SET are

1. Safety.
2. Readability.
3. Standardization.
4. Quicker results from treatment.
5. Safe co-seasonal (i.e., during the height of a pollen season) testing and treatment.
6. Individualization of mixes for each patient.

The single characteristic that most clearly distinguishes SET from other techniques is the use of consecutive 1:5 dilutions (1:5, 1:25, 1:125, 1:625, 1:3125, and so on), which are injected intracutaneously in a standardized manner, proceeding from a weak, nonreactive skin response to increasingly positive skin reactions.

PREPARATION OF THE ANTIGEN DILUTIONS FOR TESTING

The testing set should contain six dilutions of each antigen on your testing board.

Diluents

There are basically four different diluents that are available commercially: (1) normal saline (0.9% NaCl + 0.4% phenol); (2) buffered saline (0.5% NaCl + 0.275% sodium bicarbonate + 0.4% phenol); (3) albumin saline (0.9% NaCl + 0.4% phenol + 0.03% human serum albumin); and (4) 50% glycerin (normal saline with 50% glycerin by volume).

The normal saline is used for the testing dilutions. The buffered saline is not used by titrationists because it interferes with the normal whealing response. The albumin saline acts to reduce adsorption of antigens to the glass vial, thereby helping to maintain antigen potency. Normal saline and albumin saline will reduce antigen degradation at room temperture; thus, testing sets must be changed every six to eight weeks. The 50 per cent glycerinated saline is a good bacteriostatic agent and keeps antigen very stable. Its only disadvantage is it stings upon injection and will interfere with normal whealing response on the #1 dilution and possibly the #2 dilution in some individuals. The #2 is one of your controls.

Begin preparation of the testing dilution with previously acquired diluent bottles. Most allergy supply houses have these in the stock sizes required for the 1:5 dilution technique. Before starting, standardize your syringe by withdrawing a small amount of the concentrate and flushing it back into the bottle of concentrate. This removes the dead space in the needle. To prepare the #1 testing dilution, withdraw 1 ml of the antigen concentrate and inject it into the vial containing 4 ml of diluent and labeled #1. Thoroughly mix the solution by pulling it into the syringe and reinjecting it into the bottle three times. The #2 dilution is prepared by withdrawing 1 ml from the #1 dilution bottle (using the same syringe) and injecting it into the #2 bottle, which again contains 4 ml of diluent. Repeat the entire procedure for each of the desired testing dilutions, withdrawing each time 1 ml from the latest prepared dilution.

The dilutions are numbered by their relation to the antigen concentrate, so that #1 is the first dilution, #2 the second, and so on. The dilution number also reflects the dilution exponent, e.g., 1:100 = #1, 1:500 = #2, 1:2500 = #3 (Table 18–1). This is actually a lowering of the dilution factor by 5 for each dilution (Fig. 18–1). Most inhalant antigens are supplied in concentrations of 1:20, except for the dust mite

Table 18–1. DILUTIONS OF ANTIGENS

Concentrate	1:20
1	1:100
2	1:500
3	1:2500
4	1:12,500
5	1:62,500
6	1:312,500
7	1:1,562,500
8	1:7,812,500
9	1:39,062,500
10	1:200,000,000

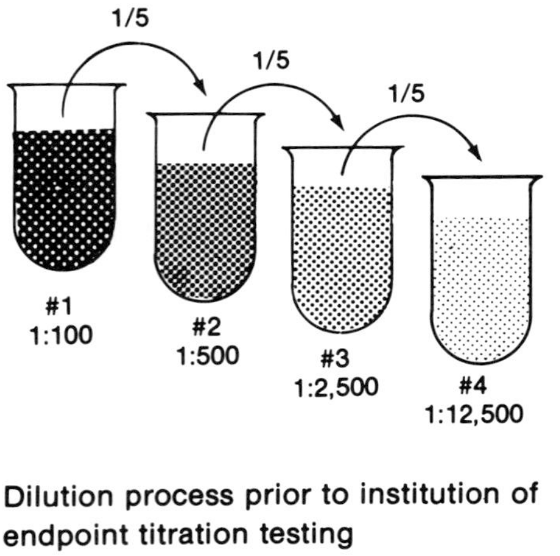

FIGURE 18–1. Dilution process before the start of endpoint titration testing.

antigen, which is a 1:100 concentrate. Conversely, food extracts are generally 1:10 concentrates, as are the mold and animal dander extracts. The concentrate becomes extremely important if you wish to have your #1 vial always a 1:100 concentration. Thus, the concentrate for the dust mite antigen can be your #1 vial without further dilution, but because it contains 50 per cent glycerin, you can expect it to give you a false-positive skin response if, for any reason, you should want to test down to the #1 level. If you are using the RAST scoring technique, it is essential to make the concentrate for dust mite(s) the #1 concentrate. Some titrationists dilute the dust mite antigen so that the #1 is really 1:500. As long as you are consistent, you may do it either way. To make dander and mold extracts 1:100 concentrations on the #1 dilution, add 0.05 ml of the antigen concentrate (1:10) to 0.45 ml of diluent or 0.25 ml of antigen to 2.5 ml of diluent.

It is vital that your syringe technique during preparation of the testing dilutions be fastidious, and that you not use the same syringe for different antigens. Whereas the use of disposable syringes eliminates the lengthy procedure of rinsing glass syringes, it must be remembered that disposable syringes are exactly that, and under no circumstances should they be reused. The testing sets are good for three months if refrigerated and for six weeks at room temperature. Dilutions greater than #2 dilution will lose their potency more rapidly than higher dilutions because you have diluted out the glycerin, which serves as a preservative. For this reason, the date on which the testing and/or treatment set is prepared must be on the label. If for any reason you are distracted during the mixing of the various dilutions or in the preparation of a vaccine, you should start over with a new syringe and fresh diluent bottles.

SERIAL TESTING

As with all diagnostic tools, it is important that SET be performed properly and interpreted properly. The patient's upper arm is used for testing. After cleansing the testing site, grasp the upper arm to put tension on the skin and, using a syringe with a 26-gauge, 3/8-inch beveled needle, slowly penetrate the most superficial layer of the skin with the bevel of the needle turned down toward the underlying muscles. Create a 4 mm wheal by slowly injecting approximately 0.01 ml (1/100) of the test dilution (Fig. 18–2). The accuracy and subsequent interpretation of the results depend on the truly intracutaneous nature of the injection. The wheal created by the injection of the test dilution should be pale with sharp, well demarcated edges, and should be exactly 4 mm in both its vertical and its horizontal diameters. If for any reason the wheal is not that size, or if pseudopod formation occurs (which means the lymphatic system has been entered), you must disregard this wheal and reapply the antigen. At the end of 10 minutes, when the tests are read, it is the diameter of the wheal that is the significant factor; the presence or absence of erythema is of no clinical significance. The original 4 mm wheal will be approximately 5 mm in diameter if it is a nonreactive or negative response, 7 mm or larger if it is a positive response. By definition, a positive reaction is at least 2 mm larger than the preceding nonreactive or negative wheal (5 mm).

Three common errors, alone or together, may

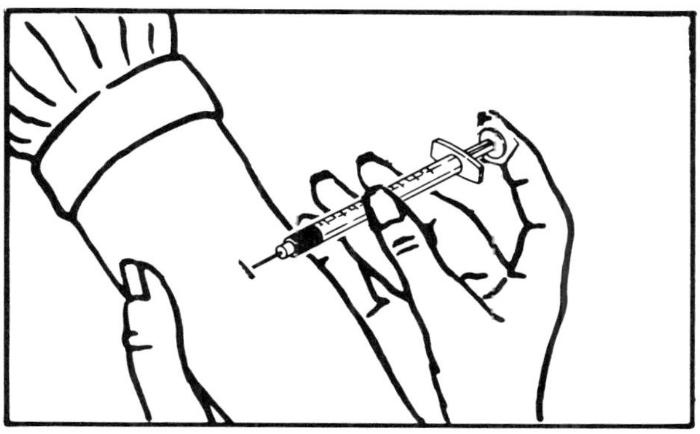

The correct way to make a wheal

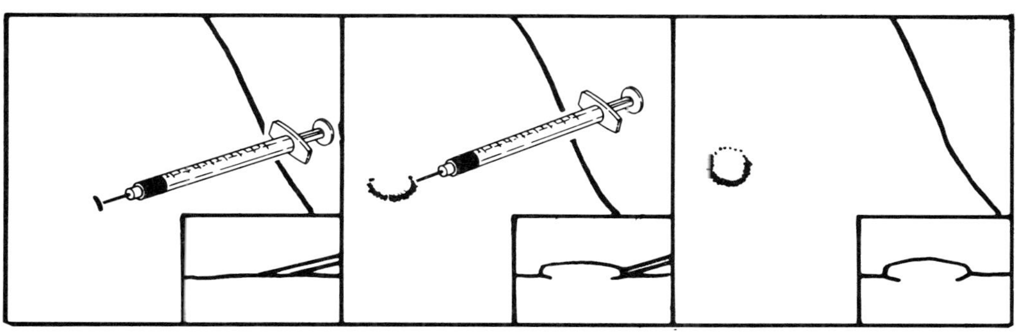

FIGURE 18–2. Intracutaneous skin test. A short-bevel, 26-gauge needle should be used. *Left,* The most superficial layer of skin is penetrated with the bevel of the needle down; *center,* allergenic extract is injected slowly with the needle and syringe held parallel to the skin; *right,* the resulting injection of allergenic extract should produce a wheal 4 mm in diameter. The wheal should be elevated and pale, with sharply demarcated margins. (Courtesy of H. C. King, M.D. Used with permission.)

occur during these injections: (1) the antigen may be injected too deeply under the skin; (2) too much or too little antigen may be injected; and (3) irritation from injection of the needle may cause the edges of the wheal to be less distinct. Obviously, greater amounts of dilution will produce a wheal larger than the desired 4.0 mm wheal and will often lead to misinterpretation in reading the test results. Since probability of error in interpretation also increases when the edges of the wheal are indistinct, you can reduce irritation by injecting the antigen as the needle is introduced. Disposable syringes with prefixed needles for testing are recommended, since their use eliminates the problem of trauma from dull, bent, or barbed needles, and use of the prefixed needles eliminates dead space in the hub of the needle.

Controls

Before beginning your testing, positive and negative controls should be applied. A positive control is a #2 or #3 histamine, prepared by using 2.75 mg of histamine phosphate as the concentrate and diluting it to 1:5 just like your antigens. The negative control is necessary to identify a positive reaction to the diluent. The most frequently used negative control is a #2 dilution of 50 per cent glycerin and the phenolated diluent. The concentrated extracts contain 50 per cent glycerin as a preservative. Thus, the #1 dilution contains 10 per cent, the #2 dilution has 2 per cent, and the #3 dilution has 0.4 per cent of glycerin. Phenolated saline diluent alone is applied to check for phenol sensitivity. On occasion, it may be necessary to check for mast cell integrity, and for this 5 per cent codeine phosphate is used in the same manner. A word of caution: a positive skin test on the #2 glycerin concentrate indicates that endpoints on the #2 dilution of the various allergens are probably false-positive results. Here, only in vitro testing can provide the answer to such a patient's sensitivity.

Antigen Screening

Many clinicians prefer initial screening for sensitivity using some of the more common allergens: for example, extracts of house dust mites, Alternaria, Hormodendrum, dog and cat dander if the patient is exposed to these animals, and one or two pollens of weeds, grasses, and trees prevalent in the patient's area. Screening wheals are typically applied vertically, one above the other, on the lateral surface of the upper arm. The primary reason for such a screen is to identify the pattern and degree of that particular patient's hypersensitivities. In addition, the screen may serve to somewhat stabilize the skin reaction.

If a particular pollen is in season, testing should begin with a #6 dilution. If a test antigen is not in season, a #4 dilution may be used safely as the starting test in most patients. For every patient with a history of severe allergic problems, such as asthma, laryngeal edema, or angioneurotic edema, the #6 dilution of all antigens to be screened must be used as the starting test. A #6 dilution of an antigen currently in season is used because an atopic person has a tendency to become hypersensitive to a specific antigen when exposed to it in large amounts; therefore, because of increased exposure during a pollen season, the patient's sensitivity may be increased.

If the #4 dilution produces a negative response, a #3 dilution and a #2 dilution can be applied simultaneously, since, at this point, an endpoint and confirming wheal can be obtained only if both dilutions react positively. All wheals should be read after 10 or 15 minutes, and all responses recorded. A response is considered negative if, during the 10- to 15-minute period, the original wheal disappears, remains unchanged, or grows no more than 1 mm in diameter. A wheal response is considered positive if the wheal has increased 2 mm or more beyond a nonreactive 5 mm wheal. A positive wheal is always confirmed by applying the next stronger dilution, which will again cause an increase in the wheal size of 2 mm or more. A normal whealing response is a 5, 7, 9 mm combination (Fig. 18–3).

SET testing is designed to identify not only the allergens to which the patient has a positive response, but also the best starting point of immunotherapy. If performed correctly, the testing may be administered either preseasonally or co-seasonally simply by beginning testing in a nonreactive zone (a dilution weaker than the patient's sensitivity), and advancing to a reactive zone (dilutions to which the patient responds

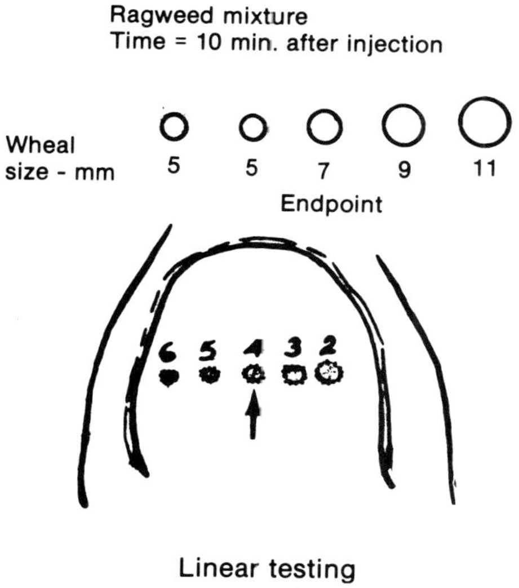

FIGURE 18–3. Normal whealing response. (Courtesy of H. C. King, M.D. Used with permission.)

positively). The purpose of the initial wheal is to determine a negative dilution from which you may proceed to stronger dilutions to arrive at a positive response. The ultimate objective of SET testing is the identification of an "endpoint" dilution for each allergen to which there is a positive response, and it is this "endpoint" that determines the safe starting point of immunotherapy.

The "endpoint" dilution is the dilution that provides the first positive wheal and that also initiates progressively more positive wheals of 2 mm or greater on application of consecutively stronger 1:5 dilutions. Cowen considers the term "endpoint" a misnomer when applied to the whealing response, since this dilution actually is the beginning point of the response and forms the beginning dilution in subsequent immunotherapy.[8] However, the term is in common use, and will probably continue to be used as it is today.

Variations in the Whealing Response

Bizarre whealing responses will occur in 5 to 15 per cent of tests applied. There are three well-recognized abnormal wheal responses, although others may occur.

Flash Response. The flash response is a huge whealing response of a very positive nature to a dilution that is weaker than the true endpoint. It is not a repeatable whealing response and may often be eradicated immediately by applying weaker dilutions and moving forward through the flash to the true endpoint and confirming wheal. The flash response usually, but not always, occurs when the antigen is out of date or the patient has a food allergy. If you cannot eradicate the response immediately, then you should repeat the test within 24 hours. An example of a flash response is a 15 mm wheal with a #6 dilution; when the test is repeated, starting with a #8 dilution (in such a case the titration or testing set must be further diluted in the same manner as the original six dilutions), the response will give you a 5, 5, 5, 7, and 9 mm wheal, making the #5 dilution the true endpoint (Table 18–2).

Table 18–2. FLASH RESPONSE TO OAK VACCINE (mm)

	Dilutions								
Day	9	8	7	6	5	4	3	2	1
1	5	5	5	5	13	18	21		
2		5	5	5	5	7	9	11	

Plateau Response. The plateau response is a 7 mm or larger wheal, followed by the same size wheal on progressively stronger dilutions until a dilution produces an increase in wheal size of 2 mm or larger. The dilution that initiates the larger wheal is close to the confirming dilution, and the preceding dilution is close to the endpoint dilution. An example would be a 7, 7, 7, and 9 mm wheal response. The dilution producing the 7 mm wheal followed by the 9 mm wheal is the endpoint, and should be seen when the test is repeated (Table 18–3).

Hourglass Response. The rare hourglass response is a large response on the initial weak dilution and subsequent smaller responses on the next few stronger dilutions until a negative response occurs, which is then followed by a

Table 18–3. PLATEAU RESPONSE TO OAK VACCINE (mm)

	Dilutions								
Day	9	8	7	6	5	4	3	2	1
1	7	7	7	9	9	9	11	11	
2	5	5	5	7	9				

normal response. Initiation of normal whealing determines the true endpoint. An example would be a sequence of 11, 9, 7, 5, 7, 9 mm wheal responses, with the dilution that produces the second 7 mm wheal being the endpoint. The hourglass response shows the inaccuracy of scratch testing and usually is seen only when very dilute solutions (#8, #9, #10) are used.

One must not be dismayed by other responses, such as 5, 5, 13, and 15 mm wheal sequences that are repeatable. The 13 mm wheal is your endpoint because it initiated a wheal that was 2 mm or larger than the negative wheal and is followed by a confirming wheal, which was 2 mm larger than the endpoint.

One of the many strong points for using SET is its value in the patient who has bizarre whealing responses, because it should prevent the physician from using a misleading skin response as the starting point for immunotherapy. The single application of an antigen with a huge response might have the unsuspecting allergist beginning treatment at far too weak a dilution, thus necessitating many weeks or months to reach a therapeutic dose. With determination of the true endpoint, a much stronger starting point for immunotherapy is possible.

Influence of Medications

Although there is little disagreement about the effects of antihistamines on the whealing response, there is considerable lack of agreement on how long the patient should abstain from antihistamine therapy before SET testing: Because some patients metabolize antihistamines more slowly than others, some physicians require an antihistamine-free period of 7 to 10 days; the author believes that testing can be successful if antihistamine therapy is discontinued for a minimum of 72 hours before testing begins. When the new antihistamines with prolonged half-lives become available, this time frame will have to be extended.

A problem in this regard is the antihistamine-like qualities of other medications the patient is taking. Patients may honestly forget to mention some medications they are taking, or they may not consider over-the-counter preparations to be "true" medicine. The widespread use of tranquilizers and mood elevators, many of which are almost identical to antihistamines in their physiologic action, is a common problem for the diagnostician. Every clinician who conducts SET testing must be familiar with all the medications a patient is taking and with their potential effects on testing. The "antihistamine effect" may range from almost total elimination of whealing to simply a decrease in erythema. In any case, the whealing response is diminished enough to prevent the "true" whealing response needed for correctly started immunotherapy.

Steroid-dependent patients are inevitable in referrals to clinicians handling severe atopic problems. Ideally, such patients should be tested at least six weeks after the last steroid dose was given. However, since steroids may not be withdrawn abruptly and thus the delay before testing and immunotherapy would be long, some practitioners find it safe and satisfactory to titrate such patients and to treat them accordingly, retesting them as they are weaned from steroids.

Influence of Ingestants

Allergic ingestants may influence the whealing response. The difficulty is in determining whether a response is due to the allergen tested or to enhancement by the ingested allergen of the response of the test injection. RAST inhibition tests have shown cross-reactivity between certain aeroallergens and certain food antigens. Concomitant foods suspected or proven are listed in Table 18–4. If only seasonal antigens exhibit atypical responses, concomitant foods should be suspected. If the initial day's testing produced relatively normal whealing and the patient returns the next day with initial test wheals raised, erythematous, and pruritic, in all probability the culprit is an allergenic dinner

Table 18–4. CONCOMITANT AND SYNERGISTIC FOODS

	Suspected or Proven Concomitant Foods
Ragweed	Milk, melons, bananas
Iva ciliata	Wheat
Sage	Potato
Pigweed	Pork
Grass	Legumes: beans, peas, soybeans, cottonseed (cooking fats)
Marigold	Milk
Cedar	Beef, yeasts (baker's, brewer's, malt)
Elm	Milk
Oak	Egg
Pecan	Corn, banana
Birch	Apple

consumed the previous evening. For this reason, it may be desirable to test the patient in a semifasting state. The patient must be instructed to have no food after dinner the evening before testing and to abstain from breakfast the morning of retesting.

Influence of Animal Danders

The influence of animal exposure on whealing response, especially exposure to cats and horses, cannot be overemphasized. Either regular or intermittent exposure to an animal should be suspected when the whealing response is consistently erratic and unpredictable.

Influence of Seasonal Allergens

The presence or absence of specific airborne allergens may be of great importance in the whealing response of some patients. Depending on seasonal exposures, multiple variations in response may be exhibited, including the "hourglass," the "flash," or other unusual "endpoint" responses. In much of the United States, tree pollens are suspected if symptoms occur between February and May; grass pollens are usually present from late April to frost, but are heaviest in May and June; weed pollens are generally present from late July to frost; molds are prevalent in the fall, but are present perennially. All pollen seasons are geographically determined.

ADVANTAGES AND DISADVANTAGES OF SET

SET has several distinct advantages over other methods of allergy testing:

1. It safely indicates the strength and amount of antigen that may be used to initiate immunotherapy.
2. It allows a larger amount of antigen to be injected following titration, which decreases the interval to successful immunotherapy and the cost of that interval.
3. It allows easy adjustment of allergen dosage in multiple allergen treatment vials. Since titration was designed for use with multiple antigen immunotherapy, treatment sets are made up according to the individual patient's degree of sensitization to the various antigens. If for any reason the suggested increase in dosage is not well tolerated, retitration may be performed to determine which antigen in the extract is too strong or too weak, thus salvaging the immunotherapy effort.
4. It may be performed at any time of the year, preseasonally or co-seasonally.
5. It allows safe testing and treatment of the patient with severe symptoms such as asthma or angioneurotic edema.

However, SET does not solve all problems in atopic management.

1. It does not show a clinically significant correlation between the degree of sensitivity exhibited and the active symptoms of the patient, so that very low sensitivities are not related to minimal symptoms and, conversely, high sensitivities do not necessarily indicate severe symptoms.
2. Sensitivity responses do not decrease consistently with clinical improvement, nor do they indicate when a patient may discontinue immunotherapy.
3. SET does not indicate the antigenic dose required for therapeutic relief of symptoms any more reliably than any other mode of testing. Rather, it simply suggests the dilution at which antigen therapy is best started. From that point on, dosage is as empirical as with other methods and is related solely to the clinical response of the individual patient.

SUMMARY

In conclusion, SET is a safe method of determining antigens to which a patient is sensitive and the patient's degree of sensitivity to those antigens. Thus, it enables the clinician to determine the amount of the respective antigens to put in the patient's treatment vial so that the dosage is adjusted to that degree of sensitivity.

SET is safe. Since it pinpoints with accuracy the dilution with which immunotherapy may safely be started, therapy can, without untoward results, be initiated with a much larger dose of antigen than with any other method of immunotherapy. Use of such a specific dosage avoids or eliminates the frequent undesirable symptoms of treatment such as arm swelling, provocation of allergic symptoms, or, in the extreme, anaphylactic shock, which can occur when antigens are all placed in the treatment mixture in the same concentration.

Over 3000 physicians in a variety of medical disciplines and in various parts of the United States and other countries are successfully using the SET technique in the diagnosis and treatment of inhalant allergies.

Acknowledgment

The author wishes to thank Mrs. Judith T. MacMillan and Miss Nina Haynes for their assistance in the preparation of this chapter.

REFERENCES

1. Hansel FK: Coseasonal intracutaneous treatment of hay fever. J Allergy 12:457, 1941.
2. Rinkel HJ: Inhalant allergy. Ann Allergy 7:639, 1949.
3. Rinkel HJ: The management of clinical allergy. Part I. General considerations. Arch Otolaryngol 76:491, 1962.
4. Rinkel HJ: The management of clinical allergy. Part II. Etiologic factors and skin titration. Arch Otolaryngol 77:56, 1963.
5. Rinkel HJ: The management of clinical allergy. Part III. Inhalant allergy therapy. Arch Otolaryngol 77:205, 1963.
6. King WP: Endpoint titration—current status. Trans Am Soc Ophthalmol Otolaryngol Allergy 10:173, 1980.
7. Cowen DE, Dixon BJ (revision by Ward WA): Skin Endpoint Titration Technique. Washington, DC, American Academy of Otolaryngic Allergy Manual, 1987, pp 1–13.
8. Cowen DE: Serial dilution titration: technique and application. ORL Allergy Digest 41:37, 1979.
9. King HC: Endpoint titration and immunotherapy. Otolaryngol Clin North Am 18:703, 1985.
10. Williams RI: Modern concepts in clinical management of allergy in otolaryngology. Laryngoscope 76:1389, 1966.
11. Williams RI: Skin titration: testing and treatment. Otolaryngol Clin North Am 4:507, 1971.
12. Willoughby JW: Serial dilution titration skin tests in inhalant allergy. A clinical quantitative assessment of biologic skin reactivity to allergenic extracts. Otolaryngol Clin North Am 7:579, 1974.

CHAPTER 19

In Vitro Tests in the Diagnosis of Allergic Disorders

Donald J. Nalebuff, M.D.

Over 60 years ago, Prausnitz and Küstner demonstrated a transferable factor in the serum of allergic patients. The formerly nonreactive recipient of this factor was found to react with a positive wheal and flare response when suitably challenged with the appropriate allergen.[1] Until that classic experiment, the allergic reaction was thought to be an altered state of individual reactivity. Their observation made it clear that allergy was closely related to the presence of a serum factor, which for lack of a better name had been called either "reagin" or the skin-sensitizing antibody (SSA). The search for the exact nature of this transferable protein continued until the mid-1960s when the Ishizakas isolated a "reagin-rich" factor from the serum of an atopic individual; it gave a P-K titer of 80,000, the reciprocal of the highest dilution of serum giving a definite positive reaction. Discovering that it was different from the other known immunoglobulins, they called it "gamma E globulin," since it appeared to mediate the erythema skin reaction.[2]

At about the same time, Johansson and Bennich in Sweden had isolated an atypical protein from the serum of a myeloma patient. The patient's initials (ND) were adopted by them as an interim label for this material, minute amounts of which were found capable of blocking the P-K reaction. They observed that similar material also was present in trace amounts in the serum of patients with hay fever and allergic asthma.[3]

Subsequent study by both groups established that the "gamma E globulin" and the "ND myeloma protein" were, in fact, the same substance. The research findings of the two teams were merged, a new class of immunoglobulins was formally established, and in 1968 it was officially designated immunoglobulin E (IgE). The long search for the nature of "reagin" was over, and the study of its properties and clinical applications of this new knowledge were launched.

THE IMMEDIATE HYPERSENSITIVITY ALLERGIC REACTION

IgE antibody does not mediate the allergic reaction alone; its most important property is its ability to sensitize homologous tissues such as blood basophils and tissue mast cells. These tissue mast cells are most numerous in the lining of the respiratory and gastrointestinal tracts as well as under the skin—loci, as might be expected, that are the main sites of both the lymphoid cells that form IgE antibody and the major organs affected in IgE-mediated allergic reactions.

We now know that specific IgE antibodies, synthesized by plasma cells in response to allergen, move through the bloodstream to these tissue mast cells and become firmly fixed to their surface receptors. The cell membrane of each mast cell is studded with between 100,000 and 500,000 receptors for IgE molecules. Electron microscopy reveals that when two similar IgE molecules are bridged by antigen, there is a change in their molecular configuration—a change believed to trigger a series of biochemical reactions, which modifies the structure of the outer cell membrane. Two important series of events then take place very rapidly:

Channels are generated in the cell membrane, causing the ingress of calcium into the cell, which in turn activates enzymes of the cyclic adenosine monophosphate (cAMP) system. Once the reaction has started and the intracellular levels of cAMP decrease, energy is released that promotes the assembly in the cell of microtubules and the contraction of threadlike microfilaments. These contractile structures cause the intracellular mast cell granules (about 1000 per cell) to move to the cell membrane, fuse with it, and release into the microenvironment its storehouse of active preformed chemical mediators: histamine, heparin, bradykinins, serotonin, and several chemotactic factors that attract blood platelets, white blood cells, and eosinophils. Each of these mediators contributes in its own way to the allergic reaction.

Another significant change set off by the interaction of IgE and antigen is that transmethylating enzymes are stimulated that produce changes in the cell membrane phospholipids with the resultant cleavage of arachidonic acid to form two important groups of potent biologic mediators—the prostaglandins and the recently characterized leukotrienes, formally called the slow-reacting substance of anaphylaxis (SRS–A). Detailed descriptions of all of these products and their individual roles in the immediate hypersensitivity allergic reaction have been reviewed in detail elsewhere.[4]

One can summarize that the net effects of the release of these mediators into tissues are increases in capillary permeability and in the secretion of nasal and bronchial mucus, contraction in the smooth muscle of the bronchi and gastrointestinal tract, and an influx of polymorphonuclear leukocytes and eosinophils to the area. These events are now recognized as the hallmarks of allergic disorders of the immediate type.

The IgE-mediated mechanism is indeed the predominant trigger for disease in atopic patients who tend to have a positive family history and to produce abnormally high levels of total and specific IgE antibody. Allergen immunotherapy is efficacious in these patients by ultimately reducing responsiveness to antigen exposure.

NON–IgE-MEDIATED REACTIONS

It is now known that the degranulation of tissue mast cells, as previously described, may be initiated by several factors other than the bridging of adjacent specific IgE molecules by allergen. Some immunologic factors (e.g., complement components such as the C3a and C5a anaphylatoxins) and several nonimmunologic factors (e.g., chemicals, physical factors, neurogenic stimulation, exercise, and infection) are all capable of inducing signals in the mast cell membrane that lead to mediator release and, therefore, produce a disease state clinically indistinguishable from IgE-mediated allergy.

Individuals whose disease is exclusively triggered by such factors are not atopic, usually do not have positive family histories, do not produce elevated levels of IgE, do not demonstrate "positive" test results for specific IgE antibody, and—most important—do not respond to allergen immunotherapy. It is essential, therefore, to distinguish between these populations.

From the time that atopy or IgE allergy was first recognized as an entity, clinical attempts to treat it have been governed by the accuracy of diagnosis, which, in the past, has been based almost entirely on patient history and the evaluation of several traditional in vivo skin test procedures. With the development and commercial availability of tests to measure both total and specific levels of IgE antibody, an extra dimension of precision in diagnosis has become possible.

THE PAPER RADIOIMMUNOSORBENT TEST

Two distinctly different methods are used for the measurement of total IgE protein, each with a different range of sensitivity. The first type is the radioimmunosorbent test (RIST), a competitive inhibition procedure that measures IgE from its capacity to block the reaction between a defined amount of radiolabeled IgE and specific antibodies to IgE; the more IgE there is in a serum sample, the less radioactivity bound to the antibody. The second type is a double-antibody sandwich assay, the paper radioimmunosorbent test (PRIST), in which there is a direct or positive relationship between IgE concentration and the binding of tracer. Whereas these diverse techniques give similar responses in the higher concentration range (100 ng and above), there are significant discrepancies in the lower ranges due to false elevations as a result of interfering serum factors in the RIST. This problem is eliminated in the PRIST, and it is possible to accurately detect 50 to 100 picograms with this procedure.

CLINICAL APPLICATION OF TOTAL IgE MEASUREMENT

There have been correlations reported with levels of IgE in cord blood and the development of atopy in later life.[5] Serum IgE levels are helpful in the diagnosis of hyperimmunoglobulin E syndrome, IgE myeloma, and Wiskott-Aldrich syndrome and in the diagnosis and treatment of parasitic infestations and allergic bronchopulmonary aspergillosis. The total IgE antibody level can be correlated with clinical allergy only in a general way; that is, patients with the higher concentrations of total serum IgE are usually positive to multiple allergens, and in these patients there is a greater incidence of extremely high levels of specific antibody detected, especially in patients with total IgE levels of 200 μ/ml or more.[6] However, in some patients with a total serum IgE level of over 400 μ/ml, no positive specific antibody is ever found. This can be because there are a number of diseases that can elevate serum IgE besides atopy (parasitic infestations, malignancies, dermatologic disorders, liver disease, and immunodeficiency states). On the other hand, 50 per cent of patients with clinical evidence of allergy and detectable allergen-specific IgE have total IgE levels in ranges usually considered to be within normal limits, and some patients with serum total IgE levels below 50 μ/ml have significant specific antibody titers to a limited number of antigens. Patients with total serum IgE levels of 10 μ/ml or less, however, rarely have detectable specific IgE levels.

THE IN VITRO DIAGNOSIS OF ATOPIC ALLERGY

In 1967, within months after IgE was discovered, Wide et al. developed the radioallergosorbent test (RAST) for the detection of specific IgE antibodies in serum.[7] This technique reliably detects the actual presence of allergen-specific IgE antibody against a particular allergen and also accurately assays its serum concentration and thus the degree of allergen sensitization; sensitivity in the range of picograms per microliter has been reported. RAST results are not altered by drugs, metabolites, irritants, contaminants, ongoing disease, autonomic nervous system imbalances, and neither highly nor poorly reactive skin. Investigators report a high correlation between the RAST scores and the allergic history, P-K transfers, the response to allergen challenge, and the results of skin endpoint titration. RAST is more quantitative than the P-K reaction, obviates the need of a recipient, and eliminates the risk of transmitting disease such as hepatitis. Large numbers of serum samples can be handled simultaneously in the RAST, and a clear differentiation among the specimens is readily achieved.

Test Principles

The basic principles of the RAST are similar to the indirect Coombs test used for the detection of Rh-positive antibodies in the serum of Rh-negative women (Table 19–1). In the RAST,

Table 19–1. PRINCIPLES OF THE RADIOALLERGOSORBENT TEST

Soluble allergens are bound to solid-phase supports (e.g., a paper disc) to create a stable immunosorbent, which then acquires the antigenicity of the allergen
The passively created immunosorbent (insoluble allergen), on incubation with a test serum, will react with specific antibody to form a solid-phase complex
Anti-human IgE serum raised in another species (e.g., rabbit) and radiolabeled will react with antigenic determinants on the Fc portion of the IgE antibody bound to the allergen-coated immunosorbent
The greater the amount of radioactivity bound to the disc, the more specific the IgE present in the serum sample under test

allergens are chemically linked to solid-phase supports—usually paper discs—that are incubated with a droplet of serum from the allergic patient. If specific IgE antibodies are present in the serum sample, they will bind with the insolubilized allergen to form a complex. After this first step, the allergen-coated paper discs are washed to remove all unattached serum protein. In a second step, the discs are incubated with radiolabeled anti-human IgE antibodies that have been raised in another species, usually the rabbit. After this second incubation, all free labeled anti-IgE is washed away. The more specific IgE initially bound to the solid-phase disc, the more rabbit anti-human IgE with its attached radioactive tag is left behind to be counted in a scintillation gamma counter. Thus, the quantity of bound radioactivity is directly related to the quantity of specific IgE present in the serum sample.

RAST in Clinical Diagnosis

Since its initial development, RAST has found worldwide acceptance for specific IgE antibody estimation; it is estimated that over 100 million tests have been performed. RAST has been applied successfully in the determination of IgE antibodies to animal dander, pollens, and stinging insect venoms; viruses, bacterial components, and chemical substances have been shown to produce specific IgE antibodies.[8–13] The RAST has also been shown to be dependable in the detection of IgE-mediated food reactions. In a study reported by Aas and Lundkvist, 56 children who could not tolerate the ingestion of codfish were compared by RAST with another 56 allergic children who could eat the fish without untoward effect. Every patient who had difficulty eating the fish had a positive test result, whereas all of the other children did not.[14] RAST has also been found helpful in confirming milk and egg white sensitivity. Monro et al. report that patients suffering from migraine headache are often allergic to several food groups and that with elimination from the diet of the RAST-positive foods, patients become symptom-free.[15]

THE MODIFIED RAST SCORING SYSTEM

Since 1977, the author has utilized a modification of the RAST that has been described in detail elsewhere.[16, 17] The modified RAST (MRT) has been shown to have an increased test sensitivity without a significant loss of specificity. In the MRT, after the second incubation period with the labeled rabbit antibody against human IgE and before counting the disc-bound radioactivity, the allergen-coated discs are removed from their original tubes and placed into fresh ones to ensure that only radioactivity immunologically bound to them is measured. Despite careful washing, a minute amount of radioactive residue adheres to the inner surface of the polystyrene carrier test tube and can take on significance in those sera with low levels of specific IgE antibodies. In this system, the lower limit of detectable levels of allergen-specific IgE averages 1.5 times the binding of negative controls. These controls are either human cord serum, serum from nonatopic patients, or serum from highly atopic patients tested against an inappropriate allergen. Improved reproducibility of assay is accomplished by "normalizing" the result by using a time or count control (i.e., the time used to count each disc matches that required by a known 25 unit IgE/ml sample to reach 25,000 counts when tested against an anti-IgE disc and run in parallel to the atopic sera under test). This step eliminates the day-to-day variation caused by isotope decay. The nonspecific binding in the system averages 300 counts. In the current MRT scoring system, 500 counts is at the 95 per cent confidence level for the detection of specific IgE antibody, but scores between 500 and 750 counts are considered to be an equivocal score (i.e., the specific IgE antibody detected may not be clinically relevant).

Scores above 750 counts are divided into distinct classes, each representing approximately a fivefold increase in the amount of serum-specific IgE antibody present in the sample (Table 19–2). MRT class 1 (751–1600 counts) is a low level positive score. Although class 1 levels are usually associated with a positive skin test reaction, only 70 per cent of affected patients will respond to a nasal or conjunctival challenge test. In contrast, MRT class 2 scores and above (1601–40,000 counts) represent positive scores with increasing levels of detectable specific IgE antibody and degrees of clinical sensitivity, and 95 per cent of patients with these scores respond to challenge test. These findings are confirmed

Table 19–2. MODIFIED RAST SCORING AND INITIAL IMMUNOTHERAPY DOSE SCHEDULES

Class	Counts*	Interpretation	0.1 ml (w/v)
1	250–500	Negative	no Rx
1/0	501–750	Equivocal	1:100
1	751–1600	Positive with increasing levels of specific IgE	1:500
2	1601–3600		1:2500
3	3601–8000		1:12,500
4	8001–18,000		1:62,500
5	18,001–40,000		1:312,500

*Counts obtained when the 25 unit time control is run at 25,000 counts.

in a study observing that patients with scores less than MRT class 2 often had skin reactivity not significantly different from a 2 per cent glycerin control;[18] 56 of 125 skin tests in patients with MRT class 1 scores and 300 of 397 in those with negative MRT scores gave a whealing response no greater than the negative control.

The major qualities of the MRT have been verified in two other reviews of the system.[19, 20] Additionally, in a 1981 study done by the In Vitro Allergy Committee of the American Academy of Allergy and Immunology, 17 participating laboratories assayed multiple positive and negative serum specimens; their results confirm the test's ability to quantify test results as well as its sensitivity and specificity.[21] Table 19–3 lists the results obtained by the laboratories investigating a birch reference serum containing various amounts of specific IgE antibody. Similar results were found with positive sera containing mite, rye grass, Alternaria, milk, and cat antibodies. In the 500 tests performed with known positive serum, there were no false-negatives recorded by any of the 17 investigators. Negative results were recorded in 116 of 119 tests with a nonatopic serum, 111 of 119 with human serum albumin, and 118 of 119 with a horse serum diluent as a negative control.

IN VITRO CLONES OF THE RAST

Recently, there has been a tendency to replace the radioactive labels used in the RAST with enzymatic markers. These enzyme labels are stable for longer periods of time and avoid the hazards of radioactive materials and the protocols for compliance with regulatory agencies. Precision and ease of operation are shown to be comparable when isotopic and enzymatic labels have been compared. In other RAST clones using enzymatic markers, plastic microtiter plates serve as the solid-phase support (Table 19–4). In these assays, individual allergens are

Table 19–3. MODIFIED RAST TEST RESULTS FROM A 1981 AMERICAN ACADEMY OF ALLERGY AND IMMUNOLOGY STUDY

Investigator	Birch-A	Birch-B	Birch-C	Birch-D	Birch-NAS
Adkinson	22,734	16,166	6497	4268	377
Baer	22,945	17,201	7444	4475	272
Bernstein	22.642	16,173	—	4044	228
Curran	22,357	15,445	6105	4068	447
Evans	24,258	18,525	8638	4939	409
Hamburger	22,231	18,293	7606	5433	556
Hoffman	23,946	17,620	7089	4321	329
Krumholz	20,756	15,442	7019	4955	394
Nalebuff	21,849	16,319	6507	4277	281
Perelmutter	21,274	16,127	6663	4447	277
Steinberg	22,536	17,398	8021	5443	350
Targan	21,095	14,831	5179	3424	326
Townley	23,263	17,869	7853	5076	342
Wypych	23,524	16,531	6168	3917	397
Yanari	23,135	14,435	6279	4317	326
Yoo	22,202	14,646	6628	4376	382
Yunginger	22,839	17,132	7443	4553	434

Note the reproducibility achieved by the 17 laboratories; 81/84 results were of the same class score. Similar results were obtained with short ragweed, rye grass, oak tree, mite, cat dander and Alternaria, and milk allergens.

Table 19–4. IN VITRO TESTS FOR THE DETECTION OF IgE ANTIBODY

Test Name	Solid Phase	Marker
RAST	Paper disc	Isotope
VAST	Paper disc	Isotope
PHADEZYME RAST	Paper disc	Enzyme
EAST	Paper disc	Enzyme
IP	Microtiter plate	Enzyme
FAST	Microtiter plate	Enzyme*
MAST–CLA	Cellulose thread	Enzyme†

*Plus fluorescence.
†Plus chemiluminescence.

adsorbed to the plastic surface by a hydrophobic interaction rather than by the chemical linkages used in the RAST. Studies utilizing an immunoperoxidase enzymatic marker (IP micro-ELISA) report that assays for serum IgE antibodies against ragweed, June grass, and Timothy grass antigens are correlated with those obtained with the RAST procedure.[22] Another micro-ELISA assay (FAST assay system) uses an enzyme/fluorogenic substrate for detecting specific IgE to common inhalant and environmental allergens; it has been reported to have good correlation with both prick testing and modified RAST.[23, 24] Identical results were found in 42 per cent of cases; a total of 82 per cent of the tests differed by one class or less. Another in vitro method for the detection of allergen-specific IgE is the MAST chemiluminescent assay system. The basis of this system is an analytical test chamber, which contains a cellulose thread as the solid-phase matrix and allows multiple test results from a single assay. Immunographic exposure onto high-speed Polaroid instant film allows quantification of results with an automatic recording infrared-transmittance densitometer.[25, 26]

As the number of commercial kits available to measure specific IgE levels increases, so does the need to evaluate their claims to efficiency in diagnosis. These newer technologies may give different values from each other, often making claims inconsistent with test performance. Until other in vitro tests are shown to perform as well as the RAST, one should exhibit caution in accepting the claims of their proponents. Emanuel compared RAST, MAST, IP micro-ELISA, and the FAST assay system kits in their ability to correlate with the results of the allergic history, positive skin test, and nasal provocation tests. Significant variations were observed in each test's sensitivity and specificity, and the RAST results had the best correlation with the clinical picture in all allergens tested.[27] These differences are likely due to a number of factors, such as the potency of the allergens used, the type of solid phase employed, the varying adsorption to the plastic surface by the allergens used, and the specificity of the anti-IgE used by the different manufacturers. Of equal importance are the quality control measures taken prior to releasing these assays for clinical and commercial use.[28] Even in the measurement of total IgE levels, in which comparisons of results should be consistently close, wide discrepancies in results are reported.[29] A comparison between three IgE antibody kits utilizing the same serum found that all gave the same scores only 30 per cent of the time. This variability in test results is of extreme importance for those physicians who use the in vitro test score as a guide in selecting initial immunotherapy dosage as described later.

SPECIFIC IgG

In vitro systems are also capable of measuring the presence of specific IgG antibody, providing an additional modality available to aid physicians in the management of their atopic patients; these tests could provide an objective measure of the effectiveness of allergen immunotherapy as described later. It has been suggested that measurement of specific IgG levels can also serve as a test to detect food intolerance. Its use for this purpose, however, remains speculative and should be regarded as experimental at this time. All individuals are exposed to large amounts of potentially immunogenic food proteins. Most people respond by producing IgG, IgA, or IgM antibodies. The presence of such antibodies in serum is a normal but not necessarily physiologic phenomenon. In certain groups of individuals, such as young infants, persons with a selective IgA deficiency, and patients with inflammatory gastrointestinal disorders, especially high levels of such antibodies are commonly found despite complete tolerance to intake of the food in question.

Obviously the finding of IgG, IgA, or IgM antibodies to food proteins in serum is of limited clinical relevance. The problem is at least partly due to failure to appreciate the great heterogeneity of IgG and differences in the biologic and antibody properties of the four IgG subclasses. However, highly specific monoclonal anti-IgG subclass reagents are now available, and it is now possible to measure these antibodies accurately. It is possible that raised levels of IgG antibodies in food intolerant patients represent a protective phenomenon; IgG_2 and IgG_4 are poor complement-fixing subclasses and could, therefore, interfere with complement fixation by other antibodies. In contrast to the case with non-IgE antibodies, the presence of IgE antibodies in serum is a nonphysiologic state of clinical relevance. High concentrations of IgE antibodies not only to classic food antigens such as egg, fish, cow's milk, nuts, shell fish, peanuts, and cereals but also to less typical allergens such as celery, some spices, and other vegetables often indicate a pronounced food allergy that can give rise to a serious reaction upon contact.

ADVANTAGES OF RAST

This test is convenient for the patient—only a single blood sample can provide enough serum for multiple tests. Other advantages are that there is no patient risk, the results are quantitative, and the results are not influenced by drugs. In vitro tests are of great benefit in apprehensive children, in patients with dermatologic problems in whom skin testing is contraindicated, and in those patients unable to stop medication that can potentially influence the test result. Although it has been shown that in vivo skin tests and in vitro RAST tend to be highly comparable in results, they do have significant differences. The RAST is less time-consuming for the patient than is the skin test. RAST is also the most reproducible procedure for identifying allergies, since the reagents can be kept for years without losing activity.

Whereas diagnostic RAST testing may initially be more expensive than skin testing on a test-for-test basis, it is only moderately so and is justifiable because the initially incurred diagnostic expenses are only a small portion of the overall cost of a chronic illness such as allergy. Effective cost containment of allergy diagnosis and treatment could be readily obtained if it were mandatory to demonstrate the actual presence of clinically important allergen-specific IgE antibodies before initiating allergy immunotherapy. Some patients continue to receive allergen injections based on suspected history of allergy coupled with false-positive skin tests. The use of screening RASTs also contributes to cost-effective diagnosis.

ALLERGEN SCREENING

The concept of employing a RAST allergen screen in diagnosis to aid in cost containment was developed when it was observed that the prevalence of sensitization to individual allergens varied widely. Some allergens such as June and Timothy grasses, for example, were commonly found associated with a positive response in allergic rhinitis patients. Other allergens, such as mold spores, were not. The incidence of positive scores for various allergens ranged from as low as 20 to as high as 80 per cent.[30] We can take advantage of this variability in the incidence of sensitization to select a suitable group of representative allergens to serve as an effective screening mechanism. This enables the physician to detect those patients who are indeed atopic (i.e., with demonstrable serum levels of allergen-specific IgE antibody) and to avoid performing multiple tests on those who are not.

The probability of a patient with atopic allergy not being sensitive to at least one of the most common offending allergens is quite low. For example, if one assumes an incidence of positive scores of only 50 per cent for each of five or six screening allergens (June grass, short ragweed, house dust mite, Alternaria, oak tree, and an animal dander when indicated), half of our atopic patients would be scored as negative and be missed if only one of these allergens were used, 25 per cent would still be missed if two allergens were both used, and 12.5 per cent if three were used, and so on. Only 3 per cent of atopic patients would be expected to be found negative to a five-allergen screening panel when the probability of each is 50 per cent; less than 1 per cent of atopic patients should be negative to such a screening panel because the prevalence of positive reactions in atopic patients to June grass (80 per cent) and short ragweed (65 per cent) is significantly higher than the 50 per cent used in the theoretical mathematical model.

Results of Allergen Screening

To confirm the efficiency of this approach, a retrospective analysis was done of the records of 100 consecutive rhinitis patients; total IgE levels had been determined in all patients and their sera had been subjected to 1784 individual MRT tests—an average of 18 suspected allergens examined per patient. Of these patients, 78 had at least one MRT class 2 score and were designated "positive atopics." Additionally, 14 patients had at least two MRT class 1 scores and were designated "equivocal atopics." Only 8 of the patients' sera were negative to all 152 allergen tests performed; these patients were then considered to be "nonatopic."

Prediction of which patients would subsequently be found positive by the MRT could not be determined from the patients' total IgE levels. Whereas those individuals classified as "positive atopics" were found to have significantly higher geometric mean levels of total IgE than the others, the range of these levels within each of the three groups was so wide that it could not adequately serve to identify an individual atopic patient. Several patients, for example, were found to have total IgE levels above 100 μ/ml, the level usually considered to be the cutoff between normal and abnormal ranges, and were still negative to as many as 25 MRT allergens. On the other hand, there were several patients with total IgE levels within the so-called normal range with high MRT scores to a limited number of the test allergens.

Had an initial attempt to demonstrate the presence of specific IgE antibody been done on these patients with an MRT atopy screen (consisting of one representative allergen from each of the major antigen groups—grasses, weeds, trees, molds, dust components, and an animal dander), all 78 of the "positive atopic" patients and 12 of 14 of the "equivocal atopic" patients (a total of 90 of the 92 patients with demonstrable levels of allergen-specific IgE) would have been detected with an overall sensitivity level of 98 per cent. Smaller miniscreens composed of three or four individual allergens would have been only 85 and 90 per cent effective, respectively. In our study, those patients classified as "positive" usually had five MRT class 2 or greater scores plus an additional five MRT class 1 scores. Patients classified as "equivocal" averaged six MRT class 1 scores and 11 negative scores with a similar panel. The major exceptions to this were in patients in whom the only positive miniscreen allergen had been either an animal dander or the house dust mite. In these situations (which represented 5 per cent of the cases), all additional MRT results were often found to be negative.

The potential magnitude of the problem of using large batteries of RASTs in the initial diagnostic workup was revealed when King reported in 1982 that 31 per cent of 100 consecutive ear, nose, and throat patients whose chief complaints were of rhinitis, asthma, urticaria, respiratory tract infections, laryngitis, serous otitis media, and recurrent headaches had completely negative MRT responses to a battery of 16 to 20 allergens.[31] He describes a screening method consisting of approximately one third the number of tests ordinarily utilized in his full battery. Of 469 responders to a full RAST battery, King notes that the screening RAST would have missed 27 patients; only four of these, however, were definite "positives" with an MRT class 2 or greater score. Of the 23 "equivocal" cases, 12 had relatively low scores of less than 1000 counts. King speculates that in these cases, a high level of total IgE may have contributed to the nonspecific background and caused an otherwise negative response to be read as an MRT class 1 score.

RAST Atopy Screening with Allergen Mixes

In a further attempt to lower the cost of using RAST as a diagnostic tool, all of the regular battery allergens were linked to a single paper disc to create a microscreen allergen disc. Initial analysis of the MRT data obtained from 85 patients in whom a complete battery of tests was also done with individual allergens revealed that the single microscreen disc worked as effectively as the routine battery in identifying both negative and positive responders at a significantly lower patient cost.

The concept of using mixes to screen for the presence of specific IgE antibody was introduced by Merrett and Merrett.[32] They report that circulating specific IgE antibody to at least one of three tested allergens (house dust mite, grass, or cat dander allergens) can be identified by a

RAST atopy screen composed of a mixture of the three individual allergens coupled together on a single solid-phase support of cellulose particles. Relative to the individual RAST, they report that the atopy screen has a sensitivity of 97 per cent.

Recently, dipstick allergen screening devices that require no instrumentation for reading their result have been made available. Although not as sensitive as the other methods, they are extremely specific. A positive result can be expected with serum taken from patients with modified RAST scores of class 2 or greater; thus, they can be used as an inexpensive diagnostic device to select patients suitable for more extensive testing.

INAPPROPRIATE AND APPROPRIATE USES OF IN VITRO TESTING

In spite of the cost effectiveness of using in vitro screens in the initial diagnostic workup, it must be recognized that there are situations in which such data may be informative and yet not significantly contribute to better patient care. There are a number of inappropriate reasons for which in vitro tests may be ordered. The author sees no valid reason for using these tests when the diagnosis is apparent from the clinical history (e.g., symptoms on exposure to cat or ingestion of a particular food) or when nonspecific therapy is found to be effective in alleviating symptoms. Furthermore, patients in whom properly performed skin tests have given negative results are not likely to have measurable levels of allergen-specific IgE antibody. On the other hand, the in vitro is extremely helpful in many situations. Many physicians have found it to be of great benefit in apprehensive children, in patients with dermatologic problems in whom skin testing is not indicated, and in those patients unable to stop medication that can potentially influence the test result. We have found RAST particularly valuable in evaluating individual sensitivity when initiating specific immunotherapy and in evaluating transfer patients now on immunotherapy and not doing well; more than one third of such patients have undetectable levels of specific IgE antibody, and immunotherapy is discontinued while other causes of their continuing complaints are searched for. The discontinuation of such therapy has been done with confidence.

SUMMARY

Advances in the development of in vitro technology to measure allergen-specific IgE antibody may continue at an exponential rate, and the otolaryngic allergist should be prepared to incorporate these changes into practice. However, it is important that we maintain a critical yet open-minded attitude toward advancing technology. As with any diagnostic procedure, the use of these procedures should be part of a complete clinical evaluation by a well-informed physician knowledgeable of their limitations. Such physicians should be capable of incorporating this information into responsible, judicious, and effective management of allergic patients. Only after the correct diagnosis has been made can appropriate treatment be started, and the net result will be improved patient care.

REFERENCES

1. Prausnitz C, Küstner J: Studien uber die ueber Empfindlichkeit. Cent Backt 86:160, 1921.
2. Ishizaka K, Ishizaka T, Hornbrook MH: Physicochemical properties of reaginic antibody. V. Correlation of reaginic activity with the E-globulin antibody. J Immunol 97:840, 1966.
3. Stanworth DR, Humphrey JH, Bennich H, Johansson SGO: Specific inhibition of the Prausnitz reaction by an atypical human myeloma protein. Lancet 2:330, 1967.
4. Wasserman SI: Mediators of immediate hypersensitivity. J Allergy Clin Immunol 72:101, 1983.
5. Kjellman N: Predictive value of high IgE values in children. Acta Paediatr Scand 65:465, 1976.
6. Zetterstrom O, Johansson SGO: IgE concentrations measured by PRIST in serum of healthy adults and in patients with respiratory allergy. Allergy 36:537, 1981.
7. Wide L, Bennich H, Johansson SGO: Diagnosis of allergy by an in-vitro test for allergen antibodies. Lancet 2:1105, 1967.
8. Johansson SGO, Bennich HH: The clinical impact of the discovery of IgE. Ann Allergy 48:325, 1982.
9. Evans R, et al: An immunologic evaluation of ragweed sensitive patients by newer techniques. J Allergy Clin Immunol 49:285, 1972.
10. Berg TLO, Johansson SGO: Allergy diagnosis with the radioallergosorbent test. J Allergy Clin Immunol 54:209, 1974.
11. Norman P: Correlations of RAST with in vivo and in vitro assays. *In* Evans R (ed): Advances in Diagnosis of Allergy: RAST. Miami, Symposia Specialists, 1975, p 45.

12. Welsh PW, et al: Preseasonal IgE ragweed antibody level as a predictor of response to therapy of ragweed hay fever with intranasal cromolyn sodium solution. J Allergy Clin Immunol 60:104, 1977.
13. Eriksson NE: Diagnosis of reaginic allergy with house dust, animal dander and allergens in adult patients. III. Case histories and combinations of case histories, skin tests, and RAST compared with provocation tests. Int Arch Allergy Appl Immunol 53:441, 1977.
14. Aas K, Lundkvist U: The radioallergosorbent test with a purified allergen from cod fish. Clin Allergy 3:255, 1973.
15. Monro J, Brostoff J, Carini C, et al: Food allergy in migraine. Study of dietary exclusion and RAST. Lancet 2:1, 1980.
16. Nalebuff DJ, Fadal RG: The modified RAST assay: an aid in the diagnosis and management of allergic disorders. Contin Educ Family Phys 10:64, 1979.
17. Nalebuff DJ: An enthusiastic view of the use of RAST in clinical allergy. Immunol Allergy Pract 3:18, 1981.
18. Radford ER, Berkowitz EC: The use of intradermal tests and relevance of negative controls in patients with negative or equivocal modified RAST test scores to inhalant allergens. Laryngoscope 97:675, 1987.
19. Hoffman DR: Comparison of methods of performing the radioallergosorbent test: Phadebas, Fadal, Nalebuff and Hoffman procedures. Ann Allergy 45:343, 1980.
20. De Filippi I, Yman L, Schroder H: Clinical accuracy of updated version of the Phadebas RAST test. Ann Allergy 46:249, 1981.
21. In Vitro Committee, American Academy Allergy Immunology Study, Feb-March, 1981 (unpublished data).
22. Ali M, Ramanarayanan MP: Correlation of a micro-ELISA assay with the skin test and the RAST assay in inhalant allergy. Ann Allergy 53:143, 1984.
23. Tsay Y, Halpern GM: IgE fluoroallergosorbent (IgE FAST) test: concept and clinical applications. Immunol Allergy Pract 6:169, 1984.
24. Seltzer JM, Halpern GM, Tsay YG, et al: Correlation of allergy test results obtained by the FAST, RAST and prick puncture methods. Ann Allergy 54:25, 1985.
25. Miller SP, Marinkovich VA, Riege DH, et al: Application of the MAST immunodiagnostic system to the determination of allergen specific IgE. Clin Chem 30:1467, 1984.
26. Ownby DR, Bailey J: Comparison of MAST with radioallergosorbent and skin tests for diagnosis of allergy in children. Am J Dis Child 140:45, 1986.
27. Emanuel I: Comparison of in-vitro allergy diagnostic methods. Immunol Allergy Pract 7:10, 1985.
28. Hamilton RG, Adkinson NF Jr: Clinical laboratory methods for the assessment and management of human allergic diseases. Clin Lab Med 6:117, 1986.
29. Perelmutter L, Emanuel I: Assessment of in vitro IgE testing to diagnose allergic disease. Ann Allergy 55:762, 1985.
30. Nalebuff DJ: Use of RAST screening in clinical allergy: a cost-effective approach to patient care. Ear Nose Throat J 64:107, 1985.
31. King WP: Efficacy of a screening radioallergosorbent test. Arch Otolaryngol 108:81, 1982.
32. Merrett J, Merrett TG: RAST atopy screen. Clin Allergy 8:235, 1978.

PART III

Therapy of Inhalant and Epidermal Allergy

CHAPTER 20

General Management of the Allergic Patient

Joseph P. Keenan, M.D., F.A.C.S.

Allergic disease is a chronic illness. It may not be realistic to believe that a patient with moderately severe allergic rhinitis treated with a combination of immunotherapy and dietary and environmental manipulation will become absolutely symptom-free. It is realistic, however, to provide significant clinical improvement to such a patient. Success in obtaining these goals varies tremendously, but approximately 90 per cent of patients receive sufficient clinical improvement to feel that continued therapy is indicated.[1]

One of the key concepts that must be stressed is the extreme importance of educating the patient to understand the underlying pathophysiologic mechanism of the disease. In other words, the patient has to be made a partner in the treatment protocol. The patient cannot feel that things are going to be done to or for him or her; rather, patients play a key role in the alleviation of their symptoms whether it is by the change in diet, the modification of the environment, or the need for regular immunotherapy. Patients must be educated about allergy and why their bodies react differently to ragweed, molds, or dust, and how they can learn different strategies to lessen their symptoms. At the beginning of therapy, different treatment options should be outlined clearly to the patient. The patient should be presented with immunotherapy not as a panacea for allergic disease, but rather as one factor in the total armamentarium to be used to combat illness.

Environmental conditions that aggravate allergic symptoms should be identified and included as part of the initial allergic management. Ideally, after the initial evaluation and identification of the offending allergens, it would be best for the patient to avoid all further contact with them. This would result in an almost complete resolution of the symptoms. From a practical standpoint, this is rarely possible. Even if it were possible, it is very likely that because of the underlying allergic predisposition, other sensitivities would develop. Since complete avoidance of the offending allergens is impossible, the next best approach to take would be to have the patient learn what the sensitivities are, to understand how pervasive the contact with them is, and to attempt to modify the everyday environment to minimize contact with these offending allergens.[2] For example, if a person is allergic to a dog or cat, it should be removed from that patient's everyday environment. If it is a family pet and the family absolutely refuses to remove the pet from the environment, then at least minimizing the allergic patient's exposure to the animal would be desirable. One should attempt to make the animal's everyday living zone and the patient's mutually exclusive. The animal should not be allowed in the patient's bedroom or other major living areas. Other family members should feed and groom the animal.

At times, modification of a patient's interaction with the environment can be carried out to minimize antigen contact. For example, even if a homeowner is grass sensitive and it is impossible for someone else to take over the job of mowing the lawn, or if hiring a professional landscaping firm is not financially feasible, he or she can still be protected. The patient should wear a mask when mowing the lawn and change outside clothes (not in the bedroom) after the work is done. Pretreatment with a systemic decongestant or prescription nasal spray may enable him or her to carry out this chore without the provocation of a severe allergic reaction.

Another very important general concept is the importance of creating an allergen-free zone.[3] The patient with multiple sensitivities should be taught the importance of creating in some portion of the living space an area that is relatively allergen-free. Many times, this would be the bedroom, since most patients sleep six to eight hours a night, and this is usually the longest time they are in one room of the house in the entire day. Dust sensitive patients are advised to have hardwood flooring in the bedroom rather than wall to wall carpeting, which tends to be a dust collector. Stuffed animals or other toys that can retain dust should be eliminated. There are hypoallergenic stuffed animals that are washable, which would be acceptable. Allergen-proof encasings are recommended for the mattress and pillows. If there is no whole-house air conditioning and air cleaning, it may be necessary to recommend the use of a high-quality air cleaner/filter in the bedroom. This air cleaner should be left running the entire night to remove dust and other indoor pollutants from the air. The regular use of the air cleaner can make a major improvement in the quality of life for the dust sensitive patient. Keeping the windows closed in this room is also important to keep out dust, pollen, and molds that might otherwise gain access by this route. In the warmer climates, if an air conditioner is used in this room, it is important to make sure the elements through which the air passes are meticulously cleaned so mold spores will not be introduced into the room air. This could sensitize a previously negatively reacting patient to these allergens.

DIETARY MANAGEMENT

Certain people who have coexisting food and dust allergies have more severe reactions at certain times of the year, depending on the total allergic load they are facing at that time. Some people can tolerate eating apples year-round except during the months of August and September when they are also being exposed to ragweed pollen. It may be the total "allergic load" on the patient rather than the presence of just one allergen that causes the provocation of symptoms. Even in patients whose major problem is inhalant allergy, it is important to diagnose and advise dietary modification for coexisting mild cyclic allergies, because these can tremendously exacerbate symptoms when certain foods are eaten during certain times of the year. The concept of the rotary diversified diet in food sensitive individuals should be stressed, since it is the monotony and repetition in diet that often leads to sensitization and results in the provocation of symptoms after the ingestion. Concepts of food allergy and the diversification of diet are covered in other chapters. The synergism between inhalant and ingestant allergy should be fully understood by the patient if the best compliance is to be obtained. For both of these types of allergy, avoidance is the prime method of treatment. Immunotherapy and dietary diversification will be of benefit in those cases in which complete avoidance is not possible.

IMMUNOTHERAPY

Immunotherapy is the mainstay of allergic management in those patients for whom avoidance is not possible. This can be carried out for both inhalant and ingestant allergies. Skin endpoint titration testing measures both quantitative and qualitative degrees of sensitivity to the various antigens. Based on the result of this testing procedure, individualized treatment sets are custom-designed for the specific patient. For those antigens to which a patient has a high degree of sensitivity, weaker initial solutions are prepared; for those antigens to which a patient has a low degree of sensitivity, stronger initial dilutions can be utilized. These are customized for each individual antigen to which the patient is sensitive. When the treatment set is administered, one starts with a dilution that is weak enough to not produce a systemic reaction or a significant local reaction. The strength of the weekly or twice-weekly injection is steadily increased to the point at which the patient enjoys relief of symptoms or serious local reactions are provoked to prevent the continuation of treatment. It is believed that the higher dose of the maintenance injection reached, the higher level of the "blocking" IgG antibody produced, correlating with better symptom control. Therefore, the dose is "pushed" until a significant local or systemic reaction prevents any further dose acceleration.

The length of treatment is generally advised to be between three and five years. Significant improvement in clinical symptoms is often reached at approximately four to six months. This approximates the time necessary to attain a maintenance dose level. If this improvement is not reached at this time, then the initial diagnosis is reexamined; coexisting food, chemical, or previously missed inhalant allergens are searched for. If the search is fruitless, it might be necessary to recommend that immunotherapy be discontinued.

There is a certain percentage of patients with true inhalant allergies who do not respond to immunotherapy. Possibly 10 per cent of allergy patients might fall into this group. Once again, following the theme that the patient should be a partner in the treatment program, the patient should understand that improvement and not total cessation of symptoms is the goal of immunotherapy. It may be unrealistic to think that a patient is going to be 100 per cent improved, but rather significant clinical improvement in terms of decrease in allergic symptoms is the realistic goal that both physician and patient should accept.

DIETARY PRECAUTIONS

Because of underlying allergic predisposition, the patient with overt inhalant allergy is at a greater degree of risk to develop cyclic food allergy than is the general population. Therefore, it is best to counsel patients undergoing immunotherapy for inhalant allergies to avoid repeat exposure to food that might be sensitizing and ultimately lead to true food allergy.

Corn, milk, wheat, and egg are the major food allergens in our culture, primarily due to the frequency of exposure. Patients should be instructed in the concept of a rotary diversified diet and its role in the treatment of cyclic food allergy. The diagnosis and treatment of food allergy are covered elsewhere.

Systemic candidiasis is the "20th century disease." Candida is a generally benign mold found in the oral cavity, vagina, gastrointestinal tract, and other areas of the body. This is the fungus that causes thrush in infants and vaginitis in some women who have been placed on repeat antibiotic or extended hormone therapy.

In the homeostatic state, bacteria and fungus maintain a balance in the different areas of the body. At times, an imbalance can develop in the allergic individual with a marked overgrowth of the candida, and it is this overgrowth coupled with the breakdown products of the metabolites of this fungus that can cause the myriad of symptoms we see in the candidiasis patient. Headache, malaise, and gastrointestinal disturbances such as diarrhea or constipation are some of the more common symptoms. Known predisposing factors are heavy and repetitious antibiotic usage, heavy refined carbohydrate diet, alcohol, and exogenous hormones, including oral contraceptives. Many of the symptoms we see in the allergic patient are also seen in the patient with possible candidiasis.[4] The inhalant sensitive patient may have increased incidence of sinus, ear, and pharyngeal infections because of impaired aeration and drainage of these organ systems. Because of these repeat infections, there is a corresponding increase in the major risk factor of systemic candidiasis, that is, repetitive antibiotic use.

SUMMARY

The general management of allergic patients includes first educating the patients and making them partners in the treatment program. They should have a good understanding of the underlying pathophysiologic mechanism of the disease and the role that immunotherapy is going to play. They must view immunotherapy not as a panacea but rather as a tool that can be used to help their chronic illness. They must be counseled to modify their environment and to create as allergy-free a zone as possible in their house to reduce the total allergic load placed on their immune system. They must understand the role of dietary management if food allergy or candidiasis is being considered and, if identified, the importance of rotating the diet and minimizing contact with the offending ingestant allergen. They should understand that the active immunotherapy will usually require three to five years, but at times it does require treatment for a much longer period of time.

REFERENCES

1. Fadal RG: Immunotherapy failures. Otolaryngol Clin North Am 18:805, 1985.
2. Druce HM, Kaliner MA: Allergic rhinitis. JAMA 259:260, 1988.
3. Rogers S: The E.I. Syndrome. Section V. Chemicals. Syracuse, Prestige Publishing, 1986.
4. Brostoff J: Food Allergy and Intolerance. London, Baillière Tindall, 1987, pp 850–872.

CHAPTER 21

Skin Endpoint Immunotherapy

Walter A. Ward, Jr., M.D.

As you will recall from Chapter 18, the endpoint is the weakest dilution that (1) will produce a 2 mm or larger wheal following nonproduction of a wheal of that size by a weaker dilution and (2) is followed by a confirming wheal 2 mm larger produced by the next stronger dilution. Skin endpoint immunotherapy for all antigens is based solely on the endpoint reactions, since the dilutions that produce the endpoints are the ones you will use to establish antigenic equivalents. Some physicians recheck endpoints within 24 to 48 hours to see if they have shifted. This second application of the endpoint is of value because the titration testing itself can result in a shift of the endpoint. The author suggests that this be routine early in your titration testing career, if possible, and routine for all patients having endpoints of a #4 dilution or higher.

PREPARATION OF TREATMENT VIAL

In titration, the endpoint is termed X, and X is always equal to 0.01 ml or 1/100 ml of the dilution producing the endpoint. Thus, a 5 mm wheal on dilution #4 of a specific antigen, followed by a 7 mm wheal on dilution #3, and a 9 mm confirming wheal on dilution #2 would establish the #3 dilution as the endpoint, and a 1X dose would equal 0.01 ml of #3 for that antigen. *Initial* immunotherapy is based on preparing a vial that is calculated to a 50X level.

In preparing a vial, you must remember that titration is based on a ratio of 1:5 for successive dilutions; therefore, a 50X dose of #3 would equal 10X of #2 (0.1 ml), or a 2X dose of #1 (0.02 ml). All volumes are initially calculated to provide 10 doses at a 50X concentration. Your computation should always reduce the 50X concentration for antigen therapy to the smallest measurable amount of the strongest dilution. This is an economical factor, since in a 10-dose treatment set, 5 ml of #3 has a much larger amount of diluent than 1 ml of #2 or 0.2 ml of #1. Obviously, 0.2 ml of #1 is the smallest amount of antigen that can be measured accurately and is the amount of antigen you could inject into a sterile vial to begin preparing your multiple antigen set.

An example of this computation for an endpoint on a #3 dilution is:

1X =	0.01 ml #3	*or*	for 10-dose vial
50X =	0.5 ml #3		5.0 ml #3
	or		*or*
	0.1 ml #2		1.0 ml #2
	or		*or*
	0.02 ml #1		0.2 ml #1

If endpoints of all antigens are not in a plus or minus 1-dilution range of each other, it is suggested that two or more multiple or single antigen vials be prepared. For example, if you have seven antigens with endpoints #4 or #3 for which you would make your treatment vial using #2 and #1, respectively, then you would not want to include two antigens with endpoint #6, nor would you include antigens with which you would begin therapy at a concentrated level.

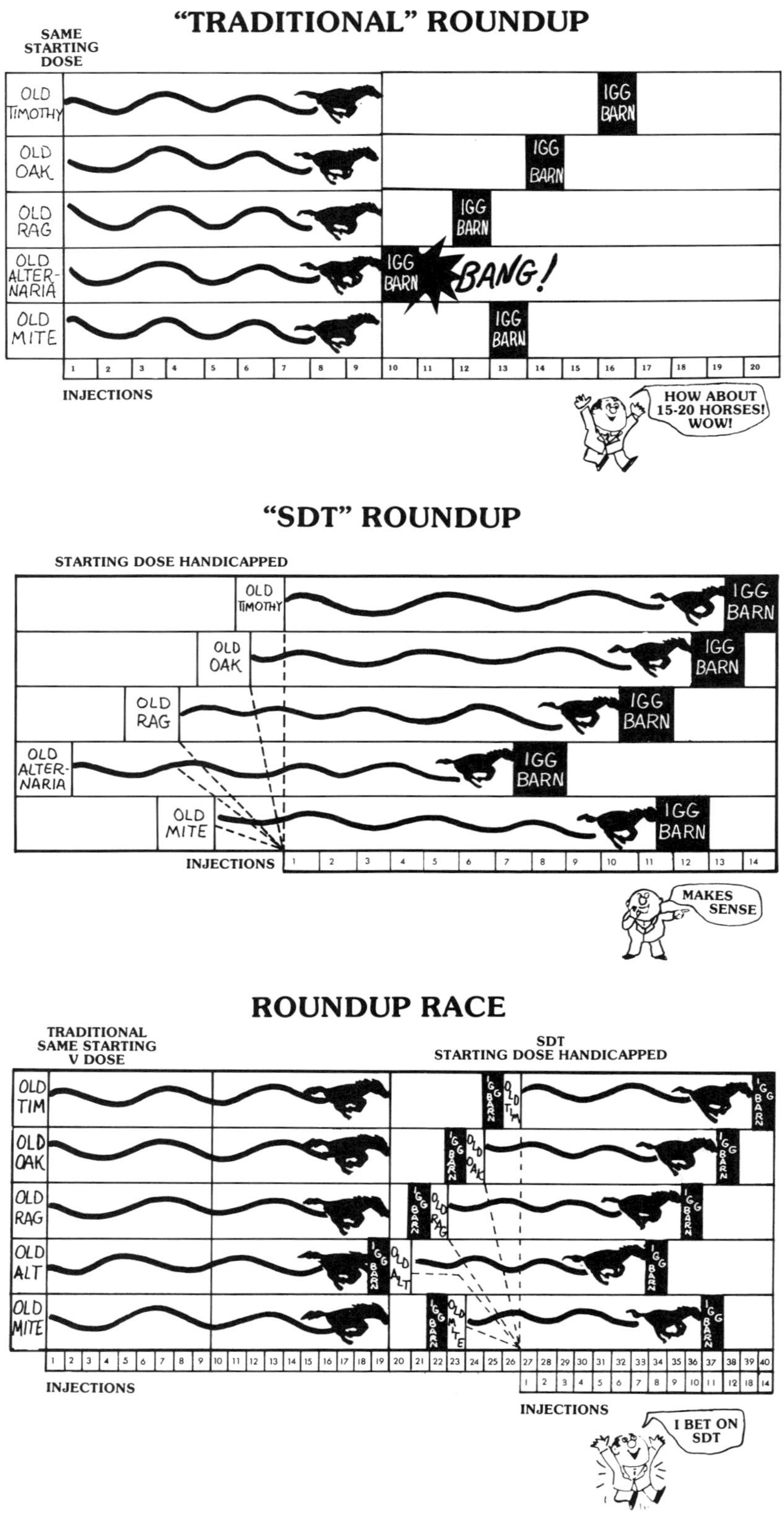

FIGURE 21–1. Race track illustrating the need for different dilutions of antigens so that all reach the goal of a symptom-free patient.

The basic reason for this separation of antigens is that one of your goals in successful immunotherapy is to move toward a dose that is in a therapeutic range of symptom relief for the patient or is that patient's maximal tolerated dose. The latter is judged to have occurred when the patient begins developing (1) an erythematous, hot injection site; (2) worsening of original symptoms shortly after injection; or (3) a systemic reaction after injection. Therefore, an antigen treated initially on a very strong concentration can keep an antigen of a weaker concentration in the same vial from reaching the desired therapeutic (maintenance) level.

This is best explained by the use of a race track as shown by King[1] and King[2] (Fig. 21–1). This maintenance level has been determined for ragweed AgE to be 2.7 to 22 μg or, for the titrationist, 0.5 ml of a #4 dilution to 0.1 ml of a #1 dilution. Traditional allergy therapy treats all allergens at the same dilution, beginning generally at a 1:50,000 weight volume to even weaker concentrations, and the point at which the antigens reach their maintenance level is determined by the allergen(s) given to which the patient is least sensitive, leaving other allergens possibly out of the therapeutic range. With titration, on the other hand, the physician is able to handicap each allergen in the treatment vial(s) so that all allergens reach the desired treatment level. This is accomplished by the titrationist's identifying the specific sensitivity to each allergen tested and beginning immunotherapy with a very potent dose, which varies according to that sensitivity. Thus, allergens to which the patient is extremely sensitive are started in the immunotherapy set at a weaker dilution than are those to which the patient has less sensitivity.

It should be noted here that Rinkel[3] taught that mold and animal dander antigens should not be treated on the basis of the 50X dose computation; rather, he recommended a 25X dose for these antigens. To accomplish this, 0.1 ml of antigen (or mold and animal dander antigens) is substituted for the usual 0.2 ml. With the improvements of antigens, many titrationists are no longer following this rule and are treating with the mold and animal dander antigens as they do with the pollen and dust antigens. The author believes it is safe to use either approach as long as you are consistent with your approach.

TREATMENT

Figure 21–2 is an example of a typical titration sheet on which the endpoints have been circled. From this titration sheet, the initial computation of dosage for each antigen can be transposed to a worksheet (Fig. 21–3). From the worksheet, you can mix your antigens in similar levels for your initial treatment vials. When you mix your initial sets, a 0.25 ml injection will equal a 25X dose, and a 0.5 ml injection will equal a 50X dose. As you prepare the various treatment vials, the amount of antigen for a 10-treatment vial is added, and then diluent is added to give a total measurement of 5.0 ml. The 50X dose will be your ultimate goal for your initial vials, unless the patient reaches his or her maximal tolerated dose before that dose is reached. Your dose schedule to reach a 50X dose is shown in Table 21–1, the schedule on the left being that for the beginning therapist or for extremely sensitive patients, and the schedule on the right being that for physicians with greater experience or for less sensitive patients.

The author does not recommend using a concentrate that will exceed a level of 0.25 ml. A simple technique to decrease the number of vials used for initial therapy is to treat the #2 endpoints at a #1 level until you get the #4 and #3 endpoints advanced past the 50X level. This would change Figure 21–3 to what is seen in Figure 21–4.

Once you have reached 50X with your initial treatment vial, you move your endpoints to one dilution stronger for your second treatment vial. You must remember, however, that your initial treatment vial was mixed using the endpoint plus two dilutions

The second treatment vial will be made using the endpoint plus three dilutions (Fig. 21–5). Obviously this vial is five times stronger than the initial vial; therefore, 0.1 ml of the new vial is equal to 0.5 ml of the initial vial, and the injection must be started at the smallest dose again (Table 21–2).

For absolute safety, it is often, but not always, necessary to skin test the treatment vial in the same manner you would skin test an individual antigen, i.e., create a 4 mm wheal with your new treatment, or endpoint plus three dilutions vial. If the skin test wheal is 9 to 11 mm or less, you may inject your initial dose based on your

Name John Doe

Allergic rhinitis

				8	7	6	5	4	3	2	1					8	7	6	5	4	3	2	1
Ragweed	0.2–2					5		⑦	9			Tree Mix											
Dock sorrell	0.2–1							5	⑦	9		Elm	0.2–1					5		5	⑦	9	
English plantain	0.2–1							5	⑦	9		Oak	0.2–2					5		⑦	9		
Lamb's quarters	0.2–C							5		⑦	9	Pecan/hickory	0.2–C							5		⑦	9
Pigweed								5		5		Box elder/maple	0.2–C							5		⑦	9
												Cottonwood								5		5	
												Sycamore/Eastern								5		5	
Grass mix												Cedar								5		5	
Johnson grass						5		5		5		Pine/Shortleaf								5		5	
Fescue	0.2–2					5		⑦	9														
Bermuda	0.2–2					5		⑦	9														
Timothy								5		5		AP dust	0.2–4					⑦	9				
Kentucky bluegrass	0.2–1							5	⑦	9		Dust mite	0.2–3					5	⑦	9			
Grass smut								5		5													
												Dog								5		5	
MMP	0.2–1							5	⑦	9		Cat								5		5	
Alternaria	0.2–2					5		⑦	9			Horse											
Hormodendrum	0.2–2					5		⑦	9														
Cephalosporium								5		5													
Aspergillus								5		5													

FIGURE 21–2. Typical titration sheet.

Vial 1
Patient Name __________
Date __________

Antigen	Endpoint	Equivalents
Lamb's quarters	#2	0.2–C
Pecan/Hickory	#2	0.2–C
Box elder/Maple	#2	0.2–C
	Antigen Total Amount	0.6 ml
	Diluent	4.4 ml
	Total	5.0 ml

Vial 2
Patient Name __________
Date __________

Antigen	Endpoint	Equivalents
Dock sorrell	#3	0.2–1
English plantain	#3	0.2–1
Ragweed	#4	0.2–2
Kentucky bluegrass	#3	0.2–1
Fescue	#4	0.2–2
Bermuda	#4	0.2–2
MMP	#3	0.2–1
Alternaria	#4	0.2–3
Hormodendrum	#4	0.2–3
Elm	#3	0.2–1
Oak	#4	0.2–2
AP dust	#6	0.2–4
Dust mite	#5	0.2–3
	Antigen Total Amount	2.6 ml
	Diluent	2.4 ml
	Total	5.0 ml

FIGURE 21–3. Typical worksheet showing computed doses.

Table 21–1. INITIAL TREATMENT SET

Schedule*				Schedule†			
Injection	*Amount (ml)*		*Dose*	*Injection*	*Amount (ml)*		*Dose*
1.	0.05	=	5X	1.	0.05	=	5X
2.	0.10	=	10X	2.	0.10	=	10X
3.	0.15	=	15X	3.	0.20	=	20X
4.	0.20	=	20X	4.	0.30	=	30X
5.	0.25	=	25X	5.	0.40	=	40X
6.	0.30	=	30X	6.	0.50	=	50X
7.	0.35	=	35X				
8.	0.40	=	40X				
9.	0.45	=	45X				
10.	0.50	=	50X				

*For therapist without long-term experience or for extremely sensitive patients.
†For experienced therapist or for less sensitive patients.

previous dose schedule. You advance this dose, still looking for the symptom-relieving dose, as judged by the patient's obtaining relief of symptoms for seven days or longer, or reaching the maximal tolerated dose. If the skin test wheal is larger than 11 mm, you need to retitrate the dose.

If the patient is giving his or her own injections rather than receiving them in your office, it is advisable to see the patient (1) when he or she reaches 0.5 ml on each vial, or (2) if that level cannot be reached. This will help you determine the patient's base dosage level, and the patient can assist you by listing his or her symptoms between each injection, or the absence of symptoms and how long these symptoms were absent.

For patients who have allergen(s) endpointing on #4, #5, #6, or higher (it is unnecessary to test above the #6 level because for these pa-

Vial 1
Patient Name ______________
Date ______________

Antigen	Endpoint	Equivalents
Lamb's quarters	#2	0.2–1
Pecan/Hickory	#2	0.2–1
Box elder/Maple	#2	0.2–1
Dock sorrell	#3	0.2–1
English plantain	#3	0.2–1
Ragweed	#4	0.2–2
Kentucky bluegrass	#3	0.2–1
Fescue	#4	0.2–2
Bermuda	#4	0.2–2
MMP	#3	0.2–2
Elm	#3	0.2–1
Oak	#4	0.2–2
	Antigen Total Amount	2.4 ml
	Diluent	2.6 ml
	Total	5.0 ml

Vial 2
Patient Name ______________
Date ______________

Antigen	Endpoint	Equivalents
Alternaria	#4	0.2–3
Hormodendrum	#4	0.2–3
AP dust	#6	0.2–4
Dust mite	#5	0.2–3
	Antigen Total Amount	0.8 ml
	Diluent	4.2 ml
	Total	5.0 ml

FIGURE 21–4. Typical worksheet showing reduction in the number of vials needed.

Vial 1
Patient Name ______________
Date ______________

Antigen	Endpoint	New Endpoints	New Equivalents
Lamb's quarters	#2	#2	0.2–C
Pecan/Hickory	#2	#2	0.2–C
Box elder/Maple	#2	#2	0.2–C
Dock sorrell	#3	#2	0.2–C
English plantain	#3	#2	0.2–C
Kentucky bluegrass	#3	#2	0.2–C
Elm	#3	#2	0.2–C
		Antigen Total Amount	1.4 ml
		Diluent	2.6 ml
		Total	5.0 ml

Vial 2
Patient Name ______________
Date ______________

Antigen	Endpoint	New Endpoints	New Equivalents
Ragweed	#4	#3	0.2–1
Fescue	#4	#3	0.2–1
Bermuda	#4	#3	0.2–1
MMP	#3	#2	0.2–1
Oak	#4	#3	0.2–1
Alternaria	#4	#3	0.2–2
Hormodendrum	#4	#3	0.2–2
AP dust	#6	#5	0.2–4
Dust mite	#5	#4	0.2–2
		Antigen Total Amount	1.8 ml
		Diluent	3.2 ml
		Total	5.0 ml

FIGURE 21–5. Typical worksheet showing changed endpoints.

tients you can safely start your vaccine at the #6 level), you may need to go to an endpoint plus four dilutions vial, an endpoint plus five dilutions vial, and so on (Table 21–3).

All allergists, no matter what their approach to immunotherapy, always want to stop treatment just before reaching a level that would cause a systemic reaction. As a titrationist, you run little risk of reaching this level by keeping your antigen in similar aliquots and by watching for skin reactions after each dose is given. You should never advance an antigen vial if a skin reaction the size of a 50-cent piece develops, and you should repeat your previous dose whenever the skin reaction is the size of a quarter.

As various antigen levels are advanced, you can add them to vials with the same antigen levels, thereby eventually reducing the treatment vials to one, or to two at the most. Once the

Table 21–2. SECOND TREATMENT SET AFTER 50X DOSE

Schedule*				Schedule†			
Injection	*Amount (ml)*		*Dose*	*Injection*	*Amount (ml)*		*Dose*
1.	0.10	=	50X	1.	0.10	=	50X
2.	0.15	=	75X	2.	0.20	=	100X
3.	0.20	=	100X	3.	0.30	=	150X
4.	0.25	=	125X	4.	0.40	=	200X
5.	0.30	=	150X	5.	0.50	=	250X
6.	0.35	=	175X				
7.	0.40	=	200X				
8.	0.45	=	225X				
9.	0.50	=	250X				

*For therapist without long-term experience or for extremely sensitive patients.
†For experienced therapist or for less sensitive patients.

Table 21–3. THIRD TREATMENT SET AFTER 250X DOSE

Schedule*				Schedule†			
Injection	*Amount (ml)*		*Dose*	*Injection*	*Amount (ml)*		*Dose*
1.	0.10	=	250X	1.	0.10	=	250X
2.	0.15	=	375X	2.	0.20	=	500X
3.	0.20	=	500X	3.	0.30	=	750X
4.	0.25	=	625X	4.	0.40	=	1000X
5.	0.30	=	750X	5.	0.50	=	1250X
6.	0.35	=	875X				
7.	0.40	=	1000X				
8.	0.45	=	1125X				
9.	0.50	=	1250X				

*For therapist without long-term experience or for extremely sensitive patients.
†For experienced therapist or for less sensitive patients.

patient has reached his or her maintenance level and is asymptomatic, you may begin lengthening the period between injections. Ideally, a patient receives an injection when symptoms recur after you reach a certain therapeutic level, but most physicians treat on a once- or twice-a-week basis until this level is reached. After that, you can eventually and gradually, depending on the patient, space your maintenance dose out to every three weeks. An interval longer than three weeks is not recommended because of possible amnesic reactions by the patient's body.

If you have reached a level at which you believe the patient should be asymptomatic and the patient still has symptoms, it is imperative that you look for possible reasons. Some are listed here:

1. Antigen(s) are being given at the concentrate or dilution #1 level, but there are still antigen(s) in the treatment vials at dilutions that are not strong enough to give the necessary relief.

2. The dosage may be closer to a maximal tolerated dose than to a symptom-relieving dose, thereby indicating overtreatment of the patient's allergy problem. Simply cut your dose in half and advance it by 0.05 ml until the patient receives relief of symptoms but does not manifest an exacerbation of symptoms.

3. The patient passed the symptom-relieving dose before the allergen came in season (again indicating overtreatment and worsening of symptoms with each therapeutic injection). To correct this problem, either retitrate or cut the present dosage in half and look for the appropriate dose by again slowly advancing the dose.

4. A concomitant food hypersensitivity has come into play. You should suspect this if antigen therapy gives relief for only a few hours rather than days, or if flares of symptoms occur postprandially or between 1:00 and 5:00 AM.

5. You have not treated for the allergen causing the symptoms. You must now go to the patient's history to find possible secondary minor pollens and molds, food hypersensitivities, and sensitivities to chemicals.

6. The antigen being given is not an active excitant in the patient. Retitration or RAST testing might help you correct this problem.

SUMMARY

Allergists are still looking for an immunotherapeutic dose that will relieve symptoms, build immunity, and not cause adverse reactions. As of this writing, the author believes the techniques using serial endpoint titration (SET) are best suited for achieving that goal. The safety of higher dose therapy of similar aliquots of antigen has been established. Furthermore, with SET you are able to test and treat co-seasonally and you can begin your treatment preseasonally. This alone provides a more rapid control of symptoms and makes this technique economically sound, not only for the patient but for cooperating third party carriers.

Acknowledgment

The author wishes to thank Mrs. Judith T. MacMillan and Miss Nina Haynes for their assistance in the preparation of this chapter.

REFERENCES

1. King WP: The role of the skin end point titration method in allergy. *In*: Goldman J (ed): The Principles and Practice of Rhinology. New York, John Wiley & Sons, 1987, pp 283–292.
2. King HC: Endpoint titration and immunotherapy. Otolaryngol Clin North Am 18:703, 1985.
3. Rinkel HJ: The management of clinical allergy. Part II. Etiologic factors and skin titration. Arch Otolaryngol 77:56, 1963.

CHAPTER 22

In Vitro–Based Allergen Immunotherapy

Donald J. Nalebuff, M.D.

The symptoms of allergic rhinitis can be relieved in most patients by using a combination of antihistamines, decongestants, inhaled cromolyn, or synthetic steroids. Of course, elimination or reduction of environmental factors such as animal danders, dust, and mold must also be implemented. When these measures do not provide satisfactory relief, allergen immunotherapy may still be effective (Table 22–1). Specific clinical situations in which the use of allergen immunotherapy is appropriate include patients having symptoms that extend over two or more seasons, those who experience unpleasant side effects from pharmacotherapy, and those who have symptoms that become progressively worse each year. Another important consideration is whether the patient is likely to comply with the selected therapeutic program, which is both time-consuming and potentially dangerous.

The efficacy of allergen immunotherapy in the management of allergic rhinitis is well documented. Proven clinical benefits have been reported in treatment-resistant patients with known sensitivity due to ragweed, grass, and mountain cedar pollens, house dust mite, and cat dander allergens. Several double-blind controlled studies have confirmed the effectiveness of immunotherapy in the care of allergic patients. For immunotherapy to be effective, one must ensure not only that the patient has IgE-mediated disease, but that the doses of allergen be given at relatively high concentrations.[1–3] Specific immune responses are the result of a complex interaction of antigen and immunocompetent cells. To ensure that a proper interaction occurs, a sufficient quantity of antigen has to be localized and trapped in lymphoid organs. A limiting factor in achieving high dosage, however, is the threat of causing undesirable systemic reactions. All of the three allergen immunotherapy techniques commonly used attempt to solve this problem.

Table 22–1. INDICATIONS FOR IMMUNOTHERAPY

The patient responds inadequately to environmental control measures and pharmacotherapy
In the treatment of allergic rhinitis triggered by inhalant allergens via IgE mechanisms
The severity, duration, and frequency of symptomatic episodes are more of a problem than the inconvenience and costs involved with immunotherapy
The patient is likely to comply with the schedule of periodic injections for up to several years

THE TRADITIONAL METHOD

In the traditional method, an arbitrary safe starting dose of allergens is administered in high dilutions (1:100,000 to 1:10,000,000 w/v). Dosage increments are increased once or twice a week over several months until a maintenance dose is reached. During the first two or three months of such treatment, the titer of specific IgE antibody rises, usually twofold or more. By the end of the year, as therapy is continued, the titer returns to or below its original level. Because therapeutically effective doses are not reached until six to 12 months, some physicians accelerate the dose schedule by administering injections several times a day—a variation called "rush therapy." Patients are started at doses of 0.1 ml of a 1:10 million w/v; subsequent doses are increased four times a day for five days of treatment, with gradually increasing doses and concentrations until the maximum tolerated dose is reached. An inherent disadvantage of this traditional method is that all patients are treated the same way. In the other major forms of immunotherapy, efforts are made to tailor the initial levels of therapy to the patient's individual sensitivities.

SKIN ENDPOINT TITRATION

For years, most otorhinolaryngologists have used an approach in which each patient's sensitivity is measured by the graded response of the skin to allergen challenge. Doses of each allergen in a treatment set mixture are individually determined by this bioassay to be inversely related to patient sensitivity. The allergen concentrations are adjusted to be in balance, which minimizes the risk of an adverse reaction during treatment. A potential weakness in this approach, however, is the selection of allergens for immunotherapy based on endpoints at low dilution and of questionable clinical significance. In the past, another problem has been the failure of advancing doses upward to effective maintenance levels. In the currently accepted method, the starting dose is approximately 10 times the volume of allergen required to cause a positive skin test reaction, and treatment doses are increased incrementally until the maintenance level is reached—which may be several thousand times the amount of allergen found to cause the original endpoint response.

TECHNIQUE OF RAST-BASED IMMUNOTHERAPY

In RAST-based immunotherapy, the recommended initial doses are given at concentrations as listed in Table 22–2. Patients are regularly started at allergen concentrations of 1:500 w/v for those allergens with low serum-specific IgE levels (MRT class 1 scores). As the serum antibody concentration rises, the suggested initial dose is proportionally decreased in fivefold increments. For those allergens in which the specific antibody score is extremely high (MRT class 5 scores), the recommended initial dose is significantly lower at an allergen concentration of 1:312,500 w/v. After the initial doses have been administered and tolerated, injections are usually increased at subsequent visits (unless the clinical response suggests it would not be safe) until the dose reaches maximum levels. Before starting such immunotherapy, however, it is mandatory that a small amount of the incriminated allergen be placed intradermally as a skin test challenge (enough of the allergen must be injected to produce a 4 mm skin wheal). The patient is then observed, and if in 10 minutes this in vivo challenge produces a wheal of 15 mm or less, the suggested dose is given subcutaneously. Whereas this challenge is performed in all patients, it is especially important for class 1 through class 3 allergens, for which the suggested RAST-based doses are high (1:500 to 12,500 w/v). With class 4 and 5 allergens, the in vivo challenges are less important because the suggested allergen doses (1:62,500 to 1:312,500 w/v) are consistent with levels considered safe even for extremely sensitive patients. Nevertheless, even in these situations, the in vivo challenge serves the useful purpose of confirming the biologic potency of the highly diluted allergen extract. Only rarely have the skin test challenge responses suggested that the RAST-based dose would be excessive. The technique of preparing stock and individualized treatment sets is described in the following.

Table 22–2. MODIFIED RAST SCORING AND INITIAL IMMUNOTHERAPY DOSE SCHEDULES

Class	Counts*	Interpretation	0.1 ml (w/v)
0	250–500	Negative	no Rx
1/0	501–750	Equivocal	1:100
1	751–1600	Positive	1:500
2	1601–3600	with	1:2500
3	3601–8000	increasing	1:12,500
4	8001–18,000	levels of	1:62,500
5	18,001–40,000	specific IgE	1:312,500

*Counts obtained when the 25 unit time control is run at 25,000 counts.

Preparation of Serially Diluted Stock Solutions

The author uses 50 per cent glycerinated allergen extracts because these maintain potency well. These are obtained at a 1:20 w/v concentration in the 30 ml vial size. To ensure a constant rotation of fresh solutions, we work with small amounts of solution in both the stock and treatment vials (2.5 ml and 5.0 ml). The stock solutions are prepared as follows: 5.0 ml of the 1:20 w/v concentrated extracts is withdrawn from the large vials (30.0 ml) and placed into an empty sterile 5.0 ml vial for subsequent use in the vial trays. Fivefold stock dilutions of this material are then prepared from the 1:20 w/v concentrate vials (Table 22–3). Preparations of stock dilution #1 (1:100 w/v) are made from the stock concentrates as follows: 1.0 ml of the 1:20 w/v concentrate plus 4.0 ml phenolated saline diluent will make stock dilution #1 and give a total volume of 5.0 ml. Preparations of stock dilution #2 (1:500 w/v) are made from the #1 stock dilution as follows: 1.0 ml of the 1:100 w/v concentration plus 4.0 ml phenolated saline diluent will make stock dilution #2 and give a total volume of 5.0 ml. Preparations of stock dilution #3 (1:2500 w/v) are made from the #2 stock dilution as follows: 1.0 ml of the 1:500 w/v concentration plus 4.0 ml phenolated saline diluent will make stock dilution #3 and give a total volume of 5.0 ml. Finally, preparations of stock dilution #4 (1:12,500 w/v) are made from the #3 stock dilution in a similar fashion: 1.0 ml of the 1:2500 w/v concentration plus 4.0 ml phenolated saline diluent will make stock dilution #4 and give a total volume of 5.0 ml. These stock solutions are then used to create individualized treatment sets for our atopic patients.

Table 22–3. CONCENTRATIONS OF STOCK VIALS

Stock Vials	Concentration (w/v)	Noon Units/ml*
Concentrate	1:20	50,000
Dilution #1	1:100	10,000
Dilution #2	1:500	2,000
Dilution #3	1:2500	400
Dilution #4	1:12,500	80

*By definition, a 1:1 allergen concentrate contains 1,000,000 Noon units per milliliter.

Preparation of Individual Patient Treatment Vials

The modified RAST (MRT) scores of a typical patient with perennial allergic rhinitis are listed in Table 22–4. An appropriate treatment set for this patient is made by taking 0.1 ml of one dilution stronger than the suggested initial concentration for each clinically relevant allergen to be included and adding enough phenolated saline diluent to a total volume of 2.5 ml; thus, a maximum of 25 allergens can be included in a single treatment vial. Allergens of low sensitivity (classes 1, 2, and 3) are placed in vial A, and allergens of high sensitivity (classes 4 and 5) are kept together in vial B. The treatment vial containing highly sensitive allergens is prepared by taking 0.1 ml of the appropriate dilution from the stock vials plus sufficient phenolated saline diluent to a total volume of 2.5 ml (Table 22–5). Once the treatment set is made up according to this technique initial treatment doses are escalated as shown in Table 22–6.

It is important to stress that these findings cannot as yet be extended to all of the newer in vitro methods available for the measurement of allergen-specific IgE. To date, dosing schemes

Table 22–4. TYPICAL RAST RESULTS FOR PATIENT "JOHN DOE" WITH ALLERGIC RHINITIS

Allergen Disc	Counts	Modified RAST Class
Bermuda grass	1250	1
Timothy grass	6200	3
June grass	7350	3
Short ragweed	19,400	5
Mugwort	1690	2
English plantain	1120	1
Lamb's quarters	490	0
Dandelion	285	0
Maple tree	375	0
Oak tree	2600	2
Birch tree	12,200	4
Elm tree	375	0
Mucor	1050	1
Penicillium	1180	1
Cladosporium	985	1
Aspergillus	1375	1
Alternaria	2465	2
House dust mite	23,500	5
Cat epithelium	6450	3
Dog epithelium	275	0

Note the high RAST scores for house dust mite, short ragweed, and birch tree pollen (classes 4 and 5). These are the allergens for which the patient is at risk in advancing doses. The patient should be advised of the importance of removing the cat from the home environment.

Table 22–5. TREATMENT SET VIALS FOR PATIENT "JOHN DOE"

Allergen	Class	Technique Take	Final Concentration of Each Allergen
Allergens of High Sensitivity—Vial A			
Oak tree	4	0.1 ml of stock #3	(1:62,500 w/v)
Ragweed	5	0.1 ml of stock #4	(1:312,500 w/v)
House dust mite	5	0.1 ml of stock #4	(1:312,500 w/v)
		add 2.2 ml of diluent	
Total Volume		2.5 ml	
Allergens of Low Sensitivity—Vial B			
Penicillium	1	0.1 ml of conc	(1:500 w/v)
Cladosporium	1	0.1 ml of conc	(1:500 w/v)
Aspergillus	1	0.1 ml of conc	(1:500 w/v)
Mucor	1	0.1 ml of conc	(1:500 w/v)
Plantain	1	0.1 ml of conc	(1:500 w/v)
Alternaria	2	0.1 ml of stock #1	(1:2500 w/v)
Mugwort	2	0.1 ml of stock #1	(1:2500 w/v)
Birch	2	0.1 ml of stock #1	(1:2500 w/v)
Timothy	3	0.1 ml of stock #2	(1:12,500 w/v)
June grass	3	0.1 ml of stock #2	(1:12,500 w/v)
Cat epithelium	3	0.1 ml of stock #2	(1:12,500 w/v)
		add 1.4 ml of diluent	
Total Volume		2.5 ml	

Class 1, 2, and 3 allergens are grouped together in vial A, and class 4 and 5 allergens in vial B.

based on serum levels of allergen-specific IgE have only been described for the RAST and IP micro-ELISA techniques.[4–7] Until the discrepancies between the various procedures have been eliminated, attempts to extend this principle are potentially dangerous.

Results of RAST-Based Immunotherapy

A review of the MRT records of patients treated in our clinic between 1979 and 1986 reveals that on an average they were sensitive to 10 of 22 test allergens; 85 per cent of the positive scores were at the lower levels (classes 1 to 3). All patients tolerated their initial high doses of these allergens and were readily advanced to doses of 0.1 to 0.25 ml of a 1:100 w/v concentration of the allergen material without untoward reaction. In these same patients, the remaining 15 per cent of incriminated allergens were associated with high levels of specific IgE antibody (class 4 and 5 MRT scores) and were started in therapy at lower dose levels. These allergens were advanced on a more deliberate schedule. We were not able to routinely raise these allergens to the high levels achievable with the others in these same patients. They commonly caused large local and even mild constitutional reactions when high dosage levels were attempted—even after a year's course of allergen immunotherapy. During the past nine years, the only constitutional reactions requiring medical intervention in our practice have occurred in patients with allergen sensitivities associated with high modified RAST scores, and in whom we attempted to raise the dose above the 1:500 w/v concentration.

In 46 allergic rhinitis patients in whom pharmacologic agents had failed to provide relief, it was noted that 41 of 46 patients obtained symptomatic improvement within 24 weeks.[4] In another study, 200 ragweed sensitive hay fever patients were also started on treatment with initial doses suggested by their MRT score.[5] These patients all had positive histories of seasonal rhinitis occurring from August through October and demonstrated skin reactivity of 3+ or more with a short ragweed extract and a positive nasal or conjunctival provocation on sequential challenge with the ragweed pollen extract at a concentration of 1:100 w/v or less. Ninety serums were scored as MRT class 1 for the ragweed allergen, and these patients were given high doses of the extract. To stress the system, the doses employed were one fivefold

Table 22–6. INITIAL TREATMENT DOSES

Schedule for Allergens of Low Sensitivity

Injection #	Volume (ml)	Route	Class 1 Units	Class 2 Units	Class 3 Units
1	0.05	Intradermal	100.0	20.0	4.0
2	0.10	Subcutaneous	200.0	40.0	8.0
3	0.20	Subcutaneous	400.0	80.0	16.0
4	0.30	Subcutaneous	600.0	120.0	24.0
5	0.40	Subcutaneous	800.0	160.0	32.0
6	0.50	Subcutaneous	1000.0	200.0	40.0

Schedule for Allergens of High Sensitivity

Injection #	Volume (ml)	Route	Class 4 Units	Class 5 Units
1	0.05	Intradermal	0.8	0.16
2	0.10	Subcutaneous	1.6	0.32
3	0.20	Subcutaneous	2.4	0.48
4	0.30	Subcutaneous	3.2	0.64
5	0.40	Subcutaneous	4.0	0.80

Note that the first injection (0.05 ml) is given intracutaneously as a skin test challenge; this is a safety measure (see text).

level more concentrated than regularly used. These patients were given, as their initial dose, 0.1 ml of a 1:100 w/v material containing 3 μg of antigen E (AgE); no systemic reactions occurred. One third of these patients did experience large local reactions that were attributed to the high concentration of glycerin remaining in the extract at the selected concentration. Fifty-two patients were started on therapy with allergen material at a 1:500 w/v concentration. Only six patients were started at the lowest dose used in this particular study, a concentration of 1:62,000 w/v. Although 70 per cent of these patients (140 of 200) received 3 μg doses of AgE within the first week of treatment, no constitutional reactions occurred in the entire group.

Similar findings were reported by Young in a study to determine whether the MRT score could safely predict a safe initial starting dose.[8] His study included 40 patients with a history of rhinitis with a seasonal exacerbation to either timothy grass or ragweed pollen. All patients had a 2+ or greater skin reaction to the study antigens; 26 of these patients had scores in class 1 through 3 and were given the suggested high doses; 14 patients were started at a modest dose because of the higher serum antibody levels; all patients were able to tolerate the initial dose without reaction. In a study reported by Santrach et al., 50 patients were started on immunotherapy with initial doses based on the MRT score.[9] All 35 patients with class 1 to class 3 scores were given their initial doses according to the more aggressive dose schedule (1:100 to 1:2500 w/v) and tolerated the dose without incident. The initial doses were withheld in 15 other patients because the preliminary skin test challenge gave greater than a 15 mm wheal. As a result, these investigators reported that 30 per cent (15 of 50) of their patients could not tolerate the suggested MRT dose. Examination of the data from these patients shows that the recommended doses were at a 1:312,500 w/v concentration—a level considered safe by most allergists even for their highly sensitive patients. In fact, they even noted that the initial dose in the RAST-based system for such patients is actually less than recommended by most traditional allergists for such patients. It is likely, therefore, that those patients who did not pass the skin test challenge could have tolerated the suggested initial dose.

Length of Treatment and Prognosis

The extent to which patients respond remains unpredictable in any given patient. Usually therapy is continued through two or three years of reduced or symptom-free seasons. It is also evident that few patients receive enough benefit from this modality to enable them to discontinue all medication. Although for some patients there is a permanent relief, permanent "cure" is rare; it has frequently been observed that relapses occur once therapy has discontinued, and such patients may require a repeat course of immunotherapy. Immunotherapy should be discontinued, however, if after two years of uninterrupted maintenance dosage the patient shows no clinical improvement. If there has been no response by then, it is unlikely that there will be, should immunotherapy be continued. The measurement of specific IgG antibody should be helpful in deciding the course to be followed in such patients. One must be sure, in those not responding, that other forms of rhinitis are not coexisting and that any physical factors contributing to symptoms, such as septal deviations and turbinate enlargement, are corrected.

REFERENCES

1. Johnstone DE: Study of the role of antigen dose in the treatment of pollenosis and pollen asthma. J Dis Child 94:1, 1957.
2. Frankland AW, Augustin R: Prophylaxis of summer hay fever and asthma: a controlled trial comparing crude grass pollen extracts with the isolated main protein component. Lancet 1:1055, 1954.
3. Rocklin RE: Clinical and immunologic aspects of allergen specific immunotherapy in patients with seasonal allergic rhinitis and/or allergic asthma. J Allergy Clin Immunol 72:323, 1983.
4. Fadal RG, Nalebuff DJ: The study of optimum dose immunotherapy in pharmacological treatment failures. Arch Otolaryngol 106:38, 1980.
5. Nalebuff DJ, Fadal RG, Ali M: Determination of initial dose for ragweed hypersensitivity with modified radioallergosorbent test. Otolaryngol Head Neck Surg 89:271, 1981.
6. Nalebuff DJ, Fadal RG: RAST-based immunotherapy. Rhinology 22:11, 1984.
7. Ali M: Immunoperoxidase-based diagnosis and selection of initial therapy dose. Otolaryngol Clin North Am 18:745, 1985.
8. Young SH: Use of the modified RAST to determine initial immunotherapy dose. *In* Fadal RG, Nalebuff DJ (eds): RAST in Clinical Allergy. Miami, Symposia Specialists, 1981, p 217.
9. Santrach BA, Parker JL, Jones LT, et al: Diagnostic and therapeutic applications of a modified radioallergosorbent test and comparison with the conventional radioallergosorbent test. J Allergy Clin Immunol 67:97, 1981.

CHAPTER 23

Pharmacotherapy in the Management of Allergic Diseases

Helen F. Krause, M.D., F.A.C.S.

The management of otolaryngic allergy involves expert diagnostic skills and technical acumen to identify causative factors. Therapy involves elimination of these factors, pharmacotherapy, and/or immunotherapy.

Pharmacotherapy must involve an understanding of immunochemical processes in the phenomenon known as allergy. It must include an understanding of how the target organs are provoked, of the pharmacologic action of the drugs presently available, and of new agents that are added to the Pharmacopeia each year. We must be aware of physiologic alterations in the field of allergy not previously recognized, such as the late or delayed allergic responses, and learn to use pharmacologic agents to the best advantage in the treatment of these as well as type I immediate reactions.

Chemical mediators produce alterations in the target organs by direct tissue reaction and indirectly by neural reflexes and vascular mechanisms as discussed in earlier chapters. These need to be short-circuited in some manner to prevent the consequences of allergic reactions. We may consider allergic rhinitis as a pathophysiologic model for drug use, recognizing that similar effects may occur in the pharynx, larynx, eyes, lungs, possibly the eustachian tube, and the ears. Drugs utilized for asthma care are discussed in Chapter 26.

Allergic rhinitis is a disease with diverse degrees of expression and morbidity. Symptoms may be transient and mild, requiring no testing and minimal drug treatment or no treatment. They may be constant and overwhelming, requiring extensive evaluation and the use of a variety of therapeutic modalities. Symptoms may vary in both severity and frequency, being seasonal or perennial. Allergic rhinitis and other expressions of allergy are influenced by factors such as the degree of allergic sensitivity, infection, metabolic changes occurring in puberty and pregnancy, stress, both active and passive cigarette smoking, and chronic exposure to allergens or to chemical sensitizers. These factors all play a role in the selection of pharmacotherapeutic choices and their clinical effectiveness. Pharmacotherapy may be used to prevent such symptoms or control them after they occur.

Drugs benefit both acute and chronic allergic diatheses by modifying or preventing the effect of mediators on small blood vessels and tissue receptors, or by short-circuiting the stimulus, blocking the release of the mediators. Such mediators may be preformed within the mast cell or the circulating basophil in the cellular matrix or the cell granules, or may be secondarily formed after a variable time delay as a membrane response. This may explain the variations in experimental and clinical nasal and pulmonary provocation responses described as immediate, delayed, or a combination of both called the dual response.

In susceptible individuals, histamine may cause edema, secondary vascular changes, and increase of thin mucus secretion. Serotonin may cause flushing, asthma, and diarrhea. The bradykinins may cause edema and urticaria. Heparin combines with histamine and serotonin to decrease the target organ stimulation. In the 1950s, Dr. David Dolowitz at the University of Utah experimentally proved the protective effect of heparin in anaphylactic shock in rats and its ability to reverse such shock. The metabolites of the arachidonic acid cascade produced by way of the cyclo-oxygenase pathway may cause both bronchoconstriction and bronchodilation. By way of the lipo-oxygenase pathway, the leukotrienes formed are primarily bronchoconstrictors. As basic research identifies the stimuli of allergic reactions, pharmacotherapeutic drugs can be developed to control or prevent them.

With mild transient symptoms, antigen avoidance or low-dose drug therapy may be adequate. With persistent seasonal or perennial symptoms, elimination of environmental factors, a variety of drugs, and/or specific immunotherapy and, occasionally, even surgery may be necessary.

The pharmaceutical industry has provided a plethora of chemicals to modulate the effect and control the symptoms of allergic rhinitis and other expressions of allergy. Four major classifications of such drugs are antihistamines, both oral and topical decongestants, systemic and topical corticosteroids, and cromolyn sodium—which is topical only at this time.

ANTIHISTAMINES

The commercial search for more effective antihistamines, that is, histamine-blocking agents that produce fewer central nervous system (CNS), parasympathetic, and other side effects, has flooded the market with single and combination preparations. Most of the presently available antihistamines are H_1 antagonists effective by competitive binding to the H_1 receptors of the target cells. There are five major classes of antihistamines plus newer ones with other actions.

1. *Ethanolamines* are potent H_1 antagonists with strong sedative effects: e.g., diphenhydramine HCl (Benadryl) and clemastine fumarate (Tavist).
2. *Ethylenediamines* are effective H_1-blocking agents with possible sedative and gastrointestinal effects: e.g., tripelennamine HCl (Pyribenzamine).
3. *Alkylamines* are the most frequently used H_1 antagonists with somewhat less sedation: e.g., chlorpheniramine maleate (Chlor-Trimeton or Teldrin); brompheniramine maleate (Dimetane); dexchlorpheniramine maleate (Polaramine). These are often combined with various decongestants.
4. *Piperazines* have prolonged H_1-blocking activity, but are less often used for other symptom control: e.g., hydroxyzine HCl for tranquilizing and cutaneous effects to decrease the wheal and flare reactions (Atarax; Vistaril, useful in chronic urticaria); and meclizine HCl (Bonine; Antivert, antivertigo drug).
5. *Phenothiazines* are effective H_1 blockers, but have exceptional sedative effects: e.g., promethazine (Phenergan); trimeprazine tartrate (Temaril, with antipruritic effects).

Additional antihistamines are now available. Azatadine maleate (Optimine) blocks histamine release from mast cells and basophils. It is useful in relieving the skin wheal and flare and itching as well as symptoms of allergic rhinitis. Terfenadine (Seldane), an H_1 antagonist, is rapidly absorbed and crosses the blood-brain barrier poorly, resulting in little or no sedation. Not yet FDA-approved drugs loratadine, mequitazine, and astemizole appear to have long half-lives and little or no sedative effects. There may, however, be untoward problems due to this prolonged half-life. Astemizole is nonsedating, and studies suggest more relief for itching eyes, sneezing, and rhinorrhea, but not of nasal obstruction. It also increases appetite and therefore weight gain.

Antihistamines act primarily by inhibiting histamines released from degranulating mast cells and basophils, preventing interaction with the histamine receptors on the target cells. There are also some anticholinergic effects. This group of drugs is best to relieve the itching sensation in the nose, throat, and eyes, the reflex sneezing, and the increased clear secretions in both the nose and the eyes.

Seasonal allergic rhinitis seems to respond more favorably than does perennial rhinitis to antihistamines, although they are useful for both. Routine use over a period of time, rather than intermittent use, is more effective in preventing symptom occurrence. Sedation is a major side

Table 23–1. ANTIHISTAMINE DRUG INTERACTIONS

MAO (monoamine oxidase) inhibitor—prolongs and intensifies	
Alcohol	
Antidepressants (esp. tricyclic)	have an additive effect
Barbiturates	have an additive effect
Other CNS depressants	have an additive effect
Oral anticoagulants—effect may be inhibited	

effect of many preparations. Tachyphylaxis, the development of tolerance with prolonged use, may occur, but can be overcome by changing to another drug class. In general, drugs with multiple mixtures of antihistamines do not seem to have any increased effectiveness. Antihistamines, except for promethazine, improve mild asthma and do not have a deleterious effect on more severe asthma, as has been previously suggested. Antihistamines may also interact with other drugs and should be avoided in their presence (Table 23–1). They may prolong the effect of MAO inhibitors, be additive to CNS depressants, and inhibit the effect of oral anticoagulants.

DECONGESTANTS

Common oral decongestants are pseudoephedrine HCl, phenylpropanolamine HCl, and also phenylephrine HCl as well as a variety of newer topical decongestant formulations. Decongestants are sympathomimetics acting as alpha-adrenergic stimulators of blood vessels, the end result being peripheral vasoconstriction and decreased edema. Overuse of topical decongestants may produce rhinitis medicamentosa locally, and all decongestants may produce systemic vascular symptoms including elevated blood and ocular pressures, tachycardia, urinary obstruction, and central nervous system stimulation. They must be used cautiously at all times and avoided in patients with heart disease, hypertension, diabetes, glaucoma, hyperthyroidism, and peptic and possibly gastric ulcers.

> CASE HISTORY: A 32-year-old nurse was admitted for evaluation of severe headaches, visual disturbance with increased intracranial pressure, and elevation of intraocular pressure. Skull films revealed sinus opacification, and an otolaryngology consult was ordered. The history revealed long-term nasal congestion and "sinusitis" untreated. However, half-hidden beneath her pillow was a nasal spray—a common over-the-counter topical decongestant. The patient admitted using this "on the average" hourly when awake, sleeping with it in her hand, and spraying her nose "off and on" all night whenever she awakened. Examination revealed severe rhinitis medicamentosa. Oral steroids and decongestants were started immediately with confiscation of her spray. Within 48 hours all the central nervous system symptoms were gone and the nasal airway was clearing. Within two weeks the sinusitis had cleared.

Multiple antihistamines and decongestants are available singly or in combination. This is one of the most common classes of drugs on the market. We are detailed on these nearly daily. With increasing frequency these drugs are becoming available over-the-counter. Some of these are new preparations, others are previously commonly prescribed preparations now considered safe enough by the Food and Drug Administration to be nonprescription items as long as warnings are on the labels. The addition of a decongestant to an antihistamine preparation may improve the clinical picture while allowing a lower dose of antihistamine to be used. It may offset some of the side effects produced by the antihistamine, especially the sedative effects. New preparations appear with great frequency. If a patient needs such antihistamines and decongestants or a combination, he or she may tolerate one preparation and not others, so a trial of more than one may be necessary. These drugs vary in degree and speed of effect by virtue of the vehicle and form in which they are produced. For example, one has a shell of antihistamine that dissolves immediately and lasts for 12 hours, while the decongestant within the shell gradually dissolves over 12 hours (Tavist-D).

CORTICOSTEROIDS

The action of steroids is nonspecific, suppressive, and palliative. It may be based on the blocking effect of the arachidonic acid cascade. It prevents the formation of arachidonic acid from phospholipids, short-circuiting both the cyclo-oxygenase and lipo-oxygenase pathways described in the immunology section. It takes longer for these effects to occur with the final blocking of the mediator release, so the therapeutic effects are slower than with the other drugs discussed. It appears also that steroids increase catecholamine responses, especially by enhancing beta-adrenergic receptor activity. Steroids influence histamine release, reduce the number of mucosal mast cells and circulating basophils, and thereby also reduce mediator effects. They reduce local inflammatory responses by stabilizing the vascular wall, reducing edema and leukocyte migration. Steroids have been found to have an important role in late allergic reactions and in nonallergic rhinitis. Most otolaryngic allergists use oral or parenteral corticosteroids for the more difficult to manage problems. High-dose burst therapy may be indicated in severe seasonal allergic rhinitis, in rhinitis medicamentosa, for aspirin sensitive patients, and pre- or postoperatively in markedly allergic patients. Because of the importance of this group of drugs, it is discussed in Chapter 25.

INTRANASAL MEDICATIONS

Topical and injectable steroids and topical cromolyn sulfate are of major importance in the management of nasal symptoms. They are discussed at length in Chapter 24, but will briefly be summarized as follows.

Intranasal topical steroids utilize the general effects of parenteral steroids for local responses in the nasal mucosa. Specifically, there is reduction in the number of mast cells in the surface mucosa; there is reduction of edema and vasodilation in the inflamed mucosa; the endothelial and epithelial barriers appear stabilized; and there is reduction in the nerve-stimulated sneeze reflex and in the glandular responses that produce the rhinorrhea. Eosinophils, goblet cells, mast cells, and the albumin content of nasal secretions are all reduced by intranasal steroids.

Intranasal cromolyn sodium (Nasalcrom 4% solution) has been available in the United States for the treatment of allergic rhinitis since early 1983. Ophthalmic cromolyn, Opticrom, became available for allergic conjunctivitis in early 1985. The mechanism of action is not entirely clear, but it appears that cromolyn prevents the release of histamine and other mediators by stabilizing the mast cell wall and inhibiting the inflow of Ca^{++} ions into the mast cell, preventing degranulation. Cromolyn is minimally metabolized and causes few side effects. It is most effective when used before the allergy challenge occurs. It will then significantly reduce the immediate reactions of rhinorrhea and sneezing and the late reaction of obstruction. Patients with seasonal allergy and high IgE levels respond the best. Those with perennial allergic rhinitis also respond to cromolyn, but somewhat less effectively.

Table 23–2. "SAFE" DRUGS FOR ALLERGY IN PREGNANCY

Antihistamines
Chlorpheniramine
Diphenhydramine
Tripelennamine
Cough suppressant
Dextromethorphan
Decongestants
Pseudoephedrine
Steroids
Beclomethasone—topical

Some patients respond well to either intranasal steroids or cromolyn and not the other. If one is not effective, the other should be tried.

Some drugs used for allergy are safer for use in pregnancy than are others (Table 23–2), although all should be avoided if possible. Of the antihistamines, chlorpheniramine (Chlor-Trimeton), diphenhydramine (Benadryl), and tripelennamine (Pyribenzamine) are considered the safest. Of the decongestants, pseudo-ephedrine is suggested. The cough suppressant dextromethorphan appears acceptable if absolutely needed, and of the steroids, beclomethasone topically is recommended. Medications are safest when taken in the mid trimester. In general, antihistamines should be avoided if possible in

Table 23–3. ANTIHISTAMINES IN PREGNANCY AND LACTATION

In general, antihistamines should not be used in the third trimester
Newborns and premature babies may react with sleep disturbances, hyperactivity, or convulsions
During lactation some antihistamines may pass to the baby, causing CNS symptoms

Table 23–4. DRUGS AFFECTING SKIN WHEALING

Drugs	Comment
Antihistamines	All antihistamines are capable of inhibiting immediate skin responses Hydroxyzine is the most potent and prolonged inhibitor
Epinephrine and other beta-adrenergic agents	Variable inhibiting activity
Theophylline	Variable inhibiting activity
Cromolyn	Inhibits delayed skin reactions May interfere with immediate skin tests in massive doses
Diethylcarbamazine	Interferes with the arachidonic acid metabolism
Phenothiazine	Antihistaminic action
Imipramine	Antihistaminic action

the third trimester of pregnancy. During nursing, the mother should be aware of the central nervous system symptoms that can be caused by the antihistamines and decongestants. Newborns, infants, and young children may react adversely to antihistamines with overstimulation rather than sedation (Table 23–3).

One additional class of drugs must be mentioned as a potential danger to allergic patients. Reports are available of severe reactions in patients on beta-adrenergic blockers used for cardiac arrhythmias, hypertension, and migraine headaches—the classic drug being propranolol (Inderal). Although rare, shock may occur in patients receiving immunotherapy, especially to ragweed. Calcium channel blockers do not affect immunotherapy. As a matter of fact, some of these chemicals may prove beneficial clinically in patients with asthma and possibly even with allergic rhinitis. Drug histories are of vital importance before testing is started, and patients must be cautioned to inform the allergist of any additional drugs prescribed by another physician while receiving immunotherapy. With the influx of new drugs for nearly every disease, we must be cautious about cross-reactions and not become complacent with our care.

Medications are essential in emergency treatment of anaphylactic shock, especially epinephrine, diphenhydramine, and steroids as discussed in Chapter 41.

As of June 1980, the FDA required labeling of dyes such as tartrazine on all commercial products. In June 1984, it was announced that there will be voluntary labeling of all inactive ingredients in most nonprescription drugs including binders, emulsifiers, flavorings, colorings, and preservatives. Products with any form of sulfite preservative must be labeled as of early 1986. The Pharmaceutical Manufacturer's Association representing companies marketing prescription drugs is moving toward a similar program beginning with the sulfites.

Many drugs affect the skin whealing response and must be avoided for varying periods of time prior to skin testing, including antihistamines, tranquilizers, and possibly steroids (Table 23–4).

The use of the simplest form of therapy that will effectively relieve the problem is wisest. Often, as specialists, we will see patients previously treated with many drugs, and may elect to test and treat with immunotherapy initially. Frequently, a combination of immunotherapy and pharmacotherapy is of special value at the beginning of treatment. It is important in rhinitis to determine if the patient is a "runner" with excessive secretions or a "blocker" with primarily congestion, or a combination of both, to tailor the use of medications to fit the specific case. Relief of allergic symptoms is possible in an effective medical otolaryngology practice utilizing proper modern diagnostic techniques, medications, and immunotherapy.

REFERENCES

1. Connell JT: A novel method to assess antihistamine and decongestant efficacy. Ann Allergy 42:278, 1979.
2. Current Pharmacotherapy for Allergic Rhinitis and Urticara (Symposium Proceedings). Journal of Respiratory Diseases Monography Series, Ciggott Publishing Co, 7:1, 1987.
3. Dockhorn RJ Shellenberger MK: Antihistamines: the new generation. Immunol Allergy Pract 9:124, 1987.
4. Drouin MA: H_1 antihistamines: perspective on the use of conventional and new agents. Ann Allergy 55:747, 1985.
5. Greenberger PA, Patterson R: Beclomethasone dipropionate for severe asthma during pregnancy. Ann Intern Med 98:478, 1983.
6. Krause HF: Allergic rhinitis. *In* Current Therapy in

Otolaryngology: Head and Neck Surgery 3. Philadelphia, BC Decker, 1987, pp 271–274.
7. Kniker WT (ed): The Nose and Sinuses. Schering Corporation, 1986, pp 42–46.
8. Metzger WJ, Patterson R: Questions and answers in immunotherapy during pregnancy. Consultant, November:106, 1978.
9. Murphy S: Cromolyn sodium: science and serendipity. ENT Technology, September 1984.
10. Mygind N: Nasal Allergy. 2nd ed. London, Blackwell Scientific Publications, 1979, pp 285–342.
11. Naclario RM, Meier HL, Kagey-Sobotlin S, et al: In vivo model for the evaluation of topical anti-allergic medication. Arch Otolaryngol 110:25, 1984.
12. Nelson MM, Forfar JO: Association between drugs administered during pregnancy and congenital abnormalities of the fetus. Br Med J 1:523, 1971.
13. Normal PS: Review of nasal therapy: update. J Allergy Clin Immunol 72:412, 1983.
14. Schatz M, Patterson R, Zeitz S, et al: Corticosteroid therapy for the pregnant asthmatic patient. JAMA 233:804, 1987.
15. Schatz M, Zeiger RS, Mellon M, et al: Asthma and allergic disease during pregnancy: management of the mother and prevention in the child. *In* Middleton E, Reed CE, Ellis EF (eds): Allergy Principles and Practice. St. Louis, CV Mosby, 1983, pp 935–986.
16. Schwartz JF: The effect of cromolyn on nasal disease. Ear Nose Throat J 65:419, 1986.
17. Toogood JH: Beta-blocker therapy and the risk of anaphylaxis. Can Med Assoc J 136:929, 1987.
18. Trzeciakowski JP, Levi R: Antihistamines. *In* Middleton E, Reed CE, Ellis EF (eds): Allergy Principles and Practice. St. Louis, CV Mosby, 1983, pp 575–592.
19. Watase T, Okuda M: The effects of autonormotropic drugs on allergic nasal mucosa. Rhinology 24:181, 1986.
20. Wilson J: Use of sodium cromoglycate during pregnancy. Acta Therapeutica [Suppl]:45, 1982.

CHAPTER 24

Intranasal Medications: Sprays and Aerosols, Corticosteroid Injection

Richard L. Mabry, M.D.

The pharmacotherapy of allergic rhinitis must be thoroughly understood by any physician treating patients with this disorder. Although avoidance and immunotherapy are the definitive measures for treating nasal allergy, severe symptomatic flares or complicating problems require the use of proper medications to afford relief to the patient. One avenue of therapy that is especially important to the otolaryngic allergist is the intranasal administration of medications.

NASAL TOILET

The use of saline nasal sprays and mixtures of these sprays with an aromatic, alkaline nasal douche such as Alkalol deserves special mention. Not only are such benign measures helpful in cleansing thick nasal secretions and combating nasal crusting, dryness (especially in winter), and irritation, but they can also be beneficial to patients exposed to such environmental irritants as smoke, chalk dust, newsprint, and dyes by cleansing the nasal passages of the particles deposited therein. A variety of saline nasal sprays are now available, and patients with nasal allergy should be urged to freely use one of these preparations.

TOPICAL VASOCONSTRICTORS

Action

Nose drops or sprays reduce turbinate engorgement and relieve nasal stuffiness by causing a closure of the blood-filled spaces within the turbinates. The resulting decrease in turbinate size (mainly involving the inferior turbinates) effectively increases available nasal airspace for a few hours. Unfortunately, after regular use of these preparations for five to seven days, a progressively severe "rebound" vasodilation of the turbinate erectile tissues follows the initial vasoconstriction. The nasal congestion that results usually prompts the patient to continue using the drops or spray (often in increasing amounts and more frequently), setting up a vicious cycle of "nose drops addiction."

Complications

In addition to rebound rhinitis, topical vasoconstrictors can cause sympathomimetic systemic effects. Thus, they should be used with caution by patients with hypertension, hyperthyroidism, or anxiety/insomnia.

Usage

Despite the potential for rebound rhinitis, topical vasoconstrictors are useful for short periods in the treatment of acute or self-limited problems (common cold, acute purulent sinusitis, acute otitis media, barotitis media). However, because of the potential for patient abuse, they should be used sparingly and with great caution by patients with a chronic or recurring condition such as nasal allergy. Indeed, when advised for use in the former conditions by patients with allergic rhinitis, a specific warning against prolonged or excessive usage must be clearly given.

CORTICOSTEROID NASAL AEROSOLS

Action

Although severe symptomatic flares of allergic rhinitis must often be treated with glucocorticoids for effective control, the risks and potential side effects of these preparations when given systemically led to the development of intranasal delivery systems. Not only does this reduce the risk of systemic effects and complications, but this mode of treatment concentrates the therapeutic effects of the medication on the diseased tissue.

Corticosteroids administered systemically do not prevent the occurrence of the allergic event or the subsequent release of vasoactive kinins. They act rather to minimize the resultant tissue responses. Although the mechanism of action of topical nasal steroids is not fully known, it is felt that they also probably act in this same fashion. Thus, their actions include protecting capillaries from increased permeability due to histamine release, stabilizing lysosomal membranes, retarding the production of arachidonic acid–derived mediators of inflammation, and inhibiting the accumulation of macrophages and leukocytes at the site of tissue reaction.

Complications

The undesirable effects of intranasal corticosteroid sprays can be due to their local effects or to systemic action. Although minimal with usual doses, systemic effects including hypothalamic-pituitary-adrenal axis suppression may occur if the recommended prescribing limits are exceeded. The degree of systemic absorption and effect varies with each preparation.

All aerosol nasal steroids share certain common potential local side effects. These may include sneezing and headache, nasal irritation and burning, dryness and crusting of the nose, epistaxis, and nasal septal perforations. Some of these problems are related to the delivery system of the preparation being used, whereas others (especially bleeding, crusting, and septal perforation) may also be related to a direct effect of the corticosteroid on nasal mucosa, especially in areas of septal spurs or previously operated septal tissue. Thus, caution must be exercised in prescribing nasal steroid aerosols, especially for long-term use. Close patient monitoring is necessary, in the form of both warnings to report any of the described symptoms and advising of the necessity for periodic intranasal examinations.

The degree of risk involved in using nasal corticosteroid sprays during pregnancy is unclear. Large systemic doses of all three of the steroids used in these sprays have been teratogenic in laboratory animals, but no correlation can be inferred with their local use intranasally. No teratogenicity was shown in a few studies in a limited number of humans receiving beclomethasone nasal aerosol at the time of conception and/or during pregnancy. No human studies have been reported for dexamethasone or flunisolide.

Preparations

Dexamethasone nasal aerosol (Decadron Turbinaire) was the first of these preparations to be marketed. Its onset of effect is rapid, with a brief duration of action. Significant systemic absorption of the drug occurs, apparently dose-related, so that prolonged courses of therapy should be avoided and patients cautioned not to exceed the recommended dosage. The usual initial dose is two sprays in each nostril three times daily (1200 μg dexamethasone total daily dose). Since the onset of effect with this preparation is rapid, patients should not continue therapy past one week without consulting their physician if no relief of symptoms occurs. Dosage may usually be tapered after improvement occurs, some patients responding to as little as one spray in each nostril twice daily (400 μg dexamethasone). Because of the risk of significant systemic absorption, prolonged therapy with aerosol dexamethasone is not usually advisable. Children over 6 years of age may be treated at about half the adult dose, not to exceed 800 μg daily, and preferably less.

Beclomethasone nasal spray (Vancenase, Beconase) is a poorly soluble powder in suspension, delivered by a Freon propellant. The risk of systemic absorption and effect is less with this preparation than with other steroid nasal aerosols. In one study, adrenal suppression was not noted after several months of therapy at doses approximately five times the recommended daily maximum. Dosage should be begun with one spray in each nostril four times daily (336 μg beclomethasone daily), and tapered to the lowest effective dose after therapeutic results are evident. However, patients must be advised that this may require from one to three weeks to occur. Thereafter, satisfactory maintenance may be achieved with as little as one spray in each nostril once daily (84 μg beclomethasone). Because of the slow build-up to therapeutic levels, patients must be educated that intermittent therapy for short periods to relieve acute symptoms will most likely be ineffective. One benefit of this characteristic, however, is noticeable symptomatic relief for several days after treatment is discontinued.

Aqueous forms of beclomethasone in a pump spray are now available. The initial dosage is two sprays in each nostril twice daily, with tapering as necessary. This delivery form seems less prone to cause local nasal irritation.

Children 12 years of age and over are treated at the adult dosage of beclomethasone, whereas use of this product to treat children below the age of 12 years is not approved. Because of the wide safety margin for systemic effect, and the existence of at least some studies demonstrating safety of this preparation used during pregnancy, beclomethasone is probably the best choice of nasal steroid aerosols if one must be used to treat a pregnant patient.

Flunisolide nasal solution (Nasalide) is supplied in a propylene glycol vehicle delivered by a pump spray, avoiding the fluorocarbon propellants of the other forms. However, up to 45 per cent of patients treated with this preparation report nasal stinging and burning. The recommended initial adult dose is two sprays in each nostril twice daily (200 μg flunisolide total daily dose). Improvement may not be noted for one to three weeks, at which point the dosage may be decreased to a maintenance level, sometimes as low as one spray in each nostril (50 μg flunisolide daily). Flunisolide is absorbed through the nasal mucosa, where about half is changed by the liver to less active 6-beta-hydroxy metabolites. Adrenal suppression has been demonstrated at doses of 700 μg per day and above. No conclusive evidence of depression of endogenous cortisol has been shown at the recommended dose of 200 μg per day. Nevertheless, although the maximum adult dosage is listed as eight sprays per nostril per day (800 μg total), if dosages this high are required, a significant risk of systemic effect would appear to exist.

Flunisolide is approved for treating children age 6 years and above, at initial doses of up to 150 to 200 μg per day, with a maintenance dose of 50 μg daily.

Usage

For a nasal steroid aerosol to be effective, it must reach the affected nasal mucosa. This often requires combining this treatment at its onset with the use of a systemic antihistamine-decongestant, using a short course of a topical nasal vasoconstrictor, or even employing systemic steroids briefly.

The patient who is given an aerosol corticosteroid for nasal use must be warned that (with the exception of dexamethasone) results may not be evident for one to three weeks. If there is no relief after treatment at full dosage for three weeks (one week for dexamethasone), a reevaluation by the physician is necessary. Patients must also be instructed not to exceed the recommended maximum daily dose. After improvement is noted, the dosage of the spray should be gradually reduced to the smallest amount that provides symptomatic relief. If symptoms recur dosage adjustment will be necessary. Patients must be strongly cautioned that simply using the spray on an "as needed" basis for occasional acute symptoms will be ineffective. Further, all persons using a nasal corticosteroid aerosol should be cautioned to consult their physician if they develop nasal irritation, crusting, or bleeding. They should also be warned to discontinue the use of their medication if they develop an active nasal or upper respiratory infection.

Nasal corticosteroids, in addition to usage to relieve nasal allergic symptoms, may be given following polypectomy and intranasal ethmoidectomy to treat reversibly diseased sinus mucosa, to diminish the likelihood of polyp recurrence, or to treat small recurrent polyps. Such therapy should not be started until two to four weeks postoperatively, when mucosal healing is well under way and crust formation does not prevent access to the area to be treated. For this purpose, the author prefers beclomethasone, started at a four times daily dose, and decreased by one dose per day each week for a total course of one month. This may be repeated in the future if needed.

CROMOLYN NASAL AEROSOL

Action

In contrast to corticosteroids, cromolyn acts by blocking the occurrence of the allergic event, inhibiting the mast cell release of histamine and other vasoactive substances, probably by interfering with calcium transport across the mast cell membrane. Cromolyn also differs from corticosteroids in its ability to protect an individual from the effect of an acute allergen challenge. Indeed, cromolyn is most effective if therapy can be started before allergen exposure. Although animal studies suggest mast cell protection (by inhibition of phospholipase A action) in nonallergic situations, cromolyn is not currently felt to be indicated in the therapy of nonallergic rhinitis. Also, cromolyn is not beneficial in the treatment of nasal polyps.

Complications

The side effects and potential complications of intranasally administered cromolyn are surprisingly few. Local problems include sneezing (10 per cent), nasal stinging or burning (4 to 5 per cent), nasal irritation (less than 3 per cent), and epistaxis (less than 1 per cent). No reported nasal septal perforations have been attributed to the intranasal use of cromolyn.

Less than 7 per cent of cromolyn administered by intranasal spray is absorbed and subsequently excreted in bile and urine. The remainder of the dose is expelled from the nose or swallowed and excreted via the alimentary tract. Although not reported for cromolyn nasal solution, the systemic side effects most often reported after inhaled cromolyn have included angioedema, joint pain and swelling, and rare instances of serum sickness and rash. Cromolyn has not been shown to be teratogenic in animal studies, even at doses up to 338 times the human clinical dose.

Usage

Cromolyn nasal solution is dispensed via a pump spray. The recommended starting dose for adults and children over 6 years of age is one spray (5.2 mg cromolyn) in each nostril every three to four hours (up to six times daily) until relief is obtained. Full effect may not be seen for four to seven days in seasonal nasal allergy, and may require up to two weeks or more in perennial allergic rhinitis. After relief is obtained, the dosage is decreased to the lowest effective maintenance level, which must be continued throughout the season of expected allergy exposure. Unlike nasal steroids, the effects of nasal cromolyn do not persist for any appreciable time after therapy is discontinued.

Because of the delayed onset of effect, and to assure more patent nasal passages to allow access of the aerosol, concomitant antihistamine-decongestant therapy is advisable at the start of cromolyn treatment. The drug is not effective in treating nasal polyps.

The protective effect of nasal cromolyn spray is especially helpful in preventing symptoms when a known heavy allergen exposure can be anticipated and therapy started beforehand. This "immediate" effect sometimes leads patients to feel that nasal cromolyn can be used sporadically as symptoms arise. They must be educated that to gain full benefit, the drug must be used regularly during the entire expected symptomatic season.

CORTICOSTEROID INJECTION

The intranasal injection of corticosteroids for the symptomatic relief of allergic rhinitis was first mentioned in the literature by Semenov in 1951. For years thereafter it was part of otolaryngic lore, passed on mainly by word of mouth and observation. In the 1960s, two reported cases of visual loss following intranasal steroid injection caused many otolaryngologists to discontinue the procedure. As more clinical research was done on the subject in the late 1970s and beyond, the mechanism of such complications was clarified as retinal embolization and vasospasm, and the technique was refined to attempt to avoid such problems. Nevertheless, any otolaryngologist performing this procedure must be aware of this potential complication and exercise caution to avoid it.

Action

Like topical nasal preparations, intranasally injected steroids act locally to block the effect of the allergic event, not to prevent it. Prior studies involving plasma cortisol measurement have indicated that systemic absorption of intraturbinally injected corticosteroids is probably not clinically significant, so that their action is primarily local. This is further borne out by the lack of effect of intranasal steroid injection on such distant symptoms as itching mucous membranes and eustachian tube obstruction. The procedure, however, does give excellent symptomatic relief of nasal congestion, and to a lesser degree the rhinorrhea and sneezing, due to allergic rhinitis (as well as other nasal disorders such as vasomotor rhinitis, rhinitis medicamentosa, and rhinitis during pregnancy).

The major advantage of intranasal steroid injection is the rapid onset (one to two hours) and prolonged duration (three to six weeks) of effect. Because systemic effect is not clinically significant, the procedure is useful in patients with conditions that might preclude systemic corticosteroid therapy. Finally, daily usage (as with sprays) and dosage adjustment and tapering (as is necessary with sprays and oral steroids) are not required.

Complications and Cautions

The most common side effects of this injection are nasal bleeding and facial flushing, each reported by about 2 per cent of patients. The nasal bleeding actually is oozing at the injection site of blood-streaked nasal mucus, which spontaneously ceases in less than an hour without attention. The facial flush, caused by steroid-induced vasodilation, occurs the day following the injection and requires no treatment. A vasovagal "needle reaction" may develop before the injection begins, requiring postponement of the procedure; one occurring with the injection in progress is managed by injecting as much of the steroid as is safely possible into the turbinate already punctured, then terminating the procedure. A rare patient may demonstrate diaphoresis and lumbar or posterior thoracic pain within a few minutes of receiving an intraturbinal injection of a repository corticosteroid. This represents a reaction to the repository vehicle and may also occur after intramuscular or intra-articular injection. The episode will normally end in less than an hour and requires no specific treatment. However, any future intranasal or intramuscular injection of a repository corticosteroid for that patient should be of a different preparation than the one producing the idiosyncratic reaction.

The rarest complication of intranasal steroid injection, but the most catastrophic, is visual loss. A review in 1981 of reported cases, anecdotal cases, and the adverse reaction files of the Food and Drug Administration and numerous drug companies documented a total of 11 such instances. In six cases, permanent partial or total unilateral visual loss followed the intranasal injection of a repository corticosteroid preparation, whereas five other instances of temporary visual blurring were reported. The mechanism of injury appears to be retinal embolization or vasospasm.

To avoid embolization and vasospasm, specific points of technique have been outlined that differ somewhat from those utilized over 30 years ago by early proponents of the procedure. Utilizing the technique described in the following, the author has safely employed this procedure in many thousands of patients with no visual complications. Many other otolaryngologists also report excellent results and lack of complications when careful detail to technique is observed.

Technique

Pledgets of cotton moistened with 5 per cent cocaine solution are placed against the anterior tips of each inferior turbinate. While these are in place, the procedure is explained to the patient, along with an assurance that it is not painful. Failure to spend a few moments doing this will result in a high percentage of "needle reactions." The material for injection is then prepared by drawing 1 ml of triamcinolone acetonide (Kenalog-40) into a tuberculin syringe. This is never mixed with a local anesthetic or a vasoconstrictor, which may cause particle clumping in the steroid solution or spasm of local vessels. The material is drawn up fresh for each patient to minimize the risk of particle conglomeration, and a repository steroid with the smallest available particle size is employed. After the cotton pledgets are removed, 0.5 ml of steroid is gently injected submucosally into the anterior tip of each inferior turbinate (Fig. 24–1) with a 1.5 inch 25-gauge needle. The "feel" of the injection should be similar to local infiltration of a septum or ear canal, and if undue pressure is necessary for injection, the needle should be moved. Proper injection produces a white blanching as the steroid infiltrates just submucosally. A dry cotton pledget is placed over the injection site for a few minutes, while any further instructions are given and prescriptions are prepared. The cotton is then removed and the patient is allowed to blow any remaining blood from the nose. Warnings are given to expect slight bloody oozing or a possible facial flush, and the patient is allowed to leave.

Other repository steroids suitable for this injection are triamcinolone diacetate (Aristocort Forte) and prednisolone tebutate (Hydeltra-TBA). Some clinicians have found dexamethasone acetate (Decadron-LA) to be acceptable.

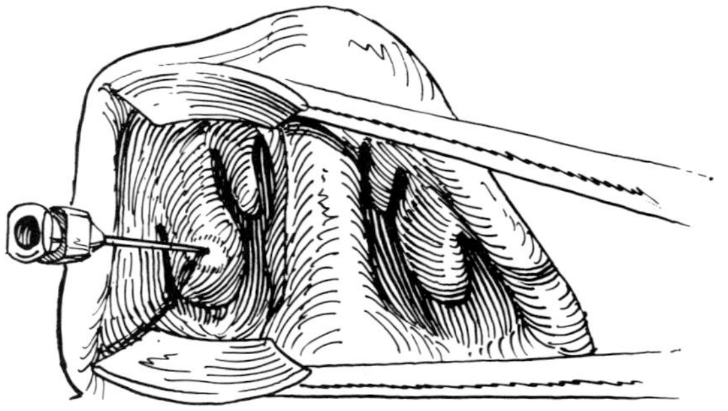

FIGURE 24–1. Injection just beneath mucosa of anterior tip of inferior turbinate, producing blanching as steroid spreads in submucosal plane. (Reprinted by permission from the Southern Medical Journal 71:789, 1978.)

The author does not use methylprednisolone acetate (Depo-Medrol) because of its somewhat larger particle size. It should be noted that only triamcinolone acetonide is listed by the USP as indicated for intraturbinal injection.

Usage

Intranasal steroid injection is beneficial to control the nasal symptoms of severe allergic flares, and since its duration of action is usually four to six weeks, some patients may experience marked relief throughout an entire pollen season after one injection. The injection is not given until symptoms first occur, nor is it repeated until symptoms return (and never earlier than three to four weeks after the last injection). The author generally tries to limit the number of injections to four a year, but has given up to seven within a 12-month period without demonstrable adrenal suppression. It should be further emphasized that if intranasal steroid injection is required more than two to three times per year to control nasal allergic symptoms, the immunotherapy program for that patient must be carefully scrutinized.

Intrapolyp injection of corticosteroids is often beneficial, especially when combined with antibiotic therapy for any associated sinusitis and management of underlying allergy. A total of 1.0 ml of triamcinolone acetonide or one of the other repository corticosteroids already listed is injected intranasally, dividing the dose between the anterior tips of the inferior turbinates (if accessible) and the most accessible polyp masses. After polyp shrinkage occurs, aerosol corticosteroid therapy may be used for further treatment of residual small polypoid tags. Polyps that do not rapidly respond to medical management including intranasal steroid injection will require surgical removal, including appropriate sinus surgery.

COMPARISON OF THERAPY

Table 24–1 shows a broad comparison of the characteristics of intranasal steroid injection, corticosteroid nasal aerosols, and cromolyn nasal spray. The rapid onset and prolonged duration of action of intraturbinal corticosteroid injection make it popular with both patients and physi-

Table 24–1. COMPARISON OF INTRANASAL THERAPY FOR ALLERGIC RHINITIS

	Intranasal Steroid Injection	Corticosteroid Sprays*	Cromolyn Spray
Onset	Hours	7–14 days	4–7 days +
Dosage	× 1 (3–6 weeks)	2–4 × daily	3–6 × daily
Local side effects	Bleeding, facial flush (caution re visual complications)	Stinging, bleeding, crusting; possible septal perforation	Rare, mild, transient
Systemic effects	Virtually nil	Possible with high doses, chronic Rx	None
Protection from acute challenge	±	−	+
Applications	Broad	Broad	IgE-mediated atopy

*Beclomethasone; flunisolide.

cians. However, it does involve an office visit and injection, whereas the sprays can be kept on hand and started by the patient whenever needed. Cromolyn is the only preparation that affords true protection from an allergic challenge when used beforehand. Corticosteroid sprays cannot do this, and intranasal steroid injection only alleviates symptoms (although if given before an exposure, its rapid onset and prolonged action afford subjective relief that is indistinguishable from "protection"). Finally, corticosteroids have a broad range of application for intranasal problems (vasomotor rhinitis, rhinitis during pregnancy, rebound rhinitis), whereas cromolyn is currently indicated only for true IgE-mediated allergic rhinitis.

Despite definitive therapy through avoidance and hyposensitization, patients with allergic rhinitis will require medications for symptomatic relief at various times during the course of their disease. To effectively manage these patients, physicians would do well to follow these three precepts: (1) make an accurate diagnosis; (2) if therapy is not effective, look for a complication; (3) be thoroughly familiar with every available therapeutic modality, and employ the one that best suits the individual patient and clinical situation. The physician who treats every patient the same way will be successful more by chance than by clinical acumen.

REFERENCES

1. Ballin JC: AMA Drug Evaluations. 5th ed. Chicago, American Medical Association, 1983, pp 887–893.
2. Mabry RL: Rhinitis medicamentosa: the forgotten factor in nasal obstruction. South Med J 75:817, 1982.
3. Mabry RL: Corticosteroids in the management of allergic rhinitis. South Med J 76:487, 1983.
4. Mabry RL: Corticosteroids in otolaryngology: intraturbinal injection. Otolaryngol Head Neck Surg 91:717, 1983.
5. Mabry RL: Cromolyn nasal aerosol. Otolaryngol Head Neck Surg 93:135, 1985.
6. USP: Drug Information for the Health Care Provider. 6th ed. Rockville, MD, The United States Pharmacopeial Convention, 1986, pp 31–34; 617–618.

CHAPTER 25

Corticosteroids: General Considerations of Systemic Therapy

Richard L. Mabry, M.D.

Although capable of producing profound changes and inducing potentially catastrophic side effects, corticosteroids constitute one of the most valuable tools in the therapeutic armamentarium of the physician treating allergic disorders. Corticosteroids should be respected, but not feared, by the practitioners who employ them. The key to successfully treating with corticosteroids is a thorough knowledge of their effects, proper usage, and potential adverse effects.

PHARMACOLOGY

Classification

Corticosteroids may be classified as glucocorticoids or mineralocorticoids, depending on their primary effects. Although the preparations employed in allergy management are of the glucocorticoid class, all have varying degrees of mineralocorticoid activity. Even those preparations said to have negligible mineralocorticoid activity can cause sodium retention, hypokalemia, and fluid retention, depending on dosage and patient predisposition. Table 25–1 lists representative corticosteroids with their equivalent dosages and relative glucocorticoid/mineralocorticoid activity.

Action

The anti-inflammatory and antiallergic actions of glucocorticoids are not due to a prevention or inhibition of the allergic event per se. Rather, these compounds diminish the resultant tissue responses (edema, aggregation of inflammatory cells, synthesis of vasoactive amines) without affecting the underlying cause.

The exact mechanisms of action by which corticosteroids exert their anti-inflammatory effects are quite complex, and in some phases are not fully understood. However, it is commonly accepted that these actions include inhibition of macrophage localization through blockage of macrophage inhibitory factor, reduction of dilation and permeability of capillaries (decreasing edema formation), and reduction of adherence of leukocytes to capillary endothelium with inhibition of leukocyte migration. Finally, glucocorticoids increase the synthesis of lipomodulin or macrocortin, which in turn inhibits the action of phospholipase A_2 to drive the arachidonic acid cascade. The end result is a reduced formation of such inflammatory vasoactive kinins as prostaglandins, thromboxanes, and leukotrienes.

HPA Axis

The negative feedback mechanism that regulates the production of corticosteroids by the adrenal cortex through the action of pituitary-secreted corticotropin (ACTH) is called the hypothalamic-pituitary-adrenal (HPA) axis. The administration of exogenous corticosteroids causes a reduction in the production of endog-

Table 25–1. RELATIVE POTENCY AND HALF-LIFE OF VARIOUS ADRENOCORTICOIDS

Preparation	Relative Potency			Biologic (Tissue) Half-life (hr)
	*Glucocorticoid Dose (mg)**	*Glucocorticoid Activity*	*Mineralocorticoid Activity*	
Short-acting				
Cortisone	25	0.8	2+	8–12
Hydrocortisone	20	1	2+	8–12
Intermediate-acting				
Methylprednisolone	4	5	0	18–36
Prednisolone	5	4	1+	18–36
Prednisone	5	4	1+	18–36
Triamcinolone	4	5	0	18–36
Long-acting				
Betamethasone	0.6	20–30	0	36–54
Dexamethasone	0.5–0.75	20–30	0	36–54

*Approximate; applies to oral or intravenous administration only.

Adapted from USP DI: Drug Information for the Health Care Provider. Vol. I. Copyright 1987. The United States Pharmacopeial Convention, Inc. Permission granted.

enous adrenocorticoids. This reciprocal relationship between exogenously administered and endogenously produced corticosteroids is quite important.

Adrenal suppression is mainly dependent on the duration, and to a lesser extent on the dosage, of corticosteroid therapy. Other factors that affect suppression and recovery of adrenal function are the timing and frequency of administration and the potency and biologic half-life of the agent used. For example, divided doses appear to cause more adrenal suppression than does a single dose, and a daytime dose results in less adrenal suppression than one given at bedtime. It is generally felt that the equivalent of 15 mg of prednisone daily for less than one month should cause no significant adrenal suppression. However, 20 to 30 mg daily of prednisone or its equivalent may produce significant adrenal hypofunction after only a week. Recovery is likewise quite variable, from as little as a week to as much as a year or more, depending on the factors already listed.

EFFECTS OF PHYSIOLOGIC AMOUNTS

Corticosteroids in physiologic (i.e., replacement) doses or in normal amounts in the body affect many organ systems. Since the side effects and complications of therapeutically administered steroids are often an extension of these physiologic effects, the latter should be familiar to the physician using these compounds.

Carbohydrate, Protein, and Fat Metabolism

Glucocorticoids increase the availability of glucose. They stimulate the catabolism of protein and mobilize fat deposits.

Water and Electrolyte Balance

The glucocorticoids have less effect in this area than do mineralocorticoids. To varying degrees, glucocorticoids promote sodium reabsorption and water retention and a depletion of body potassium.

Cardiovascular and Hemic Systems

Adrenocorticoids are felt to be necessary for the vasoconstrictor action of epinephrine on small blood vessels. In the absence of glucocorticoids, one may see inadequate vasomotor responses with hypotension and increased capillary permeability. These hormones affect the hematopoietic system by increasing the number of erythrocytes and polymorphonuclear neutrophilic leukocytes, while decreasing the number of other types of leukocytes.

Central Nervous System

Corticosteroids influence mood and sleep patterns, and lowered levels are associated with irritability and depression. Glucocorticoids lower seizure thresholds, whereas mineralocorticoids raise them.

Skeletal Muscle

Glucocorticoids maintain muscular strength mainly by their effect on circulation, carbohydrate metabolism, and electrolytes.

Bone

Glucocorticoids decrease bone formation and increase bone resorption.

SIDE EFFECTS AND COMPLICATIONS OF PHARMACOLOGIC DOSES

General Principles

The risk of side effects and complications resulting from therapy with pharmacologic doses of corticosteroids generally increases with the duration and frequency of dosage, and to a lesser extent with the amount administered. Other factors that influence the development of untoward effects include the preparation and route of administration, age and condition of the patient, and underlying diseases. The complications of therapy may be due to the action of glucocorticoids on a number of organ systems, and are quite often an extension of the physiologic effects of these preparations. The areas listed are by no means all of those possibly affected, but represent the most common or most serious adverse consequences of corticosteroid treatment.

Gastrointestinal Effects

Glucocorticoids decrease protection by the gastric mucus barrier, increase the production of gastric acid and pepsinogen, and hinder tissue repair. Thus, they may either cause or contribute to peptic ulcer development. In addition, steroids may mask the symptoms of an ulcer so that bleeding and/or perforation occur suddenly and without warning. As a result of this problem, antacids are sometimes routinely given to patients on long-term corticosteroid therapy. However, it should be pointed out that antacids decrease the absorption of orally administered steroids. Periodic examinations of stools for blood are recommended in monitoring patients receiving long-term corticosteroid therapy.*

Edema and Hypokalemia

Even the glucocorticoids considered to have little or no effect on fluid and electrolyte balance can cause sodium and fluid retention and/or hypokalemia, depending on dosage and patient predisposition. Limitation of sodium intake plus monitoring serum potassium levels and providing potassium supplementation when indicated must be considered when corticosteroids are given, especially in large doses or for extended periods.

Osteoporosis

This condition is commonly seen (although often ignored or forgotten) following long-term, high-dose glucocorticoid therapy. The problem is most likely to occur in postmenopausal females, especially those not on calcium supplementation. Unfortunately, radiographs often do not show osteoporosis until late in its development. A much rarer complication is aseptic necrosis of the femoral head, usually seen after high-dose therapy, and more common in younger age groups. Patients receiving corticosteroids should be warned to report hip pain, and radiographs should be performed in such instances.

Carbohydrate, Protein, or Lipid Metabolism Disturbances

The most common such disturbance is aggravation of diabetes mellitus (since glucocorticoids raise blood sugar). Protein breakdown may cause muscle atrophy and a negative nitrogen balance. Mobilization of fat often results in elevated serum lipid concentration.

Central Nervous System Effects

Large doses of steroids may produce behavioral and personality changes, most often eu-

*Some gastroenterologists now also suggest the use of H_2 suppressors for ulcer prophylaxis in selected patients on long-term steroid therapy: cimetidine (Tagamet), ranitidine (Zantac), or the newer famotidine (Pepcid).—Ed.

phoria. These compounds may also produce hyperkinesis, irritability, insomnia, and even frank psychosis. The development of these problems does not appear to depend on the presence of any preexisting psychiatric illness. The symptoms are dose-related, and diminish or disappear with dose reduction.

Ocular Effects

The most common such complication is the development of posterior subcapsular cataracts in patients undergoing prolonged systemic corticosteroid therapy. The phenomenon appears to be dose-related, but may occur even after alternate-day therapy. Because of this problem, patients on long-term treatment with corticosteroids should undergo periodic ophthalmoscopy and should be warned to report any visual blurring. Corticosteroids have also been reported to increase intraocular pressure in some cases of open angle glaucoma, although this is apparently more likely with topical than systemic administration. The phenomenon of retinal embolization or vasospasm after intraturbinal corticosteroid injection is discussed in Chapter 24.

Infection

The reactivation of quiescent pulmonary tuberculosis by systemic corticosteroids is no longer a common problem, but must be kept in mind when treating patients with a history of ill-defined pulmonary infection. Impairment of host defense mechanisms in patients receiving corticosteroid therapy may increase the risk of developing (or lessen the patient's ability to handle) bacterial, viral, or fungal infections. Also, since steroids tend to mask the symptoms of infection, treatment may be delayed in such instances. Systemic corticosteroids should be used with caution in patients with herpetic lesions that may involve the eye, because of the risk of perforation of herpetic corneal ulcers.

Miscellaneous

Other side effects or complications of the administration of pharmacologic amounts of corticosteroids include menstrual aberrations, cushingoid changes, weight gain, headache, hypertension, and impotence.

PREPARATIONS AND EQUIVALENT DOSES

Dosage Forms

Corticosteroids for systemic administration are available in a multitude of preparations. The clinician may choose from a number of glucocorticoids, each of which is usually available in forms for oral, intravenous, and intramuscular administration. The intramuscular type is usually subdivided into those preparations that are freely soluble in water (esters of phosphate and succinate) and rapidly absorbed after intramuscular injection, and those that are relatively water-insoluble (acetates, diacetates, acetonides, hexacetonides, tebutates) and slowly absorbed, which are referred to as "repository" preparations. Onset, peak, and duration of action depend on the route and site of administration, the solubility of the dosage form, the dose administered, and such individual factors as the patient's status and the condition being treated. After oral or intravenous administration, onset is rapid, while the duration of action depends on the biologic or tissue half-life. Onset and duration of action after intramuscular administration depend on both the solubility and the biologic half-life of the dosage form.

Comparisons and Classifications

The relative potency, glucocorticoid activity, and tissue half-life of representative adrenocorticoids appear in Table 25–1. The classification into short-, intermediate-, and long-acting compounds is based on the biologic half-life of the water-soluble preparations and does not reflect the slow absorption and prolonged action of repository intramuscular preparations. As noted previously, even the compounds listed with no mineralocorticoid activity can cause sodium and fluid retention and/or hypokalemia under some circumstances (depending on dosage and patient status).

Table 25–2 lists the characteristics of several forms of various adrenocorticoids. Note that a dose of oral medication usually has a peak effect in one to two hours and lasts from 1 1/4

Table 25–2. CHARACTERISTICS OF SELECTED CORTICOSTEROID PREPARATIONS

Drug and Route	Onset of Action	Peak Effect	Duration of Action
Betamethasone			
Oral		1–2 hr	3¼ days
Sodium phosphate			
IV/IM	Rapid		
Acetate/sodium phosphate			
IM	1–3 hr		1 week
Dexamethasone			
Oral		1–2 hr	2¾ days
Acetate			
IM		8 hr	6 days
Sodium phosphate			
IV/IM	Rapid		
Hydrocortisone			
Oral		1 hr	1¼ to 1½ days
IM		4–8 hr	
Sodium phosphate			
IV/IM	Rapid	1 hr (IM)	
Sodium succinate			
IV/IM	Rapid	1 hr (IM)	Variable
Methylprednisolone			
Oral		1–2 hr	1¼ to 1½ days
Acetate			
IM	6–48 hr	4–8 days	1–4 weeks
Sodium succinate			
IV/IM	Rapid		
Prednisolone			
Oral		1–2 hr	1¼ to 1½ days
Acetate			
IM	Slow		
Acetate/sodium/phosphate			
IM			up to 4 weeks
Sodium phosphate			
IV/IM	Rapid	1 hr	
Prednisone			
Oral		1–2 hr	1¼ to 1½ days
Triamcinolone			
Oral		1–2 hr	2¼ days
Acetonide			
IM	24–48 hr		1–6 weeks
Diacetate			
Oral		1–2 hr	
IM	Slow		4 days–4 weeks

Adapted from USP DI: Drug Information for the Health Care Provider. Vol. I. Copyright 1987. The United States Pharmacopeial Convention, Inc. Permission granted.

to 3 1/4 days, depending on the steroid chosen. Preparations for intravenous administration and aqueous intramuscular forms give a rapid onset of action, whereas various repository intramuscular forms produce a slower onset and longer duration of effect. As a practical matter, a single therapeutic dose of a repository corticosteroid given intramuscularly can produce therapeutic effects (and concomitant depression of endogenous cortisol) for up to four to six weeks. The therapeutic effect of acetonide forms of adrenocorticoids is more prolonged than a similar preparation complexed as an acetate, diacetate, or tebutate owing to the difference in speed of the enzymatic degradation necessary to release the active glucocorticoid moiety.

ROUTES OF ADMINISTRATION AND DOSAGE REGIMENS

General Dosing Information

Before corticosteroids are used, a proper diagnosis should be established. Other than for severe or life-threatening situations, adrenocorticoid therapy should be considered only after less drastic measures have failed. Corticosteroids should generally be administered in the lowest effective dosage and for the shortest period of time necessary to achieve the desired control, keeping in mind that complete abatement of symptoms is not always a realistic expectation. Finally, local administration is preferable to systemic therapy when feasible, to concentrate therapeutic effect at the target site and to minimize systemic effects.

Oral Therapy

Except in severe or emergency situations, corticosteroid therapy should be instituted with small doses, which may be increased as necessary to provide the desired effect. Dosage adjustment should be more dependent on the disease process than on the age or body weight of the patient. After a favorable response is obtained, the dosage should be decreased gradually to the smallest dose that maintains the desired clinical response. Remissions, exacerbations, and changes in the status of the patient will necessitate dosage adjustment during therapy.

To lessen the likelihood of significant HPA suppression, oral corticosteroids are often given as a single morning dose, rather than in divided doses or as a single evening dose. Alternate-day therapy (ADT) utilizes a single dose of an intermittent-acting preparation administered every other morning, usually in a quantity equivalent to or slightly higher than twice the usual or established daily dose. This regimen is normally employed in long-term therapy to minimize adrenal suppression. A changeover to ADT is usually made only after initial therapy has achieved remission of symptoms. Some patients with asthma or severe perennial rhinitis may experience symptomatic flares on the off-day of ADT.

When medication has been given for five days or longer, discontinuing corticosteroid therapy should be done by gradually tapering the dose given each day. The longer treatment has been in progress, the more gradual should be the tapering process. Too-rapid withdrawal (especially after prolonged adrenocorticoid therapy) can lead to adrenal insufficiency (which can be life-threatening) or to a withdrawal syndrome (not related to HPA suppression) manifested by low-grade fever, myalgia, arthralgia, headache, nausea, vomiting, and a return of the symptoms for which steroids were originally given.

It should be noted from the preceding remarks that the commercially available tapered-dose corticosteroid packs for oral therapy fulfill only one criterion for oral steroid therapy—gradual tapering. They begin with large, divided doses, which by the fourth or fifth day are more physiologic than pharmacologic, rather than the preferred method of a single morning dose that is increased daily as needed until relief occurs. These tapered-dose preparations are helpful in acute, short-lived situations, such as for nose drops withdrawal or to treat symptoms due to an acute pollen or irritant exposure. However, the physician using oral corticosteroids in an active allergy practice will most often need to tailor a dosage regimen for each patient, carefully monitoring dose versus symptoms.

Intravenous Therapy

Corticosteroids given intravenously are usually reserved for severe or life-threatening situations. A single-dose or short-term intravenous administration of a very large dose of steroid ("pulse") therapy has been used for such situations as organ transplant rejection, acute nephritis, adult respiratory distress syndrome, and shock. However, the rapid intravenous administration of large doses of adrenocorticoids has been reported to cause seizures, angioedema, or sudden death associated with cardiac arrhythmias. Also, pulse corticosteroid therapy can increase susceptibility to infection and cause psychic disturbances.

In otolaryngic allergy, the principal use for intravenous glucocorticoid therapy is as an adjunct in the treatment of anaphylaxis. The primary treatment of such an event involves epinephrine (or heparin), oxygen, an antihistamine, and the other measures described in Chapter 41 to treat allergic emergencies. In addition, patients with reactions that do not promptly respond, those requiring respiratory and/or cardiovascular resuscitation, or those with a significant risk of relapse should also be given a rapid-acting corticosteroid intravenously or intramuscularly (e.g., 4 mg dexamethasone).

Intramuscular Therapy

Corticosteroids for intramuscular injection are available in rapid-acting aqueous and slowly absorbed repository forms. The former are chosen for therapy of anaphylaxis (see earlier) and similar acute situations (e.g., drug reactions). Most intramuscular therapy for allergic disorders involves the use of extended-action preparations. These are slow in onset of effect (eight hours to one to two days) and produce gradually decreasing therapeutic effects for up to four weeks. A combination of betamethasone acetate and phosphate (Celestone Soluspan) is unique in that it provides both soluble and repository corticosteroids in a single injection, giving an initial therapeutic burst within one to three hours and providing demonstrable therapeutic effects for over a week. All these repository preparations are useful in providing prolonged pharmacologic glucocorticoid therapy without the necessity of daily dosage adjustment or terminal tapering. However, they may produce significant HPA axis suppression for up to several weeks, and their repeated use should be avoided. Because of the local glucocorticoid effect of muscle wasting, repository corticosteroid should be injected deeply into the gluteal muscle, never into the deltoid, and injections should not be repeatedly given at the same site.

SPECIAL CONSIDERATIONS

Pregnancy

Adrenocorticoids cross the placenta. Animal studies have indicated that corticosteroids administered during pregnancy can increase the observed incidence of cleft palate, placental insufficiency, spontaneous abortion, and intrauterine growth retardation. Adequate studies have not been done in humans, and teratogenic effects in humans have not been confirmed, although some studies indicate that therapeutic doses of adrenocorticoids may increase the risk of placental insufficiency, decreased birth weight, or stillbirth.

Pediatrics

Caution is necessary in administering long-term systemic corticosteroids in pediatric patients because of the risk of growth suppression. Pediatric patients on prolonged steroid therapy also have a greater risk of developing osteoporosis, aseptic necrosis of the femoral head, and cataracts.

Geriatrics

Older patients on long-term adrenocorticoids are more likely to develop hypertension. This age group is also particularly vulnerable to glucocorticoid-induced osteoporosis, especially postmenopausal females.

General

When corticosteroids must be used in treating any of the above groups, careful attention to the general prescribing cautions listed in the preceding section is important. Also, local usage should be considered for these situations when possible.

SPECIAL NEEDS OF THE STEROID-DEPENDENT PATIENT

As already noted, adrenal suppression may occur after administration of exogenous corticosteroids for even a short time. Both the development of and recovery from this condition are highly variable, and the possibility of adrenal hypofunction must always be considered in patients who are receiving (or have recently received) pharmacologic doses of glucocorticoids. Also, even after steroid therapy has ceased and circulating levels of cortisol have returned to normal, the adrenal cortex may not be able to respond normally to stress (such as surgery or overwhelming infection) by producing the larger amounts of adrenocorticoids necessary for such a situation.

When considering surgery in a patient who has received systemic corticosteroids in high dosages and/or for long periods of time, it is often necessary to administer supplemental corticosteroids. The doses of steroid required will vary with each case. Close cooperation with an internist or endocrinologist and good preoperative communication with the anesthesiologist are important in such situations.

REFERENCES

1. Ballin JC: AMA Drug Evaluations. 5th ed. Chicago, American Medical Association, 1983, pp 887–911.
2. USP: Drug Information for the Health Care Provider. 7th ed. Rockville, MD, The United States Pharmacopeial Convention, 1987, pp 56–81.

CHAPTER 26

Management of Asthma

Shirley Murphy, M.D.

Advances in the treatment of asthma in the 1960s were largely devoted to the prevention of death from status asthmaticus. In the 1970s attention was turned to the prevention of acute severe asthma through increased understanding of the pharmacokinetics of around-the-clock administration of theophylline. In the 1980s we are in a period of refinement in the treatment of asthma.[1]

The goal of pharmacotherapy in asthma is to achieve bronchodilation and reduced airway reactivity, allowing the patient to lead a normal life with the least medication side effects. Currently available medications allow the entire disease to be modulated, the inflammation decreased, the airways stabilized, and the asthmatic's life and activity level improved. An asthma medication treatment scheme (Fig. 26–1) suggests medications to use for varying degrees of asthma severity.[2] The classes of medication used in the treatment of asthma are discussed in the following.

BETA-ADRENERGIC AGENTS

Adrenergic agents, such as epinephrine (adrenalin), have been used for over 80 years in the treatment of asthma. Recently, these compounds have been modified to be safer, longer acting, and more site specific. The major chemical structural change has been modification of the ethanolamine side chain to produce greater $beta_2$ selectivity, thus increasing bronchodilation without increasing side effects. The adrenergic agonists can be administered via several routes (Tables 26–1 to 26–3) including parenteral, inhaled, or oral.

Traditionally, in acute asthma the parenteral route has been preferred because of concerns that severe bronchospasm would limit lung disposition of an inhaled medication. However, multiple studies[3–6] have shown inhaled $beta_2$-agonists to be as effective in relieving bronchospasm as parenteral delivery, with less side effects. The inhaled route is also preferred by the patient.

When using beta-agonists for chronic asthma therapy, a decision arises as to which is preferred, oral or inhaled therapy.[7] Onset of action

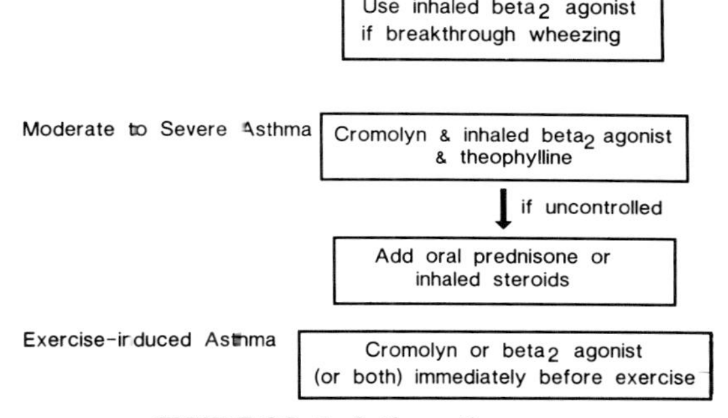

FIGURE 26–1. Asthma therapy.

Table 26–1. SELECTED SYSTEMIC BETA-ADRENERGIC AGENTS

Drug	Formulation	Dose
Epinephrine HCl	1:1000 (1 mg/ml)	0.01 mg/kg up to 0.5 mg subcutaneously every 20 minutes for 3 doses
Sus-Phrine (Berlex)	1:200 (5 mg/ml) suspension	0.005–0.01 mL/kg not to exceed 0.15 ml every 6–10 hours subcutaneously
Terbutaline Bricanyl (Merrell Dow) Brethine (Geigy)	1 mg/ml solution for injection	Subcutaneous 0.01 mg/kg up to 0.5 mg every 2–6 hours as needed. Intravenous 10 μg/kg over 10 minutes loading dose, followed by 0.2 μg/kg/min, increasing as necessary. (Close monitoring necessary.)
Albuterol	(Not available in U.S.)	10 μg/kg intravenously over 10 minutes, followed by 0.2 μg/kg/min. Increase by 0.1 μg/kg steps every 15 minutes according to response. (Close monitoring necessary.)

of medication is more rapid by the inhaled route, occurring in three to six minutes, peaking in 20 to 60 minutes, and lasting four to six hours. When given orally, the onset of action occurs in 30 minutes, peaks at one to two hours, and lasts three to six hours. When taken by inhalation, a smaller dose can be used to achieve the same degree of bronchodilation. For example, two puffs of a dose of 0.01 mg per puff would give approximately the same clinical bronchodilating effect as a much larger 2 to 4 mg dose taken by the oral route.

Side effects of the beta-adrenergic agents have been a concern, and recent warnings by the FDA concerning possible synergistic toxicity of combining beta-agonists with theophylline have added to the concern.[8] The major safety issues center on the development of tolerance with the long-term administration of beta$_2$-adrenergic agents, and the potential increased cardiotoxicity when these compounds are used in combination with theophylline. Both aspects have been implicated and widely debated as possibly contributing to deaths from asthma. Because of these concerns, it is important to be aware that the side effects of the beta$_2$ agents, including tachycardia, palpitations, arrhythmias, and tremor, are markedly less with the inhaled route of delivery of beta-adrenergic agents. In fact, many physicians caution against the use of the oral beta-adrenergic agents for patients over 45 years of age.

Clinical studies[9] have indicated that the two most important factors for a good clinical response from beta$_2$ agonists delivered by a metered-dose inhaler are good coordination and a four-second breath-holding period. Coordination problems can largely be overcome by the use of a spacer device[10] and proper demonstration.

Inhaled beta$_2$-agonists are the drug of choice for patients with infrequent episodic bouts of asthma and for relieving acute bronchospasm.

METHYLXANTHINES

For around-the-clock therapy of chronic asthma, theophylline has been shown to be as

Table 26–2. SELECTED ORAL BETA-ADRENERGIC AGENTS

Oral Preparation	Size and Form	Dosage: *Pediatric*	Dosage: *Adult*
Albuterol Ventolin (Glaxo) Proventil (Schering)	2 and 4 mg tablets 2 mg/5 ml syrup	0.1–0.2 mg/kg every 6–8 hr	2–4 mg every 6–8 hr; may increase as tolerated
Metaproterenol Alupent (Boehringer)	10 and 20 mg tablets 10 mg/5 ml syrup	0.5 mg/kg every 4–6 hr; increase by 0.25 mg/kg as tolerated	20 mg every 4–6 hr; may increase as tolerated
Terbutaline Brethine (Geigy) Bricanyl (Merrell Dow)	2.5 and 5.0 mg tablets	0.075 mg/kg every 6 hr; may increase by 0.025 mg/kg as tolerated	5 mg every 6–8 hr; may increase as tolerated

Table 26–3. INHALED ASTHMA MEDICATIONS

Inhaled Preparation	Size and Form	Dosage: Pediatric	Dosage: Adult
Beta$_2$-Agonists			
Isoetharine			
Isoetharine HCl Inhalation (Roxane)	0.1%, 0.125%, 0.2% nebulizer solution	0.1–0.2 mg/kg every 2–4 hr	3–5 mg undiluted via nebulizer with O_2 at 4–6 L/min over 15–20 min
Bronkosol Unit-dose (Breon) (Various)	0.25%, 0.5%, 1% nebulizer solution		0.5% and 1% solutions diluted 1:3 with 0.9% sodium chloride
Bronkometer (Breon)	340 μg/spray metered-dose inhaler	1–2 puffs every 4–6 hr; may increase to every hour for acute attacks	1–2 puffs every 4–6 hr; may increase to every 2 hr for acute attacks
Metaproterenol			
Alupent (Boehringer-Ingelheim)	5% (50 mg/ml) solution for nebulization	0.25–0.5 mg/kg every 2–4 hr; maximum 15 mg	5–15 inhalations of 5% undiluted from hand bulb nebulizer or 0.3 ml (15 mg) diluted with 2.5 ml 0.9% sodium chloride in nebulizer every 2–4 hr
Alupent Metered-dose inhaler (Boehringer-Ingelheim)	0.65 mg/puff MDI powder suspension	1–2 puffs every 4–6 hr and prior to exercise	2–3 puffs every 4–6 hr and prior to exercise
Albuterol			
Ventolin (Glaxo) Proventil (Schering)	90 μg/puff MDI	1–2 puffs every 4–6 hrs and prior to exercise	1–2 puffs every 4–6 hr and prior to exercise
	0.5% (5 mg/ml) solution for nebulization	0.05–0.15 mg/kg every 2–6 hr Acute attack: every 20 min in hospital with monitoring	2.5–5 mg every 2–6 hr as needed
Terbutaline			
Brethaire (Geigy) Inhaler	0.2 mg/puff MDI	1–2 puffs every 4–6 hr and before exercise	1–2 puffs every 4–6 hr and prior to exercise
Brethine (Geigy) Bricanyl (Merrill Dow)	0.1% (1 mg/ml) solution in 0.9% sodium chloride (for injection); not approved for this use	0.1–0.3 mg/kg inhaled every 2–6 hr as needed Acute attack: every 20 min in hospital with monitoring	5–7 mg (5–7 ml) undiluted inhaled every 4–6 hr as needed
Bitolterol mesylate			
Tornalate (Breon)	0.37 mg/spray MDI	1–2 puffs every 4–6 hr	1–3 puffs every 4–6 hr
Anticholinergics			
Atropine sulfate ophthalmic solution	0.5% (5 mg/ml)	0.05–0.075 mg/kg every 4–6 hr	0.025–0.05 mg/kg every 6 hr
Ipratropium bromide Atrovent (Boehringer-Ingelheim)	18 mg/puff MDI	1–2 puffs every 4–6 hr	2–3 puffs every 4–6 hr
Cromolyn NA			
Spinhaler	20 mg/capsule	1 capsule 4 times daily	1 capsule 4 times daily
Metered-dose inhaler	800 μg/puff MDI	1–2 puffs 4–6 times daily	1–2 puffs 4–6 times daily
Nebulizer solution	20 mg/2 ml ampule	1 ampule nebulized 3–4 times daily	1 ampule nebulized 3–4 times daily
Corticosteroids			
Beclomethasone dipropionate	42 μg/puff MDI	1–2 puffs 3–4 times daily	1–2 puffs 3–4 times daily
Flunisolide	250 μg/puff MDI	1–2 puffs b.i.d.–q.i.d	1–2 puffs b.i.d.–q.i.d.
Triamcinolone acetonide	100 μg/puff MDI	1–2 puffs every 6–8 hr	1–2 puffs every 6–8 hr

effective as cromolyn[11]; however, both its efficacy and toxicity are directly related to its serum concentration. Because the therapeutic index is low (the range of serum concentration optimal for bronchodilator activity and that which is toxic is narrow, 5 to 20 μg/ml), agents that affect the metabolism of the drug in the liver can markedly affect the safety and clinical efficacy of the drug. Also, substantial intersubject variation in elimination rate occurs, and therefore the dose needs to be individualized.[12]

Starting theophylline therapy with a small dose of theophylline and increasing the dose by about 25 per cent at four- to five-day intervals will cause less side effects and better patient tolerance.[13] Ideally, all patients who are treated with chronic theophylline therapy should have a serum concentration measured initially and at six-month intervals. Many factors can affect serum theophylline levels, and the level only gives one point in time.

In dosing theophylline, the patient's lean body weight is multipled by the number of recommended milligrams per kilograms for the patient's weight. This gives the total milligrams of theophylline for a 24-hour period, which must be divided again by the duration of action of the product. For example, short-acting theophyllines must be given every six hours, so the 24-hour total would have to be divided by four and that amount given every six hours. A 12-hour product would be given twice a day, so the total 24-hour dose per kilogram would be divided by two and that amount administered every 12 hours. With a 24-hour preparation, the entire dose would be given once a day (Table 26–4).

Short-acting or immediate-release theophyllines are used to treat occasional acute exacerbations of asthma, and sustained-release or long-acting theophyllines are used for chronic maintenance therapy. The short-acting preparations are available as liquids, tablets, and a rectal solution that give an immediate blood level of theophylline decreasing gradually over a four- to six-hour period. Somophyllin Rectal Solution may be useful in the vomiting child and has been shown to have reliable release characteristics. This rectal solution should not be confused with rectal suppositories, which are erratically absorbed and are potentially very dangerous.

Sustained-release products are formulated to release theophylline gradually at a constant rate over an extended period of time; however, they differ in the speed and completeness of their absorption and, therefore, cannot be used interchangeably.[12] Slow-release products should not be dissolved, crushed, or chewed, but bead-filled capsules can be sprinkled over soft food for children. Table 26–5 describes selected theophylline preparations. Table 26–6 presents guidelines in the choice of a theophylline preparation.

Table 26–4. THEOPHYLLINE DOSAGE

Patient Type	Mean Theophylline Clearance	Oral Theophylline Dose
Children		
Neonate	0.020 L/hr/kg	3–9 mg/kg/day
1 mo–6 mo	0.033 L/hr/kg	10 mg/kg/day
6 mo–1 yr	0.067 L/hr/kg	15 mg/kg/day
1–9 yr	0.094 L/hr/kg	24 mg/kg/day
9–12 yr	0.084 L/hr/kg	20 mg/kg/day
12–18 yr	0.077 L/hr/kg	18 mg/kg/day
Adults		
Nonsmoking	0.055 L/hr/kg	12–15 mg/kg/day
Smokers	0.080 L/hr/kg	20 mg/kg/day
Cor pulmonale	0.030 L/hr/kg	6–10 mg/kg/day
Hepatic cirrhosis	0.020 L/hr/kg	2–5 mg/kg/day
Congestive heart failure	0.030 L/hr/kg	6–10 mg/kg/day

Hint:
1. Start lower than usual recommended dose. Obtain blood level after three days and increase slowly.
2. Always use ideal body weight to calculate dose.

Concerning their use, *The Medical Letter* states:

> Sustained-release theophylline preparations can be effective for the treatment of asthma, particularly in children and adult smokers, but variability in absorption and metabolism may require monitoring of serum concentrations. There is no convincing evidence that any FDA-approved theophylline is clinically superior to any other. More evidence is needed to confirm the reliability of sustained-release products taken only once every 24 hours.[14]

Of increasing concern are side effects occurring with theophylline therapy. In many patients these are related to the serum concentration. Theophylline is eliminated mainly by biotransformation in the liver, with adult smokers and children metabolizing theophylline rapidly with a serum half-life of approximately four hours or less. In nonsmoking adults, the half-life of theophylline may be eight hours or longer. Many disorders, including cirrhosis, congestive heart

Table 26–5. SELECTED THEOPHYLLINE PREPARATIONS

Form	Name	Dosing Interval		Advantages
		Pediatric	*Adult*	
Liquid	Somophyllin oral liquid (18 mg/ml)	q 4–6 h	q 6–8 h	No sugar No alcohol Most concentrated Dye-free FDA-approved Used as scientific standard
Rectal solution	Somophyllin (51.4 mg/ml)	q 6 h	q 6–8 h	Reliable, rapid absorption Useful in vomiting child Useful in acute asthma when p.o. meds not tolerated
Sustained-release tablets	Theo-Dur 100, 200, 300, 450 mg (scored)	q 12 h	q 12–24 h	Consistent release characteristics Unaffected by food q 24 hr dosing possible in nonsmoking adults
	Quibron-T/SR 300 mg (multiscored)	q 8–12 h	q 12 h	Consistent release Handy multiscored tablet allows titration up and down with one size
Sustained-release capsules	Slo-bid 50, 100, 200, 300 mg	q 12 h	q 12 h	Consistent release q 12 hr in children Can be sprinkled

failure, severe obstructive pulmonary disease, and viral infections such as influenza, decrease the rate of theophylline clearance. The metabolism of theophylline may also be slowed by the concomitant use of cimetidine, propranolol, allopurinol, and macrolide antibiotics such as erythromycin. Use of these medications with theophylline may result in toxic serum levels. On the other hand, Dilantin and barbiturates increase theophylline clearance.

Besides the potential life-threatening neurologic and cardiovascular side effects of theophylline, there are increasing reports of soft neurologic symptoms occurring in children, including decreased attention span, concentration, and short-term memory.[15]

Theophylline is an effective drug for the treatment of asthma, but because of potential for toxic effects, serum levels should be carefully monitored.

CROMOLYN SODIUM

The allergy section of the American Academy of Pediatrics issued a position paper on the management of asthma in childhood stating, "Theophylline in a dose that maintains serum concentrations between 10–20 mg/ml or cromolyn is the drug of choice for managing asthma when symptoms are continuous or recur frequently."[16] The major advantages of cromolyn over theophylline are its lack of side effects, its ease of administration (no serum levels), and its unique properties of modulating lung inflammation leading to a decrease in nonspecific bronchial hyperreactivity.

Cromolyn sodium was discovered as a result of investigations with the naturally occurring antispasmodic khellin. This furanochromone, derived from the Mediterranean plant *Ammi*

Table 26–6. GUIDELINES FOR CHOICE OF THEOPHYLLINE

Single entity theophylline	Combinations have no advantages and may have greater toxicity
No salts of theophylline	May not be able to correctly interpret blood levels
No alcohol	Liquids with alcohol may lead to toxic effects in children
FDA-approved form	Assures preparations have had adequate evaluation and continued quality control
Consistent release characteristics	Alterations may occur with food → toxic or subtherapeutic levels
Convenient dosage forms	Bead-filled capsules or scored tablets give dosing flexibility

Choose one liquid, one sustained-release tablet, and one bead-filled capsule, and gain experience with them!

visnaga, was studied because its seeds had been used since ancient times as a smooth muscle relaxant. It was observed that, although khellin derivatives in which the 2-methyl groups had been replaced by a carboxylic acid moiety had no bronchodilating properties, they inhibited bronchoconstriction induced by antigen challenge.[17]

Cromolyn sodium was synthesized in 1965 and became available for use in the United Kingdom in 1968 and in the United States in 1973.

Despite intensive research, a precise mechanism explaining the clinical activity of cromolyn sodium has not been completely delineated. Its primary mode of action is considered to be that of stabilizing mast cells, which prevents the subsequent release of mediators.[17] Cromolyn sodium inhibits mast cell degranulation produced by immunoglobulin E (IgE) antibody reactions and nonimmunologic substances.

Prior administration of cromolyn sodium blocks both antigen-induced bronchospasm and also the rise in serum chemotactic activity.[16] In a clinical study, three months of cromolyn sodium therapy in asthmatic patients resulted in a significant decrease in the number of eosinophils recovered from bronchoalveolar lavage fluid.[17]

The cellular mechanisms by which cromolyn sodium inhibits mast cell mediator release have not been definitely established. Like many other secretory systems, the antigen-induced release of histamine and other mediators from mast cells requires extracellular calcium. Incubation of mast cells with cromolyn sodium inhibits calcium influx through the mast cell's membrane, probably by phosphorylation of a specific protein with a molecular weight of 78,000 daltons representing an off switch to mast cell mediator release.[18, 19]

Cromolyn also inhibits the activation of other cell types, such as peripheral blood leukocytes, monocytes, and platelet activating factors. Cromolyn sodium inhaled before antigen challenge will block the depressive effect that antigen has on mucociliary clearance.[20] Cromolyn sodium has not demonstrated significant smooth muscle relaxant properties. However, some trials have demonstrated an acute improvement in pulmonary function tests following cromolyn administration. In vitro cromolyn attenuates the contractile responses to acetylcholine, histamine, serotonin, bradykinin, and PFG_a in a dose-dependent fashion. In addition, cromolyn potentiates the isoproterenol, epinephrine, PGE_2, and salbutamol-induced relaxation responses.[17]

Cromolyn has been shown to inhibit bronchoconstriction induced in humans by a number of nonimmunologic triggers, including exercise, inhalation of cold air, sulfur dioxide, and ultrasonically nebulized distilled water or fog.[17, 21] Cromolyn sodium inhibits excitatory responses of C fiber sensory nerve endings in the dog lung that initiate reflex bronchoconstrictor responses.[22]

In addition to the immediate bronchoconstriction following inhalation challenge with antigen, many asthmatics will undergo a second bronchoconstrictive response four to 12 hours later, known as the late asthmatic response (LAR). This is a more prolonged response, is less responsive to reversal with bronchodilators, and is associated with more severe asthma and increased bronchial hyperreactivity.[17]

Cromolyn sodium blocks both the immediate bronchospasm and the LAR when administered prior to challenge.[23] $Beta_2$-agonists will block the early response but not LAR, whereas steroids have no effect on the early response but will block the LAR. Cromolyn is unique in blocking both the early and late asthmatic response. Because the LAR is associated with severe asthma and also correlates with increased bronchial hyperreactivity, the role of cromolyn in preventing the LAR may be one of the keys to its ability to control and improve chronic asthma.

One interesting aspect of the pharmacology of cromolyn sodium is its long-term effect on reducing bronchial hyperreactivity. Airway hyperreactivity is the characteristic feature of bronchial asthma, and the degree of bronchial responsiveness as measured by histamine challenge has been shown to correlate with the severity of asthma, the diurnal fluctuations in peak flow rate, and the amounts of medication needed to control symptoms.[17] Cromolyn was first shown to decrease airway reactivity in a 10-year follow-up of severe asthma in children in 1975[24] and confirmed in other clinical trials.[17, 25]

There are hundreds of published clinical trials demonstrating the clinical effectiveness of cromolyn sodium in controlling mild to moderate chronic asthma.[17, 26–32]

In 1969 the Drug Committee of the American Academy of Allergy instituted a double-blind, placebo-controlled trial of cromolyn sodium in 252 asthmatic patients (adults and children) in the United States. The study's objective was to determine the short-term (four weeks) therapeutic effectiveness and safety of cromolyn sodium 20 mg qid via Spinhaler. Cromolyn sodium was significantly better than placebo in patient symptom scoring, physician evaluation, and concomitant medication reduction, with 72 per cent of the patients improved after active treatment. No significant side effects were encountered in the study.[17]

In 1972 the Brompton Hospital/Medical Research Council evaluated the efficacy and safety of cromolyn sodium in severe adult extrinsic and intrinsic asthmatic patients in a one-year, double-blind, placebo-controlled, parallel-group study. By the end of 52 weeks, 9 of 35 patients taking cromolyn had failed, and 31 of 39 taking either beta-agonists or placebo had dropped from the study. Treatment with cromolyn sodium was statistically better from the fourth week of treatment to the end of the study. Patients who received cromolyn sodium twice daily had the same control of their asthma as those who received it four times daily. No factors were predictive of response to cromolyn sodium, including FEV_2, eosinophilia, allergy history, skin test results, and age. Among 20 patients classified as extrinsic asthmatics, 3 (15 per cent) failed cromolyn therapy, and 4 of 9 (44 per cent) classified as intrinsic asthmatics failed. No evidence of toxic effects or adverse reactions was seen during the study.[27]

Long-term clinical trials in humans have not demonstrated any tachyphylaxis. In addition, the dosage of cromolyn sodium can be decreased after one month of therapy to three times a day and further tapered to twice a day, supporting the theory that tachyphylaxis does not occur during therapy.

Cromolyn sodium as a 1 per cent solution has been studied in several clinical trials in very young asthmatics. Mellon et al. studied cromolyn sodium 1 per cent nebulizer solution in 19 young asthmatic children (mean age 5 to 9 years) who required daily oral bronchodilators but not corticosteroid maintenance. During the eight-week active treatment phase, significant reductions in asthmatic symptoms, physician assessment of asthma severity, and concomitant bronchodilator usage were observed in 16 of 19 children. These 16 patients continued to receive nebulizer cromolyn sodium treatment for at least one year after completion of the study. During the six-month interval of cromolyn maintenance, there was a marked reduction in emergency visits, corticosteroid courses, and hospitalizations.[28]

Several short-term trials evaluating cromolyn sodium 2 mg qid delivered by pressurized metered-dose inhaler have recently been conducted. Rubin et al. compared cromolyn with placebo in a 12-week, double-blind, crossover trial in 31 adult asthmatic patients. Those who received cromolyn sodium showed significant improvement in breathlessness at rest, breathlessness on exertion, and morning peak expiratory flow rate (PEFR). Usage of bronchodilators (theophylline and aerosol $beta_2$-agonists combined) significantly decreased during cromolyn sodium therapy.[29]

Three therapeutic forms of cromolyn sodium are available in the United States: 20 mg powdered capsule delivered via Spinhaler apparatus; 1 per cent solution containing cromolyn sodium 20 mg in 2 ml distilled water delivered by a compressor-driven nebulizer; and a pressurized metered-dose inhaler that releases 1 mg per actuation (800 μg delivered).

The Spinhaler was developed to overcome coordination problems in aerosol therapy. It is a small open plastic tube containing a propeller-like rotor that revolves at high speed through the device. Fast air flow breaks up the cromolyn from a 20 mg capsule into respirable particles.

The Spinhaler delivery system can be utilized by any patient older than about 4 years of age. Being a breath-activated system, it requires a little coordination, no spacer devices are necessary, and there are no fluorocarbons. The starting dose is usually one 20 mg capsule four times daily. When symptoms are in control, usually after one to two months of therapy, the schedule can be decreased to three times a day and then twice daily.

Cromolyn sodium has been available in the United States as a 1 per cent nebulizer solution since 1982. It contains cromolyn sodium 20 mg in 2 ml purified water with no preservatives and is packaged in 2 ml unit-dose glass ampules. The clear, colorless solution has a pH of 4.0 to 7.0 It is delivered with a power-operated nebulizer via face mask or mouthpiece. The face mask has the potential of delivering the medication to the entire upper airway, which may be an advantage in patients who also have allergic rhinitis.

Cromolyn sodium nebulizer solution has been shown to be physically and chemically compatible for up to 60 minutes when mixed in vitro with metaproterenol sulfate solution, isoproterenol hydrochloride solution, isoetharine hydrochloride 0.25 per cent inhalation solution, epinephrine hydrochloride solution, terbutaline sulfate sterile aqueous solution, and 20 per cent acetylcysteine solution. Similarly, cromolyn sodium did not adversely affect the stability of the individual bronchodilator/mucolytic drugs in the admixtures. Therefore, it is possible to make a mixture of medications that can be simultaneously nebulized to the patient.

Cromolyn sodium nebulizer solution has proved especially useful for (1) children under 4 years of age, (2) patients who are unable to tolerate the powder formulation because of extremely hyperreactive airways, (3) more severely ill patients who benefit from the bronchodilator/cromolyn sodium mixture, (4) the prevention of virus-induced wheezing in children, and (5) patients who have cough variant asthma. With the nebulizer solution, when the patient is experiencing bronchospasm, a bronchodilator may be added directly to the solution.

Cromolyn sodium became available in a pressurized metered-dose aerosol unit in 1986. Each canister contains micronized cromolyn sodium, sorbitan trioleate, with dichlorotetrafluoroethane and dichlorodifluoromethane as propellants. Each 1 mg metered spray delivers approximately 800 μg cromolyn sodium to the patient, with most of the individual particles of cromolyn sodium having a diameter not greater than 5 μ. The recommended dosage is two inhalations or 1.6 mg qid at regular intervals. To prevent acute bronchospasm following exercise or exposure to cold, dry air or environmental agents, the usual dose is two metered-dose sprays 10 to 15 minutes but not more than 60 minutes before exposure to the precipitating factor.

Because of the unique prophylactic and safety properties of cromolyn sodium, it is recommended as a first-line agent in the management of mild to moderately severe asthma. As with all inhaled medications, it is important that patients learn proper inhalation techniques. The starting dose of cromolyn is 20 mg via Spinhaler or nebulizer or 2 mg delivered by pressurized metered-dose inhaler taken at regular intervals four times daily. When the patient is stabilized, the Spincaps or nebulizer may be tapered to three times daily and then twice daily (Table 26–7). If the results are equivocal after a four-week trial, the clinical trial period should be doubled during the last six weeks of the trial.

Because there is a correlation between the degree of airway patency and the amount of cromolyn reaching the lungs, it is important that the airways are patent for maximal drug delivery. Depending on the degree of obstruction, this can be achieved with concomitant bronchodilator and/or corticosteroid therapy. It is important not to stop cromolyn if the patient is wheezing; the nebulizer solution may be used during wheezing episodes and the Spinhaler may be continued during an exacerbation of asthma by preceding it with a bronchodilator.

In acute situations, cromolyn sodium is effective in blocking an encounter with a known allergen (animal or pollen exposure), exercise-induced asthma, cold air– or fog-induced asthma, and reflex-induced bronchospasm (SO_2 exposure). Cromolyn sodium is most effective in blocking pollen-induced asthma if started one week before the anticipated pollination, although it may be started at any time during the season.

Long-term use of cromolyn is appropriate for patients of any age with mild to moderately severe asthma requiring continuous medication, patients with dual or late asthmatic responses,

Table 26–7. USE OF CROMOLYN IN CHRONIC ASTHMA

Mild to moderate asthma in patients *older* than 5 yr	Mild to moderate asthma in patient *younger* than 5 yr
↓	↓
One 20 mg Spincap or 2 puffs Intal Inhaler qid for one month then decreasing to tid and bid	One 20 mg ampule cromolyn nebulizer solution via power-driven compressor nebulization qid for first month then may reduce to tid and then bid
↓	↓
If exacerbation occurs, may add $beta_2$-agonist before cromolyn	May be mixed with any bronchodilator
	↓
	May also be used in older patients and adults with severe asthma or during exacerbations

and patients with excessive airway hyperreactivity.

CORTICOSTEROIDS

Corticosteroids are powerful and important drugs in the treatment of asthma. When first introduced for the treatment of asthma, they were hailed as miracle drugs. As experience with these compounds was extended, so was the appreciation of the severity of the side effects. Advances in understanding of the physiologic properties of the oral agents has led to the discovery of compounds that can be delivered by the aerosol route with decreased adverse effects. When used appropriately in the treatment of asthma, corticosteroids can be very safe and effective.

Corticosteroids have basically three indications in the treatment of asthma:

1. The treatment of status asthmaticus.
2. The treatment of severe, acute exacerbations.
3. Chronic maintenance therapy in patients who are not controlled on cromolyn and/or bronchodilators.

In status asthmaticus, corticosteroids restore beta-adrenergic responsiveness and decrease the lung inflammation and edema. Clinical trials in status asthmaticus have shown that patients treated with steroids have better arterial oxygenation and pulmonary functions than do those treated with placebo.[33–35]

Although there is no agreement as to the proper dosage for use in status asthmaticus, 1 to 2 mg/kg of methylprednisolone may be given every 6 to 12 hours for the first 24 to 48 hours and then rapidly tapered.[36] There is no doubt that the potential benefits of corticosteroids, given during an acute severe asthmatic attack, greatly outweigh the unfounded concern regarding side effects. There is no evidence that short-term therapy will induce a state of steroid dependency. Additionally, steroids should always be used during episodes of stress such as in status asthmaticus if they have been employed during the previous year. Corticosteroids are also useful in high-risk patients treated as outpatients who are having acute exacerbations, when bronchodilators only partially reverse the acute episodes. This often occurs in young children whose asthma is exacerbated by viral upper respiratory infections. These patients may benefit from keeping oral steroids at home and taking them at the first sign of an exacerbation of their asthma. Patients who are on chronic or oral steroid therapy will often need an increase in their steroid dosage during an acute exacerbation.

Corticosteroids are also useful in the management of chronic severe asthma and should be considered in patients whose pulmonary function testing shows moderate airway obstruction despite maximum therapy with cromolyn and bronchodilators. Also, patients who have a repetitive pattern of steroid-responsive acute attacks of asthma may need chronic oral corticosteroid therapy. This cyclic pattern of multiple burst or oral steroids can often be interrupted by the use of chronic steroid therapy administered either as a metered-dose aerosol (MDI) or as oral prednisone given every other day.[37]

Corticosteroid side effects vary with the duration and timing of the administration as well as the type of steroid preparation used. The least side effects occur when steroids are given in short courses with intervals of several weeks or months without steroid treatment. Alternate-day therapy, that is, a single morning dose every other day, is the next preferable regimen. The third preference is daily therapy given as a single morning dose. If these methods are not successful, multiple doses can be given throughout the day. Long-acting corticosteroids, such as triamcinolone, dexamethasone, or betamethasone, should not be given to asthmatic patients in whom alternate-day therapy will eventually be recommended. Prednisone, prednisolone, and methylprednisolone are short-acting preparations that are appropriate for alternate-day therapy.

Topical corticosteroid aerosols were introduced approximately 10 years ago to decrease side effects. Aerosol preparations are highly active topically, but are poorly soluble in water. Although they are systemically absorbed, they are rapidly degraded by the liver. Experience with the use of beclomethasone dipropionate for a decade has demonstrated that a standard dose of 400 μg/day is not associated with clinical side effects. A study by Wyatt et al.[38] demonstrated that adrenal suppression may be detected when therapeutic doses are taken if both urinary cortisol and plasma cortisol are measured. However, doses of 400 to 600 μg/day did not result in gross suppression or interfere with the HPA axis in most studies. Toogood et al.[39] have advocated using larger doses of steroids than those initially recommended. However, these larger doses may result in a higher incidence of side effects. The concurrent administration of intranasal steroids may have an additive effect on adrenal suppression.

Adrenal suppression has been reported with the continued inhalation of beclomethasone but physical changes of hyperadrenal corticism have not, and children maintained on the aerosol for three to five years have grown normally. Deaths due to adrenal insufficiency have occurred in asthmatic patients during and after the transfer from systemic to inhaled corticosteroids. Because months may be required for recovery of the hypothalamic-pituitary-adrenal function after withdrawal of systemic steroids, large doses of systemic steroids should be administered during severe asthmatic attacks or other periods of severe stress. The single most important side effect is oral candidiasis. In the literature, its occurrence varies from 0 to 77 per cent. Recently, a new side effect of inhaled corticosteroid therapy that is of interest to otorhinolaryngologists has been reported. Dysphonia, or hoarseness, of the voice was found in patients using inhaled steroids. When these patients were examined with fiberoptic laryngoscopy, 9 out of the 14 patients demonstrated a bilateral adductor vocal cord deformity characterized by bowing of both cords on phonation. The authors felt this was due to a muscle paresis. In a prospective study, this same disorder was found to develop in 3 out of 9 patients examined monthly after the institution of inhaled steroid therapy.

There are many adverse consequences of corticosteroid usage. However, these adverse effects can be minimized by observing certain precautions, such as considering the plasma half-life of the particular steroid agent used, the duration of therapy, the time of day that the steroid is administered, the total dose, and the route of administration. Corticosteroids are very important in the management of severe asthma, but need to be treated with great respect and caution.[40]

ANTICHOLINERGIC AGENTS

One of the oldest forms of therapy for respiratory disorders is the inhalation of anticholinergic drugs. Interest in these drugs has been revived in the last 10 years with the introduction of synthetic compounds with few side effects. The anticholinergic drugs currently available to treat airway disease are atropine sulfate, atropine methyl nitrate, and ipratropium bromide. Unlike atropine sulfate, the last two drugs are quaternary ammonium compounds and they are long-lasting, are poorly absorbed from mucosal surfaces when given locally, and do not readily penetrate the blood-brain barrier. Consequently, they have few of the undesirable side effects of atropine sulfate. This class of drugs competes with acetylcholine on smooth muscle receptors, and only inhibits acetylcholine on nicotine receptors in very high concentrations.[41] Single-dose studies with ipratropium bromide and atropine methyl nitrate demonstrate that both are effective bronchodilators without major side effects when given in the usual therapeutic doses. However, in most investigations the anticholinergics have been found to be less potent bronchodilators than the sympathomimetics. The chief disadvantage of the anticholinergics is their slow onset of action, as 60 to 90 minutes are frequently required before maximum bronchodilation is achieved.[42]

Anticholinergics are frequently quite helpful in the treatment of asthma that has resisted other forms of therapy, and also in cough variant asthma. In addition, reports have suggested that patients with chronic bronchitis show greater bronchodilation after inhaled anticholinergics than with sympathomimetics.[42, 43]

There has been a recent interest in the use of ipratropium bromide in the treatment of childhood asthma. Ipratropium bromide has been shown to be effective in infants at least 3 to 30 months of age.[44] Studies by Davis et al. have determined that a dose-dependent bronchodilation becomes significant at the 75 μg dose level with this compound.[45] Significant effects on FEV_1 were observed 15 minutes after drug administration, with maximal effects at 45 minutes. A plateau was reached at a dose of 75 to 250 μg, and this is therefore the recommended dose range for ipratropium in this patient population. All doses were associated with essentially no side effects and no changes in either heart rate or blood pressure.[45] These investigators have further examined the combined use of salbutamol and ipratropium bromide in the treatment of severe, acute asthma and have demonstrated that inhaled ipratropium produced a significant additional increase in FEV_1 after maximal effect from salbutamol had been reached.[46] This would imply that many children have a significant cholinergic component to their bronchospasm, and this may be responsible for some of the residual airway obstruction seen after treatment with salbutamol alone (salbutamol [UK] = albuterol [US]). The magnitude of this response appears to be less in children than that reported for adults, suggesting that cholinergic-mediated bronchospasm is a more prominent component in adults than in children with asthma.[45, 46]

SUMMARY

The clinician has a wide variety of pharmacologic agents for use in the treatment of asthma. Asthmatics differ in their response to medication, so therapy must be individualized. An approach to the management of acute and chronic asthma is given in Figure 26–1.

REFERENCES

1. Mansman HC: The evaluation, control, and modification of continuing asthma. Clin Chest Med 1:339, 1980.
2. Mansman HC Jr: Bronchodilation or bronchoregulation; the role of cromolyn vis-a-vis theophylline. Clinical Proceedings CHNMC, July/August and September/October, 39:271, 1983.
3. Schwartz AL, et al: Management of acute asthma in childhood. Am J Dis Child 134:474, 1980.
4. Pancorbo S, et al: Subcutaneous epinephrine versus nebulized terbutaline in the emergency treatment of asthma. Clin Pharm 2:45, 1983.
5. Tinkelman DG, et al: Comparison of nebulized terbutaline and subcutaneous epinephrine in the treatment of acute asthma. Ann Allergy 50:398, 1983.
6. Becker AB, et al: Inhaled salbutamol (albuterol) vs. injected epinephrine in the treatment of acute asthma in children. J Pediatr 102:465, 1983.
7. Shim C, Williams H: Bronchial response to oral versus aerosol metaproterenol in asthma. Ann Intern Med 93:428, 1980.
8. Nicklas RA, Whitehurst VE, Donolhue RF, et al: Concomitant use of beta adrenergic agonists and methylxanthines. J Allergy Clin Immunol 73:20, 1984.
9. Newman SP, Pavia D, Garland N, et al: Effects of various inhalation modes on the deposition of radioactive pressurized aerosols. Eur J Respir Dis 63 [Suppl 119]:57, 1982.
10. Kelly HW: New B_2 adrenergic agonist aerosols. Clin Pharm 4:393, 1985.
11. Furukawa CT, Shapiro GG, Kraemer MJ, et al: A double-blind study comparing the effectiveness of cromolyn sodium and sustained-release theophylline in childhood asthma. Pediatrics 74:453, 1984.
12. Szefler SJ: Practical considerations in the safe and effective use of theophylline. Pediatr Clin North Am 30:943, 1983.
13. Weinberger M: Theophylline. J Allergy Clin Immunol 73:525, 1984.
14. Sustained-release theophyllines. Med Lett 26:1, 1984.
15. Furukawa CT, Shapiro GG, DuHamer T, et al: Learning and behavior problems associated with theophylline therapy. Lancet 1:621, 1984.
16. Easton J, Hilman B, Shapiro G, Weinberger M: Management of asthma. Pediatrics 68:874, 1981.
17. Murphy S, Kelly HW: Cromolyn sodium: a review of mechanisms and clinical use in asthma. Drug Intell Clin Pharm 21:22, 1987.
18. Theoharides TC, Sieghart W, Greengard P, Douglas WW: Anti-allergic drug cromolyn may inhibit histamine secretion by regulating phosphorylation of a mast cell protein. Science 207:80, 1980.
19. Atkins PC, Norman NE, Zweiman B: Antigen-induced neutrophil chemotactic activity in man: correlation with bronchospasm and inhibition by disodium cromoglycate. J Allergy Clin Immunol 62:1491, 1978.
20. Wanner A: The role of mucociliary dysfunction in bronchial asthma. Am J Med 67:477, 1979.
21. Sheppard D, Saisho A, Nadel JA, Boushey HA: Exercise increases sulfur dioxide-induced bronchoconstriction in asthmatic subjects. Am Rev Respir Dis 123:486, 1981.
22. Harris MG, Parkes PEG, Lessof MH, Orr TSC: Role of bronchial irritant receptors in asthma: a collaborative study. Lancet 1:5, 1981.
23. Booij-Noord H, Orie NGM, deVries K: Immediate and late bronchial obstructive reactions to inhalation of house dust and protective effects of disodium cromoglycate and prednisolone. J Allergy 48:344, 1971.
24. Dickson W, Cole M: Severe asthma in children—a 10 year follow up. *In* Pepys J, Edwards AM, Little JC (eds): The Mast Cell—Its Role in Health and Disease. Tunbridge, Wells, England, Pitman Medical Publishing Co, 1979, pp 343–352.
25. Lowhagen O, Rak I: Modification of bronchial hyperreactivity after treatment with sodium cromoglycate during pollen season. J Allergy Clin Immunol 75:460, 1985.
26. Bernstein IL: Cromolyn sodium. Chest 87 [Suppl]:68, 1985.
27. Brompton Hospital/Medical Research Council Collaborative Trial. Long-term study of disodium cromoglycate in the treatment of severe extrinsic or intrinsic bronchial asthma in adults. Br Med J 4:383, 1972.
28. Mellon MH, Harden K, Zeiger RS: The effectiveness and safety of cromolyn nebulizer solution in the young childhood asthmatic. Immunol Allergy Pract 4:168, 1982.
29. Rubin AE, Alroy G, Spitzer S: The treatment of asthma in adults using sodium cromoglycate pressurized aerosol: a double-blind controlled trial. Curr Med Res Opin 8:553, 1983.
30. Newth CJL, Newth CV, Turner JAP: Comparison of nebulized sodium cromoglycate and oral theophylline in controlling symptoms of chronic asthma in preschool

children: a double-blind study. Aust NZ J Med 12:232, 1982.
31. Godfrey S, Balfor-Lynn L, Konig P: The place of cromolyn sodium in the long term management of childhood asthma based on a three to five year follow up. J Pediatr 87:465, 1975.
32. Settipane GA, Klein DE, Boyd GK: Adverse reactions to cromolyn. JAMA 241:811, 1979.
33. Santa CHJ, Rossing TH, McFadden ER Jr: Glucocorticoids in acute asthma: a critical controlled trial. Am Rev Respir Dis 125[Suppl]:94, 1982.
34. Kattan M, Gurwitz D, Levison H: Corticosteroids in status asthmaticus. J Pediatr 96:596, 1980.
35. Shenfield GM, Hodson ME, Clarke SW, et al: Interaction of corticosteroids and catecholamines in the treatment of asthma. Thorax 304:430, 1975.
36. McFadden ER, Kaiser R, deGroot WJ: Acute bronchial asthma: relation between clinical and physiologic manifestations. N Engl J Med 288:221, 1973.
37. Spector SL: The use of corticosteroids in the treatment of asthma. Chest 87[Suppl]:73S, 1985.
38. Wyatt R, Waschek J, Weinberger M, et al: The effects of inhaled beclomethasone diproprionate and alternate-day prednisone on pituitary-adrenal function in children with chronic asthma. N Engl J Med 299:1387, 1978.
39. Toogood JH, Baskerville JC, Gennings BH, et al: Optimal dosage in steroid dependent asthma. *In* Mygind N, Clark TJH (eds): Topical steroid treatment for asthma and rhinitis. London, Bailliere Tindall, 1980, pp 107–122.
40. Corticosteroid aerosols for asthma. Med Lett 27:5, 1985.
41. McFadden ER Jr: Bronchodilator therapy in obstructive lung disease. N Engl & Regional Allergy Proceedings 6:241, 1985.
42. Gross NJ, Skorodin MS: Anticholinergic antimuscarinic bronchodilator. Am Rev Respir Dis 129:856, 1984.
43. Gross NJ: SCH 1,000: a new anticholinergic bronchodilator. Am Rev Respir Dis 112:823, 1975.
44. Stokes GM, Milner AD, Hodges IGC, Henry RL: Nebulizer ipratropium bromide in wheezing infants and young children. Eur J Respir Dis 64:[Suppl]:494, 1983.
45. Davis A, Vickerson F, Worsley G, et al: Determination of dose-response relationship for nebulized ipratropium in asthmatic children. J Pediatr 105:1002, 1984.
46. Beck R, Robertson C, Galdes-Sebaldt M, Levison H: Combined salbutamol and ipratropium bromide by inhalation in the treatment of severe acute asthma. J Pediatr 107:605, 1985.

CHAPTER 27

Pathogenic Fungi Therapy

Walter A. Ward, Jr., M.D.

TREATMENT FOR THE "ID" REACTION

Treatment failures are usually due to overtreatment, to undertreatment, or to a misdiagnosis. Factors other than your initial testing and treatment regimens that may change the endpoint are other inhalant allergies that have not been controlled and concomitant food hypersensitivities. Most patients with a fungal hypersensitivity also have concomitant yeast ingestant problems.[1, 2] Therefore, it is necessary to place these patients on a yeast-free diet, eliminating not only foods that actively contain yeast, but also foods that contain a yeastlike substance (cheese, fermented beverages, vinegar, and so on) or that may be derived from yeast (vitamins). Yeast-free diets are readily available from allergy supply companies or in recent articles on candidiasis.[3–9] In addition, you should prescribe a diet low in carbohydrates, restricting especially the simple and refined sugars and frozen, sweetened fruits. Once your patient has his or her inhalant allergy under control and is following the proper diet, it is imperative that you recheck the endpoint because it will likely move to a higher concentration (stronger dilution).

Once you have established a stable endpoint, the classic approach to treatment is to add two dilutions to the endpoint and begin therapy with 0.3 ml of that dilution. (Szymula believes that Microsporum allergen can be used in this manner to treat the patient with psoriasis.[10]) If this dosage does not relieve the symptoms, you may repeat it or begin increasing the dose in increments of 0.05 ml on a daily or every-other-day basis. If 0.5 ml of this dilution is reached and the patient has not had a remission of symptoms, then you may retitrate or immediately move to the next stronger concentration, which would be the endpoint plus one dilution, and start treating with 0.1 ml, again advancing in 0.05 ml increments.

> Example: 7 mm wheal on #3 dilution; use 0.3 ml of #5 dilution for your first dose.
>
> Your next doses will be 0.35 ml, then 0.40 ml, then 0.45 ml, and then 0.50 ml.
>
> If there is no relief of acute symptoms, then your next dose should be 0.1 ml of a #4 dilution.

If at any point the patient has a clearing of symptoms, you should stop at this dosage and not advance it further. The maximal optimal dose is always that dose at which the "id" reaction has subsided. If the patient has an exacerbation of symptoms, it is imperative that you immediately retitrate the dose before the next injection.

More than 10 years ago the author successfully treated a patient using 0.1 ml of the endpoint as the first injection. Since that time, this regimen has been successfully continued, and the classic method of advancing treatment has been resorted to in less than 5 per cent of more than 1000 patients. If the patient does not obtain relief on 0.1 ml of the endpoint *on an every-other-day schedule* after three to five injections, then the dose is advanced to 0.15 ml of the endpoint. Rarely has it ever advanced past 0.2 ml of the endpoint before either the maximal optimal dose is reached or the symptoms are exacerbated. Whichever treatment method you choose to use, always remember that if the dose given exacerbates the symptoms, you must re-establish the endpoint.

Antibiotic therapy, especially the broad-spectrum antibiotics such as ampicillin, the tetracyclines, and the cephalosporins, and corticosteroid therapy will tend to exacerbate the "id" reaction. These flares can occur months after the problem has been under control and the patient has stopped injection therapy. The author always advises patients that if they are placed on antibiotic or steroid therapy, they ask their physician to also place them on a concomitant systemic antifungal regimen.

TREATMENT FOR THE PRIMARY INFECTION

For eradication of mucosal lesions, *nystatin*, which is available in a purified powder, tablet, capsule, or suspension form, is readily available by prescription. Each dose of the tablet, capsule, or suspension form is 500,000 units, which is given four times a day. However purified nystatin powder at the recommended four times daily dose of 1/2 teaspoonful is equivalent to three of the tablets, capsules, or tablespoons of suspension. Remember, nystatin is not absorbed from the digestive tract, but rather it coats the mucosa of the intestine, thereby preventing the fungus from multiplying. It is one of the safest of the prescription drugs. If you prescribe the powder form, you should warn the patient of its bitter taste, and when treating small children it may be necessary to mix the drug with applesauce.

At the present time, *ketoconazole* is the drug of choice for eradication of fungal infections, whether mucosal, cutaneous, or elsewhere in the body. The usual dose is one 200 mg tablet taken daily with the biggest meal. It is absorbed from the small intestine. Ketoconazole has one particular side effect about which the patient must be warned: ketoconazole may elevate the liver enzymes, and if this possibility is not monitored on a regular basis it can lead to serious toxic effects in the liver. Routinely, a monthly test of liver enzymes (e.g., AST and ALT) should be ordered. If at any time those enzymes are elevated above normal, the drug should be withdrawn until they return to the normal range.

Before the introduction of ketoconazole, *griseofulvin* was the drug of choice for eradication of primary fungal infections. It is still available on the market and is very safe for all but the penicillin sensitive patient, who may also be sensitive to griseofulvin. This drug has in vitro activity against the Microsporum, Epidermophyton, and Trichophyton species, but has no effect on bacteria or other fungi. Treatment with griseofulvin or ketoconazole must be continued until all signs and symptoms of the primary infection have disappeared.

Caprylic acid is a short chain, saturated fatty acid that is complexed with a special resin for slow release in the gastrointestinal tract. It coats the walls of the gastrointestinal tract without disturbing intestinal flora other than pathogenic fungi. It has been reported to lead to complete sterilization of fungal cultures, but this is yet to be proved. Some caprylic acids are not of a pure state and may have potential antigenic impurities. This should be checked before recommending a particular brand of caprylic acid. Some caprylic acids have a coconut base, and of course these cannot be used in patients with a sensitivity to coconut.

More nonspecific measures of value in treating pathogenic fungal infections are aimed primarily at improving nutritional status. Galland[9] has recommended dietary supplementation with the omega-3 essential fatty acids, a combination of calcium and magnesium, vitamin C, the eight essential amino acids, and an acidophilus preparation. The author has found this supportive therapy to improve the ability to treat some patients.

For topical assistance in eradicating the primary lesions, there are a number of over-the-counter and prescription preparations available. With future developments, the treatment for this condition, except from an allergic standpoint, is bound to change.

SUMMARY

When testing and treating for fungal allergy, you will quickly learn that endpoints change rapidly once treatment begins. Schedule the patient for frequent retreating until the problem is under control. Once you have established a stable treatment dose, symptoms of the "id" reaction, such as pruritus, cough, headache, and others, should subside rapidly.

REFERENCES

1. Crook WG: Yeast-connected immune system disorders: a commonly and usually unrecognized cause of chronic illness. J Holistic Med 6:38, 1984.
2. Crook WG: The Yeast Connection. A Medical Breakthrough. Jackson, TN, Future Health, Inc, 1986.
3. Crook WG: The coming revolution in medicine. J Tenn Med Assoc 76:145, 1983.
4. Lorenzani SS: Candida: A Twentieth Century Disease. New Canaan, CT, Keats Publishing, 1986.
5. Trowbridge JP, Walker M: The Yeast Syndrome. New York, Bantam Publishing Company, 1986.
6. Truss CO: Tissue injury induced by Candida albicans: mental and neurological manifestations. J Orthomol Psychiatr 7:17, 1978.
7. Truss CO: Restoration of immunologic competence to Candida albicans. J Orthomol Psychiatr 9:287, 1980.
8. Zwerling MH, Owens KN, Ruth NH: "Think yeast"—the expanding spectrum of candidiasis. J SC Med Assoc 80:454, 1984.
9. Galland LD: Nutrition and Candida albicans. 1986. A Year in Nutritional Medicine. Monograph. New Canaan, CT, Keats Publishing, 1986.
10. Szymula N: Personal communication.

CHAPTER 28

Stinging Insect Therapy

Hueston C. King, M.D., F.A.C.S., F.A.C.A.

Any substance as lethal as stinging insect venom deserves extraordinary consideration from the point of view of therapy. Bad planning can result in no second chance. It has been noted that an allergic response to an insect sting may result in death within seconds. This indicates the necessity of considering therapy on two different levels: emergency treatment immediately following a sting, and preventive therapy to keep disastrous sting results from occurring.

AVOIDANCE

Whereas most insect stings occur without warning and without apparent provocation, some routine precautions may reduce the likelihood of stings by reducing exposure. Bees are pollen gatherers, and avoidance of bright colors in clothing and of perfume, especially of the floral type, reduces the bee's incentive to investigate. Wasps are nectar drinkers, and the wasp sensitive person should avoid orchards and garbage collection areas. Fire ants present a different problem, being quite cosmopolitan in their preferences. The mounds are easily seen, however, and the sensitive patient should develop a line of alertness to their appearance and take care in placing his or her feet.

EMERGENCY THERAPY

It is quite possible for an insect sting in a sensitive individual to result in death within seconds; however, most hypersensitivity reactions develop over a period of several minutes, allowing the properly prepared victim time to take swift definitive action. A trip to the emergency room of the nearest hospital is not the answer. By the time the patient reaches the facility, the die has been cast. The patient is either dead or on the road to recovery. Action must be taken immediately by the patient himself.

Any insect sting sensitive patient should have epinephrine on hand at all times. This may be in the form of an Anakit containing epinephrine in a syringe, a tourniquet, and a chewable antihistamine; an EpiPen, an autoinjection device designed to inject a measured amount of epinephrine on contact; or a preloaded syringe of plain epinephrine.

Epinephrine is the drug of choice. Neither antihistamines nor steroids react fast enough to be of value, although both may be useful in controlling delayed reactions. These reactions, however, are not life-threatening. Epinephrine should always be in the patient's possession and should be administered immediately upon receiving a sting. Delay may result in death.[1]

It is the very nature of the time factor that makes immunotherapy so critical in the control of stinging insect allergy. No matter how alert to the problem a patient may seem to be, there is an excellent chance that at the critical time, the emergency supply of epinephrine will not be available. This is the reason that hyposensitization to insect sting reactions has been vigorously pursued for three generations.

BACKGROUND

A look at the history of stinging insect allergy provides an interesting insight into the vagaries of medical science. Stinging insect allergy has been recognized as somewhat of a separate field since early in the century. The toxic effects of venom alone were known not to be responsible for the deaths witnessed, as literally hundreds of stings would be required to kill a normal adult, and most deaths resulted from one or two. A specific hypersensitivity to the venom was known to be necessary. Also recognized was the difficulty of acquiring venom in sufficient quantities to be used in therapy. A more practical method of treatment was sought.

In 1929, comparative studies were made on skin sensitivity of a single beekeeper known to react to bee stings.[2] The skin sensitivity was the same to venom as to whole body extract of honey bee. The conclusion was drawn that treatment with whole body extract would be as effective in preventing adverse reactions as would treatment with venom, and would be much safer and less expensive. The study went unchallenged, and resulted in 50 years of treating known sting sensitive individuals with whole body extract. Over this period, the American Academy of Allergy kept a retrospective file in an attempt to confirm the effectiveness of treatment, and in over 4000 reported cases, an apparent improvement in the victim's resistance to stings was noted.

Not until 1979 did a group at Johns Hopkins University seriously challenge the concept with a controlled study.[3] In this study, 60 patients known to be sensitive to insect stings were divided into three groups. One group was treated with venom, one with whole body extract, and one with placebo. When the desired treatment level had been reached, each was challenged with a sting. The study showed that excellent protection (97 per cent) was present in the group given venom therapy, whereas 50 per cent of those in both the groups treated with whole body extract and those treated with placebo reacted badly to the test sting. Certain conclusions were apparent: first, venom therapy gave far superior protection to that offered by whole body extract; second, since 50 per cent of the placebo group showed no reaction to a test sting, sensitivity to a sting apparently declined rather rapidly in the absence of subsequent stings. Whether whole body extract gave any real protection could not be determined, but it was definitely far inferior to venom. Several subsequent studies have confirmed these results. Here was born the mystique of the venom therapy microcosm, a clearly superior form of treatment capable of being highly refined and quantitated since insect allergy is measurable by both in vitro and in vivo testing, with results able to be quantified. The results of the current approach have been rewarding, but many problems still remain and may be expected to do so for many years.

TREATMENT FORMAT

In otolaryngic allergy, most therapy patterns are based on the quantitative method of titration or one of its variations. Of all aspects of allergy, the highly potent venoms with their inherent danger in treatment should be the most in need of quantification in treatment. In the foreseeable future this may indeed be the case; already studies in the use of titration in stinging insect care are appearing in the literature. As of this writing, however, this most sensitive form of allergy treatment relies upon a very basic form of institution and progression of care. Since this too is changing with new studies and different locations, only the principles need be discussed in a textbook.

The criteria for initiating immunotherapy are (1) accurate identification of the insect causing the reaction; (2) a definite systemic reaction as opposed to a large local reaction; and (3) a skin test positive reaction of 1+ or greater.

Certain problems are immediately apparent. First, few victims are able to accurately identify the insect producing the reaction. Honey bee and fire ants may be identified, although even in these cases the victim often feels the sting and brushes the insect off without a careful look. The wasps, however, look very similar to the nonentomologist. Under current recommendation, an accurate diagnosis, although difficult, is necessary for therapy to be recommended. In view of the risks and cost of therapy, this is clearly indicated.

A second problem is that in some cases a skin test will not be positive in spite of a definite identification of the insect. This is especially likely during the immediate refractory period following the sting, which may last six weeks and during which time the victim may be at greatest risk. These are problems still in need of a better solution.

The objective of stinging insect therapy is to start venom treatment at a safe dose and to progress as rapidly as possible consistent with safety to the highest dose tolerated. This is necessary, since unlike inhalant allergy the patient is not exposed to stings with any regularity, and it is hoped not at all. No optimum dose need then be considered, but only the highest dose tolerated giving the greatest degree of protection. At present, this is considered to be 100 μg of any individual venom, but 200 μg is under consideration. It is also recognized that not all patients are able to tolerate this dosage. The individual variations in the immune system dictate a limitation in dosage in many individuals. The long-term significance of this limitation has yet to be determined. The protection provided may be fully adequate in such patients, or it may not. In addition, the degree of protection given by 100 μg has been calculated only for a single sting. The effect of multiple stings is as yet unknown.

The starting point for treatment is also determined by a rather complex pattern at present. The recommendations of the Committee on Stinging Insects of the American Academy of Allergy and Immunology are, first of all, to identify the insect producing the problem, then to initiate skin testing with a prick test performed at a strength of 10^{-3} level. If this is positive, treatment should be started at a level of 10^{-5}. If the prick test is negative, an intradermal test is performed at a level of 10^{-3} (0.001). If this is positive, treatment is initiated at this level and raised progressively according to a schedule to be discussed to a level of 100 μg of venom.

A positive test is defined as follows:

Wheal	*Erythema*
1+ = 0.5–1 cm greater than control	1.1–2 cm
2+ = 1.5–1 cm greater than control	2.1–3 cm
3+ = 1–1.5 cm greater than control	3.1–4 cm
4+ = over 1.5 cm greater than control	Over 4 cm

This definition may be reliable, but it is frequently difficult to evaluate by one conditioned to quantitative reading of allergic responses. It should also be noted that a period of six weeks may be needed following a sting before the skin again becomes reactive enough for reliable testing. This is frequently the most dangerous time for the patient, since during this period the patient's IgE level for the venom is at its peak, and a second sting should be most disastrous.

Once a definite sensitivity has been determined, therapy may be instituted. Various treatment schedules are in use today.[4] All strive for a maintenance dose of 100 μg of venom, all reaching those doses at different rates of speed. Adverse reactions to treatment increase with the speed of progression, but so does arrival at an adequate level of protection.

Three schedules are reproduced in Tables 28–1 to 28–3.

It should be noted that as of this writing, all schedules aim for a maintenance dose of 100 μg, a level providing 97 per cent protection from a single sting. Studies are in progress on the use of a 200 μg dose, and no well-established studies exist concerning protection from several stings received simultaneously.

Table 28–1. CONVENTIONAL REGIMEN FOR VENOM IMMUNOTHERAPY

Week	Injection	Total Dose (μg)
1	1	0.01
	2	0.02
2	3	0.03
	4	0.04
3	5	0.06
	6	0.1
4	7	0.2
	8	0.3
5	9	0.4
	10	0.6
6	11	1.0
	12	2.0
7	13	3.0
	14	4.0
8	15	6.0
	16	10
9	17	20
	18	30
10	19	40
	20	60
11	21	80
	22	100
12	23	100
13	24	100
15	25	100
18	26	100
Monthly		

Table 28–2. RUSH REGIMEN FOR VENOM IMMUNOTHERAPY (JOHNS HOPKINS)

Day	Total Dose (μg)
1	0.001, 0.01, 0.1
8	0.1, 0.5, 1.0
15	1.0, 5.0, 10
22	10, 20
29	20, 30
35	30, 30
43	40, 40
50	50, 50
57	100
64	100
78	100
99	100
Monthly	100

Maintenance treatment is advised at a dosage of 100 μg every four weeks. Studies are under way on the safety of extending this schedule to 100 μg every six weeks after one year. Also under study is the safety of discontinuing treatment when RAST tests for the insect venom involved become negative. Until these are complete, treatment for adults must be considered a lifetime proposition in patients with life-threatening reactions.[4]

In non–life threatening cases, 1987 studies[5] indicate a degree of safety in stopping therapy for a period of at least two years. This period may be extended as studies progress.

Table 28–3. SLOW REGIMEN FOR VENOM IMMUNOTHERAPY (WALTER REED)

Week	Injection	Total Dose (μg)
1	1	0.01
2	2	0.02
3	3	0.03
4	4	0.04
5	5	0.06
6	6	0.1
7	7	0.2
8	8	0.3
9	9	0.4
10	10	0.6
11	11	1.0
12	12	2.0
13	13	3.0
14	14	4.0
15	15	6.0
16	16	10
17	17	20
18	18	30
19	19	40
20	20	60
21	21	80
22	22	100
23	23	100
24	24	100
25	25	100
26	26	100
Monthly		

Since insect sting allergy is predominantly an IgE-mediated mechanism, levels of IgE and IgG during immunotherapy have been closely followed over the years since 1979.[6] It has been hoped that changes in those levels would provide a reliable guide to the success of immunotherapy and a safe point at which treatment could be discontinued. To date this has not been the case. Clinical responses have not followed immunologic changes in a reliable manner. At this time, treatment must continue to be based on clinical studies.

Recent longer term evaluation studies have resulted in recommending against immunotherapy in children with systemic reactions at less than life-threatening level. This is in consideration of the generally milder reactions shown by children, and the high cost of therapy.[7] To further confuse the possibility of controlled evaluation, ongoing studies indicate the tendency of most patients to lose venom sensitivity when not stung for a prolonged period in any case.[4]

Complications of Therapy

A treatment modality in use for only a few years cannot be expected to show a realistic pattern for long-term complications. As has been noted, immediate complications of the anaphylactic type occur in proportion to the speed of the schedule of immunotherapy from 0 per cent to 17 per cent. Delayed reactions have been reported as late as three hours after an injection. Local reactions are common and severe, making it difficult for the patient to raise his or her arm above shoulder level. These are considered acceptable in treatment of a life-threatening problem. In prolonged therapy, serum sickness and wristdrop have been reported.[8] The current position of the American Academy of Allergy and Immunology is that venom treatment is "relatively safe given by an experienced physician prepared to treat possible systemic reactions."[9] It may be expected that improvement will appear and problems will be reduced as experience increases in venom therapy.

Cost

Treatment with stinging insect venom is expensive. It will probably continue to be expensive, since producing venom for therapy is far more difficult than is producing other antigens for treatment. Time and improved technology will in all probability lower the cost to a degree, but the limited demand will keep it high. Potential patients must be made aware of the cost and the need for continued therapy. At the present state of the art, this is all that can reasonably be said about this aspect of the problem.

SUMMARY

Just as stinging insect allergy is unique in the field by virtue of both its purity and severity, so is stinging insect therapy. Venom is probably the most potent antigen in use now or likely to be used in the near future. On the favorable side, the problem is clearly life-threatening and treatment is indicated. The basic outlines of treatment have been clearly spelled out. In following the recommended tenets of treatment, the physician is well within the standards of the community; his or her results should be predictable. On the unfavorable side, the recommendations are continually changing as new knowledge appears. The physician must keep abreast of new material. Designating treatment as "reasonably safe" indicates the distinct likelihood of untoward reactions occurring during therapy. Possible long-term complications of therapy are as yet unknown. Finally, stinging insect treatment is prolonged and expensive.

Clearly, stinging insect therapy is not a job for the novice. When it is considered, the patient must be fully apprised of all the risks and benefits, and must be free to make his or her own decision. Regardless of the decision as to immunotherapy, the patient should be fully acquainted with the nature and habits of stinging insects, and how to best avoid stings. In all cases, the patient should have emergency treatment immediately available for self-administration.

REFERENCES

1. Frazier A: Emergency first aid for allergic reactions to insect stings or bites. Cutis 19:770, 1977.
2. Sobotka AK: Diagnosis of insect hypersensitivity. J Allergy Clin Immunol 60:213, 1977.
3. Lichtenstein JM, et al: Insect allergy. The state of the art. J Allergy Clin Immunol 64:5, 1979.
4. Gillman A, et al: Venom immunotherapy—comparison of "rush" vs. "conventional" schedules. Ann Allergy 45:351, 1980.
5. McLean DC: Insect sting allergy. Immunol Allergy Pract 9:5, 1987.
6. Golden DBK, Schwartz HJ: Guideline for venom immunotherapy. J Allergy Clin Immunol 77:727, 1986.
7. American Academy of Allergy and Immunology Meeting, Washington, DC, 1987.
8. American Academy of Allergy and Immunology Meetings, Hollywood, FL, 1983.
9. Schuberth KC: Report of American Academy of Allergy and Immunology Meetings, Hollywood, FL, 1983.

CHAPTER 29

Management of Problems and Immunotherapy Failures

Joseph P. Keenan, M.D., F.A.C.S.

Not all patients with allergic disease respond to immunotherapy. Approximately 5 to 10 per cent of patients in a practice with true inhalant allergy will not respond to immunotherapy with significant clinical improvement in their symptoms. At times there will be some minor degree of improvement, but the major symptom that brought the patient to treatment in the first place, such as nasal obstruction caused by swelling of the mucous membranes, is unaffected by the treatment.

There is a definite protocol to follow with such immunotherapy failures. The physician must be consistent and methodical in application so nothing is overlooked that might benefit the patient.

When a patient has less than ideal control of his or her allergic symptoms by immunotherapy, assuming that there have been no changes in environment, and he or she has been consistent in receiving immunotherapy injections, one should begin by rechecking the endpoints, preferably by skin endpoint titration (SET). An error may have been made in the initial interpretation of the intradermal test that could be related to variations in the strength or quality of the testing solution. A technical error could have been made in the mixing of the different dilutions, or cross-contamination of the dilutions during the testing procedure by some technical mistake in the mixing or subsequent application of the test could have led to treatment with the incorrect antigen. Such inappropriate treatment could cause exacerbation of symptoms or lack of improvement in the original presenting symptoms.

Another reason to retest the endpoints would be if the patient inadvertently took an antihistamine or other medicine prior to the original test procedure and failed to report this to the nurse at the time of the test. This, too, could result in an erroneous test result and possibly account for the lack of response to immunotherapy.

Factors, if unusually strong, that may interfere with the original testing procedure are environmental exposure, stress, or coexisting food allergy or sensitivity. If the patient had a coexisting food allergy and had eaten that particular food prior to the testing procedure, the results could have been influenced by this. Environmental exposure to indoor or outdoor pollutants could have placed stress on the immune system, which could have led to erroneous interpretation of the original test results. Increased emotional stress, such as the start of a new job or exam time for a college student, could place an additional burden on the immune system as evidenced by abnormal skin whealing response, which will lead to erroneous interpretation of skin test results. All these factors should be considered when the patient is not responding as expected to immunotherapy. It goes without saying that a careful history is of paramount importance in elucidating these different possible causes of failure of response to immunotherapy. It is just as important to obtain additional history repeatedly to ensure that nothing of importance was missed when the original history was obtained. Also, new sensitizations to common allergens may develop after the first testing, so additional tests may be necessary.

One should also investigate fully the possibility of a coexisting cyclic food allergy. Most fixed (i.e., IgE-mediated) food allergy is not difficult to identify, but a dose-related food allergy might actually become unmasked or more evident after the inhalant allergies have been treated. For example, some patients can tolerate apples year-round except during the ragweed season. If this is not revealed by the history, then symptoms may become worse during the fall while the patient is on maintenance or is just reaching the maintenance immunotherapy dose. In such a case, increased clinical symptoms might improperly be attributed to failure of response to immunotherapy, rather than to the effects of the coexisting food allergy. It is problems such as these that make the search for the etiologic factor of immunotherapy failure difficult. The sine qua non of correct diagnosis and treatment is accurate, adequate, and complete history.

A change in home or work environment occurring after the start of treatment might also be the cause of the treatment failure. A cat or dog might have been introduced into the home since the initial testing was carried out. Perhaps the patient started a new hobby such as painting or photography and is now exposed to new chemicals, such as those used in developing films, that are aggravating his or her symptoms. New medications prescribed by other physicians or self-administered ones may cause adverse reactions mistaken for allergy. Once again, it is important to make the patient a partner in the treatment process and to educate him or her to the effects that different exposures might have, either in an immediate or delayed fashion.

Coexisting systemic diseases might also impair the success of immunotherapy. Hypothyroidism can cause edema of the mucous membrane lining the nose and thereby cause nasal obstruction. Coincidental development of the disease might impair the correct determination of the cause of the symptoms. Perhaps since the commencement of immunotherapy the patient's internist diagnosed hypertension and instituted beta-blocker therapy. If a careful review history is not obtained, the patient might inadvertently fail to spontaneously report this to the physician. In this case, the nasal stuffiness might be incorrectly ascribed to the failure of immunotherapy, rather than to introduction of the antihypertensive agent into the patient with the resulting production of the aggravating side effect.

Coexisting chemical exposure that could exacerbate the patient's symptoms to inhalant allergens must be sought.[1] Carefully review the history when the symptoms are worse and try to correlate any chemical exposures either at home or at work or in the course of a hobby. Some people with allergic rhinitis have a marked increase in their allergy complaints due to exposure to chemical fertilizers, weed sprays, and insect repellants placed by commercial companies on the lawns of their neighbors or on municipally owned property, especially parks. Given in a liquid/spray form, the smell and odor can permeate an entire neighborhood when only a single lawn is being fertilized or treated with the pesticide. Repaving of roadways may fill the air with chemicals also. These are some of the obvious occurrences to be sought. There are other more subtle exposures.

On occasion, the physician is deceived by the problems of a patient whose symptoms related to allergy are interfering with everyday activities, but in whom immunotherapy has not produced the desired result, and the reevaluation has proved to be nonproductive. At this point, the patient and physician should cooperatively review the patient's symptoms and decide exactly what is causing the most discomfort. Is it the nasal stuffiness, the thick tenacious secretions, the pain/pressure resulting from intermittent maxillary sinus ostia blockage, or the intermittent fullness and popping sensations in the ears relating to faulty eustachian tube function? Therapies can be devised that, although not addressing the nasal allergy directly, are helpful in relieving at least some of the distressing symptoms.

Such an ancillary approach can be classed under medical or surgical therapies. With the former approach, one can choose between different antihistamine/decongestant combinations to relieve symptoms. Although the underlying allergy is not attacked directly, significant chemical improvement can sometimes be gained. In the case of the medication, the side effects are generally the major problem. The aggravation of incipient glaucoma, prostate obstruction, and unwanted cardiac stimulatory effects as well as drowsiness are some of the undesired effects of this class of drug.

The application of medicine topically on the nasal membrane is also of great benefit in decreasing nasal airway obstruction as well as, at times, the copious nasal discharge of which the patient may bitterly complain. The topical sprays can be of the steroidal (Beconase, Vancenase, Nasalide) or nonsteroidal (Nasalcrom) classes. It should be pointed out that Nasalcrom is the only topical nasal spray that is FDA-approved for use in children as young as 4 years old. Patients are advised to avoid using over-the-counter nasal sprays, which are chiefly potent topical vasoconstrictors. Generally, the patient is told that there are drops that work but at a great price for the relief. This relief is immediate but very traumatizing to the nasal mucus membranes, and the resultant rebound phenomenon, rhinitis medicamentosa, is often worse than the original obstruction. Patients who chronically abuse these nasal sprays become "addicted" to them and, at times, will carry a bottle of spray with them and use it several times during the day. As always, educating patients of the physiologic mechanism involved is necessary to convince them of the need to avoid totally this class of medication in their overly sensitive airways.

Eye drops may also be utilized if the major complaints are itchy, irritable, red, teary eyes—allergic conjunctivitis. These topical medications require the same instructions and restrictions as the topical nasal sprays. They may contain antihistamines, vasoconstrictors, steroids, or sodium cromolyn. Any irritation of the eye that does not respond quickly to this medication should also be referred for ophthalmologic consultation to avoid overlooking any severe ocular disease.

Many surgical approaches may be undertaken with the allergy patient. Some of these procedures attempt to modify the allergic symptoms directly, whereas others are geared to alleviate the secondary pathologic process resulting from the untreated underlying chronic disease, which uncontrolled allergy certainly is.

If the initial reevaluation is completed and the endpoints are correct, and there is no suspicion of coexisting food allergies or chemical sensitivities determined to be interfering with the result of the immunotherapy, then the role of surgery may need to be introduced. Generally, although not always, surgery should be thought of as a treatment of last resort. The general role that surgery can play is to improve drainage of the sinus and nose and improve respiration. The exact type of surgery that is recommended depends on the existing pathologic process. Certainly, facilitating the drainage of the sinus by correction of a deviated septum and hypertrophic turbinates might sometimes do away with the need for later sinus surgery. Obviously, with a person with severe nasal polyposis and chronic sinusitis, polypectomy with exenteration of the involved sinuses is indicated to remove the diseased obstructing tissue. The goal of surgery should be viewed primarily as a mechanical means to restore normal physiologic drainage and aeration of the upper airway and those structures that drain into it.

SPECIFIC PROBLEMS

In spite of every attempt to educate the patient in the role he or she must play in treatment, a small number of patients will obtain less than ideal response to immunotherapy because of noncompliance. An example of such a patient is one who complains bitterly about the symptoms of nasal allergy yet does not maintain a regular schedule for injections. As soon as these patients notice some improvement in symptoms, they skip injections and become lax in maintaining environmental control at home and work. Perhaps a patient who is sensitive to dogs gets a new pet or refuses to get rid of an old one. At times, a patient who subjectively reports that exposure to pesticides and fertilizers tremendously aggravates his symptoms persists in having his lawn sprayed with these chemicals because the desire for a green lawn overwhelms the desire for a clear nose.

The common thread that runs through all these different types of noncompliant patients is that they do not take responsibility for their illness. They expect the physician to "cure" them, and when that does not happen, they will often blame the physician for their lack of satisfactory response to immunotherapy. Education, in a repetitive fashion, attempting to make it understood by the patient that noncompliance is the major source of the continued allergic symptoms, is the proper approach for the physician.

On occasion, because of protocol and continued noncompliance on the part of the patient, the physician may be well advised to recommend stopping immunotherapy. It is best for the physician to recommend cessation of injections rather than having an unsatisfied patient continue to be "half-treated" for years. Physicians will be judged by their results, and a high success rate in treatment of allergic disease is not obtained with noncompliant patients. When this course is necessary, complete documentation on the patient's records is most important.

Another class of potential problems in allergy treatment is the pregnant patient. In the past, there has been considerable controversy surrounding the performance of allergy skin testing or immunotherapy in the pregnant woman.[2] There are two components to the problem of testing and treating allergic patients who are pregnant. The first revolves around the safety of administering the test or treatment antigen to such a patient. It has been well established that it is perfectly safe to administer the antigen to both the mother and fetus. In fact, some results seem to indicate that good immunotherapeutic management of a severely allergic mother through her pregnancy might give a beneficial effect to the fetus in terms of allergic predisposition later in life, and it certainly helps the symptomatic mother through what might, otherwise, be a severely traumatic experience.

The second component to the problem of testing and treating the pregnant patient revolves around the fact that in a small minority of patients, severe local or systemic reactions, precipitated by the antigen injections given for testing or therapy, might necessitate the administration of other drugs. Those drugs such as antihistamines, steroids, and epinephrine are well tolerated in the nonpregnant patient, but in the pregnant patient, the potential injury to the fetus is small but real.

If the pregnant patient is treated as a "brittle" patient in terms of both testing and treatment, it is perfectly safe to treat via SET technique. The major value of SET in handling the "brittle" patient is that it allows both a quantitative as well as a qualitative measurement of allergic reactivity. As a matter of courtesy to our obstetrical colleagues as well as for medicolegal consideration, getting their advice prior to testing or treating one of their pregnant patients is strongly suggested.

A rare problem encountered in allergic management in the office setting is the occurrence of local or systemic reactions during testing or treatment. The chance for life-threatening anaphylactic reactions is extremely remote with titration but possible, so the full resuscitative measures must be in place in your office. This means that supplies, instruments, medications, and training for the involved personnel must be available prior to the start of testing or treatment. After an emergency has occurred is not the time to start looking for a certain medication.

For the patient sustaining a severe local or systemic reaction after immunotherapy has been started, the dose of the last injection should be checked. There could have been a planned increase in the dosage, and the reaction merely tells you that the maximum tolerated dose has been reached. If the patient is on maintenance dose and the level has not been changed from the previous month, then the reason for the untoward reaction may have been concomitant exposure to an antigen, either inhalant or ingestant, to which the patient is sensitive. The patient with dust and related sensitivities may have just finished cleaning and dusting at home and then had the injection, thereby becoming overdosed.

Concomitant food allergies should always be sought in the patient who experiences recurrent local reactions after immunotherapy injections. At times, local reactions after injections will be the first evidence of possible cyclic food allergy. These patients should maintain a food diary for an extended period of time, concomitantly with receiving immunotherapy injections. Often, close examination of the food diary will be very helpful in uncovering a low-grade food allergy. At times, a causal connection will be seen between the ingestion of certain foods in a 24-hour period preceding the injection and the production of local reactions subsequent to the administration of immunotherapy.

Another source of adverse reactions to immunotherapy is the remote but theoretical possibility of medication error. Perhaps the wrong antigen or antigen dilution was incorporated into the treatment set during the preparation in the office setting. A nurse can accidentally confuse the identity of two patients and give the wrong injection to one of the patients. These errors can be minimized only by selecting a highly qualified professional nursing staff who understand the necessity of meticulous preparation and handling of allergy extracts. Constant attention to detail, a deep interest in the welfare of the patients, and being constantly attuned to the slight nuances of the patient's response to immunotherapy are some of the traits absolutely required in a professional and competent allergy nursing staff. If the injections are given in another physician's office, in a school infirmary setting, or when on maintenance at home, detailed instructions, clearly and concisely written, are absolutely essential.

If the physician is certain that no medication error has been made and there has been no dietary or environmental exposure, other techniques may be necessary to minimize local arm reactions and prevent systemic symptoms. First, the dose may be split into two to three different injections. At times, the arm reaction is caused by volume of injected material, and splitting the volume into two separate injections is all that is needed. At times, separating the pollens from dust and molds and giving one injection in each arm will do away with local reactions. Sometimes it is helpful, especially in the frail patient or child, to give the injections in the buttocks rather than in the arm. The larger mass of tissue in this area minimizes the chance for local reactions. The depth of injection will also have impact on whether a local reaction will develop. The injection should be given in the subcutaneous plane and not intramuscularly.

If a patient has experienced a mild systemic reaction after injection, all the previous steps should be reviewed, and the patient should be observed longer in the office after the next injections. With these patients, it may be important to prescribe a kit containing epinephrine to have on hand at home for emergencies as well as an antihistamine such as Benadryl. It is important to teach the patient to recognize the beginning of a reaction, even a very mild one, and report it to the nurse prior to the next injection so that the injection dose might be modified if necessary.

Another concern in allergic management when less than ideal results are obtained is the role that stress can play in the aggravation of allergic symptoms. Increased levels of stress can modulate intensity of allergic symptoms via the autonomic nervous system. The key step in dealing with this problem is getting the patient to recognize and deal with the sources of stress in the everyday work/home environment. Short-term pharmaceutical management of this problem is helpful if the source of anxiety/stress is short-lived or transient. If the source of the stress is more permanent or serious, then the otolaryngic allergist is well advised to refer the patient for appropriate counseling from a qualified practitioner. Once the level of stress is minimized in the patient's life, the allergy control will be more manageable with the usual technique.

At times, the successful management of the allergic patient is hindered when the patient has associated or concomitant systemic illnesses that aggravate the underlying allergic symptoms. This interference can be a direct result of the disease state itself, such as asthma, or it can be the result of the medications that are required for the management of the associated illness, as with some of the medications used in the treatment of cardiac abnormalities (i.e., beta-blockers). These pose significant problems to the otolaryngic allergist and sometimes cannot be overcome but only minimized. It is incumbent upon the physician to ensure that the patient understands the underlying pathophysiologic mechanism and how the associated illness or medication can aggravate symptoms.

Candidiasis is being recognized more commonly as a source of chronic medical problems than in the past. Although the exact mechanism is not clearly understood, there is a definite effect on the immune system in those patients with chronic candidiasis.[3] There seems to be a decreased effectiveness of the immune system, which can lead to a whole myriad of somatic complaints. Some of the predisposing factors are excessive use of antibiotics in the past, history of birth control pill use, high refined carbohydrate diet, and alcohol use. This illness is dealt with in Chapters 12 and 27; suffice it to say that the possibility of chronic candidiasis should be considered in allergy patients, especially those with the predisposing factors listed.

SUMMARY

It must be recognized that not all truly allergic individuals will receive benefit from immunotherapy. A clearly thought out plan must be followed before advising the termination of immunotherapy. Technical errors in the testing or treatment protocol must be investigated as the possible culprit when less than ideal response to treatment is obtained. The recognition that coexisting food allergy or exposure to chemicals can also impair maximum response to treatment should be understood by the otolaryngic allergist. Systemic illness, newly occurring or preexisting, or pharmaceuticals introduced for its treatment can also lead to a less than ideal response. Noncompliance with environmental modification suggested for the patient might be a factor. Medical or surgical approaches can be offered if these inquiries prove fruitless. A key concept to stress is that the patient must be made a partner in the treatment protocol.

REFERENCES

1. Boyles JH: Chemical sensitivities: diagnosis and treatment. Otolaryngol Clin North Am 18:787, 1985.
2. Middleton E: Asthma and Allergic Disease during Pregnancy. St. Louis, CV Mosby, 1983, p 94.
3. Kroker GF: Chronic candidiasis. *In* Brostoff J: Food Allergy. London, Baillière Tindall, 1987, pp 850–872.

SECTION THREE

FOOD ALLERGY

CHAPTER 30

Introduction to Food Allergy: History and Characteristics

John H. Boyles, Jr., M.D.

After being ignored for 30 years, adverse reactions to foods are finally being recognized as an important etiologic agent in a vast number of clinical disorders. The physiologic basis for these reactions and their extent have been matters of considerable controversy in medicine, with few topics gathering so vigorous a group of supporters and critics. This reluctance to accept the importance of food allergy causing serious disease of many organ systems probably results from a misunderstanding of the natural history of food sensitivity, and our inability to totally understand the biochemical mechanisms involved. In Chapter 31 an attempt will be made to explain both the nonimmunologic mechanisms as well as those of immune dysfunction. Although Dr. Von Pirquet first coined the word allergy to "denote a stage of abnormal reactivity to a foreign antigen," general allergists now restrict the word "allergy" to systemic or local anaphylactic reaction produced by IgE antibodies. In spite of this conflict of terminology, it is apparent that food allergy is probably the most common cause of chronic symptoms in medicine today.

Food allergy can be encountered in any organ system and, therefore, may be a problem for every practicing physician irrespective of his or her specialty. In otolaryngology, the ear, upper respiratory system, skin, and nervous system are common shock organs for food reactions. The term "food allergy" refers to foods that produce repeated, definite clinical manifestations when tested under correct conditions. In other words, a correctly performed challenge feeding test should exhibit a high degree of specificity and consistency. Over 60 per cent of any given population will have some symptoms of food allergy and in the majority of these, symptoms will be severe enough for the person to seek medical aid.

It is important to remember that food allergy and chemical sensitivity are dynamic processes. The propensity to develop a food or chemical sensitivity is an inherited factor, but one must usually be exposed repetitiously to the food or chemical to develop sensitivity, the rule being that sensitization develops parallel to the frequency of usage. For this reason, the foods appearing most commonly in our modern diet and the ones that have entered our food chain most recently are those that most commonly cause clinical problems. In most syndromes the common foods involved are wheat, corn, egg, milk, yeast, and soy followed by coffee, cola, chocolate, and cane. In different communities the order of frequency will vary as do the eating habits of its citizens, but one must remember that there are no nonallergenic foods.

TYPES OF FOOD ALLERGY

Food allergy may be fixed or cyclic. A fixed food sensitization implies that the frequency of usage does not modify the occurrence of the degree of sensitization. This constitutes approximately 5 per cent of total cases. Even when such foods have not been eaten for many years, the first ingestion is followed by definite, often severe symptoms. A reaction that has not subsided following absolute elimination for a period of two years may be considered a fixed or permanent food allergy. There are rare exceptions to this rule.

The remaining 95 per cent of food reactions fall in the category of cyclic food sensitization. In contrast to fixed food allergy in which a cause and effect relationship is obvious to the patient, the development of cyclic food allergy may take years, and because this abnormality develops very slowly to foods that are constantly in the diet, a definite cause and effect relationship is lost and the patient seldom, if ever, is able to self-diagnose the problem. Although the gastrointestinal passage time for food may be as short as a period of hours, the biochemical reactions usually last from three to six days. For this reason, a food eaten infrequently by the patient poses no self-diagnostic problem. Each time the ingested food enters the gastrointestinal tract it will find an unaltered patient, and a cause and effect relationship will be obvious. In contrast to this, the frequently eaten foods will constantly be in the intestinal tract or involved in various biochemical reactions, so that the obvious cause and effect phenomenon is lost and the patient slowly becomes more and more symptomatic, unaware that his or her ingestion habits are the basic cause of the symptoms. To further complicate the problem of self-diagnosis, the food allergic patient will often exhibit the phenomenon of bipolarity. This means that the initial abnormal reaction to ingestion of the food may be stimulatory before it becomes depressive. This stimulatory phase usually occurs in the central nervous system and in effect "turns on" the patient, and the patient perceives this as a beneficial reaction. The symptom progression, however, is always one of stimulation preceding depression, so that when the patient then sinks into the depression or unpleasant feeling, he or she remembers unconsciously the stimulatory phase and again ingests the food to achieve the "upper" or stimulated state. These phenomena of bipolarity and constant ingestion totally obscure or "mask" food reactions so that patients with cyclic food allergy seldom, if ever, self-diagnose their problem.

The term "cyclic food allergy" was first described by Rinkel in 1951 and refers to the dynamic circle that patients may exhibit depending on repetitious use of a specific food or omission of that food. Cyclic food allergy exists in a series of six stages: masking, short periods of omission, the hyperacute reaction, the acute reaction, the latent reaction, and tolerance. Masking is a term also coined by Dr. Rinkel and refers to the reduction or ablation of symptoms by ingestion of a specific food within the period of time that the patient is reacting to a previous ingestion of this same food. It may be perfect or imperfect. In perfect masking, the symptoms are eradicated, and there is no delayed reaction. In imperfect masking, the symptoms are controlled for a few hours, and then there is a recurrence of the reaction. Chronic food allergic patients present to the physician in the stage of "masking" or, as described by Randolph, "food addiction."

If the food is omitted from the diet for at least 96 hours, the patient's reaction to the food will usually change from the stage of masking to the stage of hyperacute reaction, an accentuated reaction compared with the previous masked reaction. When eliminating a food from a patient' diet, it is important to explain to the patient that during the period of omission symptoms may become quite severe (a withdrawal reaction), and then there will be a complete remission of symptoms. In other words, the patient may get worse before getting better. This combination, in a short period time, of masking, the period of omission, and the re-eating of the food, which produces hyperacute reaction, collectively constitutes phase I of food allergy. This series of reactions becomes quite useful in performing the challenge feeding tests and is responsible for the high degree of accuracy of this diagnostic procedure.

If a food to which a patient is sensitive is omitted totally from the diet, it will be found that the patient passes through three successive stages, i.e., the stages of active sensitivity, latent sensitivity, and, finally, tolerance (Fig. 30–1).

Active sensitization implies that the food causes symptoms every time it is eaten.

Latent sensitivity, which usually develops between three and nine months after omission, is typified by the fact that ingestion of a food produces only mild symptoms if the food is not ingested repeatedly.

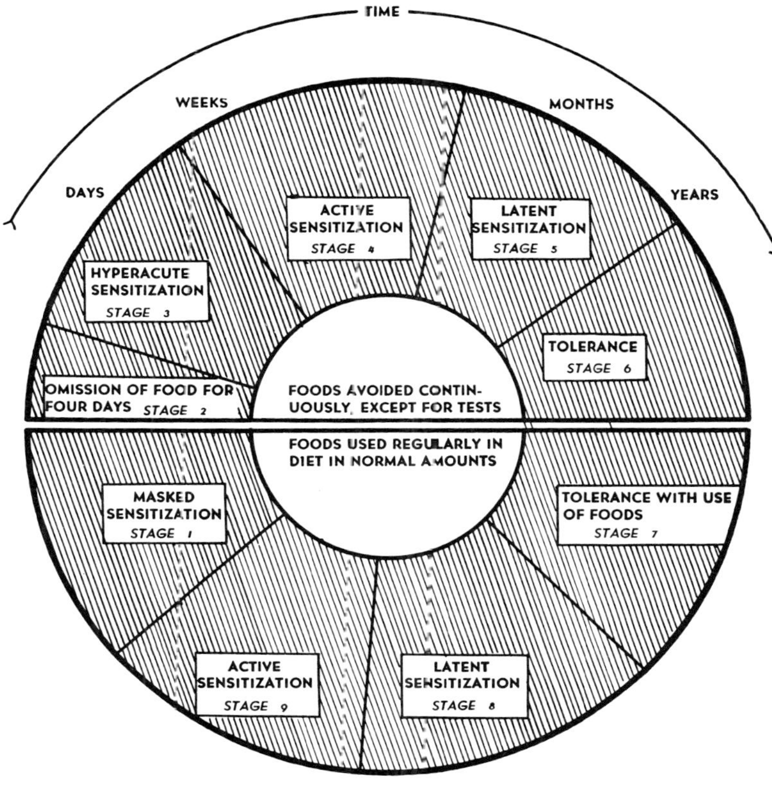

FIGURE 30–1. The changes in the degree of sensitization in cyclic food allergy. (From Rinkel HJ, Randolph TG, Zeller M: Food Allergy. Springfield, IL, Charles C Thomas, 1951. Courtesy of Charles C Thomas, Publisher. Reproduced by permission.)

Continued omission of the food will eventually lead to tolerance in most cases, but in some patients this stage is never reached regardless of the length of time the food is left out of the diet. These last three stages collectively constitute phase II of cyclic food allergy.

If the stage of tolerance is to be maintained, the food must not be eaten more than once every three or four days. If the food is ingested with the original frequency, the patient will pass through three stages: tolerance (usually lasts for two or three weeks), latent sensitization, and active sensitization. These constitute phase III. If ingestion continues to be frequent, the patient may then return to the masking stage.

The patient then has passed through a complete cycle of the various phases of sensitization; hence, the term "cyclic food allergy."

The duration of time necessary to complete this cycle will vary from patient to patient. The development of a new food allergy is usually faster in a child, as is the regaining of tolerance. Several additional factors must also be considered. Concomitant allergy refers to food that produces a reaction only in the presence of an inhalant, usually pollen. The same reaction can also happen in the presence of a dust allergy.

Maintaining tolerance is most important in the cyclic food allergic patient. The patient is advised to leave an offending food out of the diet for at least three to six months. Usually the allergy will not develop again if the food is not eaten more frequently than once in four days. A safe interval, however, may vary with different foods, and the patient must be warned about establishing safe intervals of ingestion. Foods that have never caused a reaction in the past may be consumed at closer intervals than foods to which the patient has become allergic. The patient who does not follow this type of rotary diet and does not diversify to include many different foods will slowly again develop the original problem.

Theoretically, food sensitivity is the only allergic disorder that can be perfectly controlled. In our modern society, complete avoidance of inhalants and chemicals is almost impossible, but one can effectively manage the ingestion of food in a cooperative and intelligent patient. If the diagnosis is correct and if the dietary therapy is appropriate, one should be able to achieve complete control of the food allergy patient. Elimination and rotary diet therapy, therefore, are the standards by which all other methods of treatment must be compared.

HISTORY

The successful diagnosis and management of a disease entity requires a thorough understanding of its presenting symptoms. Allergy is no exception to this rule, but may be paradoxically misleading to both patient and physician if the natural history of food allergy is not understood, particularly the phenomenon of bipolarity. Conversely, understanding this phenomenon may simplify the diagnosis and subsequent treatment.

In taking a food allergic history, one must also remember the allergic load phenomenon. In many patients, the combination of an inhalant with a food or chemical will produce severe symptoms, whereas singular exposure will produce only a mild reaction. For this reason it is most important to diagnose and treat inhalant allergy before a food or chemical workup is started. It is helpful to have patients fill out screening questionnaires for food (Fig. 30–2) and chemical problems while the inhalant workup is in progress.

The past history is often of help, since a high percentage of adults with food allergies have a history of feeding problems in infancy as well as croup, colic, eczema, frequent upper respiratory infections, bronchitis, and chronic serous otitis media in early childhood. In addition, the food sensitive person often is an inordinately fatigued person and functions best as the day wears on. Symptoms that vary in severity from day to day and that tend to involve many organ systems are also suggestive of food allergy.

In presenting the occurrence of symptoms by systems, our first consideration would be the skin. Here we find that foods may produce pruritus, urticaria, eczematous eruptions, and urticarial pigmentation.

Otologic symptoms from foods are usually found in the inner ear and predominantly result in fluctuating tinnitus, nonspecific vertigo, and true Meniere's syndrome. Hyperacusis and fullness can also be found as isolated symptoms due to food allergy.

The most common central nervous system symptom of food allergy is headache; however, there have been well-documented reported cases of epilepsy, paresthesia, personality changes, and psychiatric disorders.

It should be emphasized that foods may produce symptoms in both the upper and lower respiratory systems. Itching of the nose, nasopharynx, and roof of the mouth are very common immediate responses in food allergy, as are nasal congestion, nasal polyps, chronic sinusitis, and rhinorrhea. Chronic cough, shortness of breath, wheezing, and recurrent bronchitis are found in the lower respiratory tract of many food allergic patients. An increase of nasal obstruction after meals is suggestive of a food allergy, as are symptoms that awaken the patient between 1:00 and 5:00 AM.

Past and current medical history are often very important in the diagnosis of food allergy. Patients who have had problems with elective surgical procedures may be allergic to corn, which is the carbohydrate found in all IV solutions. Those patients diagnosed as hypoglycemic are often allergic to one or all of the three common sugars (corn, beet, cane). A list of current medications including vitamins and food supplements is extremely important. These pharmaceuticals contain a wide range of petrochemical dyes, corn starch, and other chemical substances that can in themselves cause allergic problems.

A detailed history of alcoholic ingestion will oftentimes indicate a specific allergy. The patient who has ingested alcoholic beverages for many years may have inadvertently eliminated the ones causing severe reactions and now drinks only beverages he or she can tolerate. In the United States, most alcoholic beverages are distilled from various grains, for example, bourbon-corn; rum-cane; beer-barley; scotch-barley, wheat, and corn; wine-grapes; tequila-cactus.

In summary, the most viable points of the history are

1. Suspicion of specific foods in direct relation to their frequency of ingestion and, to a lesser extent, the amount per "dose."
2. The nature of the patient's complaints, which should be multiple, chronic, and unrelieved by common medical management. The necessity of eating frequently and regularly to remain relatively well and, conversely, the tendency to become ill if one or two regular meals are omitted are pathognomonic of food allergy.

Name ______________________________ Date ______________

Please read each question carefully. Then circle Yes or No to indicate your answer. If yes, please explain.

Yes No 1. Are there any foods or beverages that you (a) crave or (b) eat frequently?
List (a) ______________ (b) ______________

Yes No 2. Are there any foods or beverages that you dislike?
List: ______ ______ ______ ______

Yes No 3. Are you awakened between the hours of 1:00 AM and 5:00 AM with the following symptoms: headache, dizziness, stomach cramps, bloating, or dry cough? (Circle which.)

Yes No 4. Do you or any member of your family have hay fever, asthma, hives, chronic skin condition, migraine headaches, or colitis? (Circle which.)

Yes No 5. During childhood did you have any of the following: eczema, hay fever, asthma, food feeding problems? (Circle which.)

Yes No 6. Do you ever have itching of the skin, palate, or roof of your mouth or skin rash? (Circle which.)

Yes No 7. Do you frequently notice swelling of your ankles, feet, hands, or face? (Circle which.)

Yes No 8. Do you have marked fatigue two to three hours after meals?

Yes No 9. Do you eat snacks frequently between meals? List examples.
______ ______ ______ ______

Yes No 10. Do you have excessive chilling when a sudden change in temperature occurs?

Yes No 11. Do you have frequent headaches or "migraine"?

Yes No 12. Do you experience belching, abdominal distention, bloating, or cramps following meals?

Yes No 13. Have you noticed numbness of the face, arms, or legs at periodic intervals for no apparent cause?

Yes No 14. Do you have drowsiness, headache, or bloating following the ingestion of a cocktail, glass of beer, or glass of wine? (Circle which.)

Yes No 15. Do you have alternating constipation and diarrhea?

yes No 16. Do you have joint or muscle pain or stiffness?

Yes No 17. Do you have fluctuating vision?

Yes No 18. Do you have recurring fungal infections (vaginitis, athlete's foot, jock itch, or ringworm)?

FIGURE 30–2. Food allergy–nutritional questionnaire.

3. The sensitivity or dislike of a basic food while eating the same food in other more subtle forms is typical of the food allergic patient.

4. The capacity of a massive dose to make one ill, or a rapidly absorbed physical form of the food such as an alcoholic distillate inducing an acute reaction, is also highly suggestive.

5. The patient will typically have multiple organ system involvement that may over a period of years switch from one system to another.

Physical findings may be similar to those in patients with inhalant allergy.

Ear	Serous otitis; fluctuating low tone hearing loss; chronic eczema.
Nose	Pale, wet, edematous swelling of the nasal mucous membranes with or without polyp formation; radiographic changes involving the sinuses; supratip crease due to the allergic salute, particularly in children.
Mouth and pharynx	Chronic lymphoid hyperplasia, especially lateral bands in the nasopharynx; furry tongue; recurrent aphthous ulcers.
Face	The chronic mouth breathing child with allergic shiners and maxillary overbite; Dennie's lines of lower eyelids.

It is often helpful to have patients fill out a diet diary; that is, have the patients write down every food and medication that they ingest during the day for an entire week and all symptoms observed. This detailed list will sometimes reveal unusual ingestants that would not be picked up by the usual history taking techniques or various questionnaires.

REFERENCES

1. Brostoff J, Challacombe SJ: Food Allergy and Intolerance. London, Baillière Tindall, 1987.
2. Brostoff J, Scadding GK: Low dose sublingual therapy in patients with allergic rhinitis due to house dust mite. Clin Allergy 16:483, 1986.
3. Dickey LD (ed): Clinical Ecology. Springfield, IL, Charles C Thomas, 1976.
4. Golos N, Goblitz FG, Leighton FS: Coping with Your Allergies. New York, Simon & Schuster, 1979.
5. Miller JB: Food Allergy, Provocative Testing and Injection Therapy. Springfield, IL, Charles C Thomas, 1972, pp 33–115.

6. Missal SC: Food allergy in ear, nose and throat disease. Otolaryngol Clin North Am 4:479, 1971.
7. Randolph TG, Moss RW: An Alternative Approach to Allergies. New York, Lippincott & Crowell, 1980.
8. Rea WJ, Podell RN, Williams M, et al: Elimination of oral food challenge reaction by injection of food extracts. Arch Otolaryngol 110:248, 1984.
9. Rinkel HJ, Randolph TG, Zeller M: Food Allergy. Springfield, IL, Charles C Thomas, 1951.
10. Rinkel HJ: The management of clinical allergy. Part IV. Food and mild allergy. Arch Otolaryngol 77:302, 1963.
11. Rinkel HJ, Lee CH, Brown DW, et al: The diagnosis of food allergy. Arch Otolaryngol 79:71, 1964.
12. Trevino RJ: Immunology of foods. Otolaryngol Head Neck Surg 95:171, 1986.

CHAPTER 31

Pathophysiology of Food Allergies and Hypersensitivities

Richard J. Trevino, M.D.

One area of clinical allergy and immunology requiring further study is hypersensitivity reactions induced by foods. This chapter presents current (1980s) data demonstrating that the entire immune system may be activated by foods to produce symptoms. Clinical testing and treatment modalities will be discussed and their immunologic bases elucidated.

In 1963, Gell and Coombs[1] classified the various immune mechanisms involved in the production of tissue damage into four basic types: I, anaphylactic; II, cytotoxic; III, antigen-antibody complexes; and IV, delayed hypersensitivity.

Type I, the anaphylactic reaction, is the classic allergic type of reaction mediated through IgE, which attaches to the cell membrane of blood basophils or mast cells in the tissues. Following a reaction between antigen and the antibody IgE, certain vasoactive amines are released from these cells producing symptoms that may be generalized or localized, depending on the mode and degree of administration of antigen. Generalized anaphylaxis may affect the respiratory tract (bronchial obstruction and laryngeal edema) the gastrointestinal tract (nausea and vomiting, cramping pain, diarrhea, bloating, and occasionally blood in the stool), the cardiovascular system (hypotension and shock), and the skin (hives). Allergic rhinitis and asthma are examples of localized respiratory reactions.

Cytotoxic reactions (type II) involve a combination of either IgG or IgM with antigenic determinants on the cell membrane. Alternatively, a free antigen or hapten may be absorbed into the tissue component of the cell membrane, and antibodies subsequently combine with this absorbed antigen. Complement fixation may then occur, frequently leading to cell damage. A typical example of this type of reaction is the hemolytic reaction induced by a mismatched blood transfusion.

Type III reactions are caused by the formation of antigen-antibody complexes circulating in the blood also utilizing complement.

Initially, there is the formation of antigen-antibody complexes, generally in antigen excess, which fix complement. Release of complement components, which are chemotactic for leukocytes, occurs. There is also damage to the platelets, resulting in release of other vasoactive amines. Increased vascular permeability and precipitation of antigen-antibody complexes occurs in capillary walls and tissues, resulting in inflammation and subsequent symptoms. Further fixation of complement and release of chemotactic factors with attraction of polymorphonuclear leukocytes may develop. Neutrophils ingest the immune complexes with release of lysosomal enzymes; this causes further tissue damage and deposition of fibrin. Finally, regression and healing of the lesion may occur if the exposure is a single dose of antigen, or chronic deposition and inflammation will result if there is continuing formation of immune complexes.

Cell-mediated immune reactions (type IV) occur as a result of the interaction between actively sensitized lymphocytes and specific antigens. Such reactions are mediated by the release of lymphokines, direct cytotoxicity, or both, occurring without the involvement of antibody or complement. The delayed skin reaction of poison oak—with its characteristic of mononuclear cell infiltrate developing over a period of 24 to 48 hours—is a typical type IV reaction.

The first requirement for any immunologic reaction to occur is the penetration of antigenic molecules through a tissue barrier of the body. It has been demonstrated that small, nutritionally insignificant amounts of antigenically intact food macromolecules are transmitted across the mature mammalian gut. For example, Danforth and Moore[2] noted that insulin injected into adult rat small intestine caused hypoglycemia, suggesting absorption in biologically active quantities. Bernstein and Ovary[3] demonstrated that haptens and larger antigens were absorbed from guinea pig small intestines in quantities that could produce passive cutaneous anaphylaxis. In human subjects, studies have shown that macromolecules, under normal physiologic conditions, can cross the mature mucosal barrier. Korenblatt et al.[4] showed that a considerable proportion, 15 to 30 per cent, of normal adults develop milk precipitins after ingestion of milk protein. In earlier studies, Wilson and Walzer[5] reported uptake and transport of undigested protein, using a passive cutaneous anaphylactic technique to measure circulating food proteins, and demonstrated precipitins to these proteins in the serum of adults. Thus, food antigens may be absorbed through the gastrointestinal mucosa into the body and stimulate immune responses.

Types of immunologic responses incriminated in the production of symptoms caused by food ingestion can be documented.

TYPE I (ANAPHYLACTIC) REACTION

The existence and mechanisms of reaginic, IgE immediate-onset food sensitivities are well established. Signs and symptoms range from anaphylaxis to urticaria, asthma, rhinitis, vomiting, and diarrhea. The onset is usually within minutes after ingestion and lasts only a few hours. In 1974, Hoffman and Haddad[6] established that RAST could be used in the diagnosis of food sensitivities. They assembled patients with unequivocal histories of food allergies (i.e., ingestion of the food produced a reaction every time it was consumed and a reaction had occurred within the previous six months), often referred to as a fixed food allergy. A number of patients with non–life-threatening symptoms were placed on a strict elimination-challenge regimen to verify the clinical histories. Prick skin testing was performed, until two severe systemic reactions resulted in discontinuation of the test. The test group displayed reactions to 14 common foods. Age-matched control sera were tested by RAST and used to determine the normal range for each allergen (Table 31–1).

Allergen systems with adequate allergenic content—that is, more than a contaminant of the extract, such as codfish, peanut, and egg white—produced excellent correlation in patients with severe symptoms; correlation with less defined allergens, such as orange and chocolate, was not as significant. Positive RASTs correlate in patients with various symptoms and unequivocal histories (Table 31–2). Note the higher correlation for the more severe symptoms.

These investigators also studied children with severe respiratory allergy without a history of food allergy, finding that 12 per cent were RAST positive to egg. Egg was removed from their diets with improvement of the allergic respiratory symptoms, suggesting that some patients previously presumed to have inhalant allergy alone might also have IgE-mediated food allergy. In 1978, May and Brock[7] reported a verification of Hoffman's findings regarding the detection of specific IgE in food sensitive patients. They found, in a large series, that those who exhibited high serum-specific food IgE levels were sensitive to those foods when challenged orally. There have now been a number of follow-up studies verifying that RAST can be used to diagnose IgE-mediated food sensitivities.[8–17]

TYPE II AND TYPE III REACTIONS

Type II or type III food sensitivity is much more difficult to diagnose than type I. These reactions are delayed rather than immediate, occurring from four hours up to several days

Table 31–1. NUMBER OF PATIENTS WITH A POSITIVE RAST/NUMBER TESTED

Foods	Anaphylaxis, Angioedema, Asthma	Eczema	Urticaria Skin Test	Other Symptoms	Control
Codfish	11/11	5/5	6/7	0/2	0/15
Cow's milk	11/12	15/15	5/5	2/8	0/15
Peanut	3/3	8/8	3/3	0/1	0/15
Orange	5/7	7/9	2/5	0/1	0/15
Egg white	8/9	7/8	9/14	0/2	3/20
Chocolate	7/12	6/10	4/8	0/4	0/20
Walnut	5/5	3/3	6/9	0/1	0/15

Adapted from Hoffman and Haddad.[6]

after food ingestion. Patients commonly do not realize that their symptoms are secondary to food ingestion. Investigation of such delayed sensitivities was initiated with the study of complement. In 1936, Lippard et al.[18] used complement fixation to detect milk protein and the subsequent appearance of antibody in the serum of infants. By this technique, small quantities of milk proteins were found in the sera of infants in the first few months of life. The appearance of complement fixation antibodies was followed by the disappearance of antigens from the sera and the presence of precipitating antibodies.

In 1962, Heiner et al.[19] described multiple precipitins to cow's milk. In 1970, Mathews and Soothill[21] demonstrated a change in C3 complement level in a group of small children after oral challenge with a small amount of milk. Some had an immediate reaction and others had a delayed reaction when orally challenged. The group with immediate reactions showed no change in C3, whereas the group with delayed reaction *did* show activation of C3.

In 1977, Sandberg[22] reported a study of children with nephrotic syndrome who had proteinuria after challenge with certain foods. When these foods were withheld from the diet, the nephrotic syndrome cleared and C3 dropped. Sandberg also measured C3c, an early detected breakdown product of C3b, documenting an increase in C3c, indicating C3 had been activated. He then studied other children, challenging them with various foods, resulting in a number of delayed symptoms and an elevation of C3c. Sandberg recommended that C3c levels be tested along with any oral challenge test performed. Although complement change may occur, it is important to remember that C3 can be activated not only by the immune system but also by the alternative system for complement activation.

In 1981, Trevino[23] demonstrated that the delayed food reaction was truly an immunologic reaction. The experimental group consisted of 55 patients, with 10 as a control group. One food showing a positive reaction on the leukocyte-cytotoxic test was chosen for each patient in the experimental group, and one food that reacted negatively was chosen for the control group. Each food was withdrawn from the patient's diet for four days. On the fifth day, the patients were instructed to ingest this food beginning with breakfast. Of the 55 patients in the experimental group, 53 reported some symptoms ranging from mild irritability, restlessness, and inability to sleep to severe migraine, nausea, vomiting, and angioedema. None of the controls reported symptoms. In those experiencing symptoms, C3 and C4 dropped significantly, with levels returning to normal the day following provocation. The control group evidenced no changes in C3 and C4. Since C4 activation occurs only by way of the classic pathway (C1–C2–C4–C3, and so on), delayed food hyper-

Table 31–2. CORRELATION OF RAST WITH SYMPTOMS FROM FOOD INGESTION IN A GROUP OF PATIENTS WITH UNEQUIVOCAL HISTORIES

Symptom	No. of Patients	% RAST Positive
Anaphylaxis	10	100
Bronchospasm	23	96
Angioedema	13	92
Atopic eczema	30	87
Urticaria	26	62
Diarrhea*	12	92
Acute gastrointestinal upset	6	33
Tension-fatigue syndrome	15	0

*Cases of disaccharidase deficiency, infection, etc. are not included.

Adapted from Hoffman and Haddad.[6]

sensitivity with complement activation is an immunologic phenomenon. Subsequent studies of delayed food sensitivities show that these early components on complement are activated by food antigens. Paganelli et al.[24] found circulating complement-fixing immune complexes bound to the specific food antigen to which their patients were clinically sensitive. Such immune complexes were seen in both normal and food sensitive subjects, but the concentrations were considerably higher and clearance was slower in the food sensitive patients.

The study of delayed food reactions has progressed from the investigations of complement, showing that complement is activated by way of the classic complement pathway stimulation, and on to the measurement of immune complexes. More recently, RAST tests for specific food IgG have been developed, and studies continue to document what correlation, if any, exists among high IgG titers, complement use, and production of symptoms.

TYPE IV REACTIONS

Type IV (delayed hypersensitivity) reactions are the most difficult to demonstrate since the T cell effect develops 24 to even 72 hours after the attachment of antigen to the target cell, and the attachment itself may not occur until several hours after ingestion. In 1971, Garcia et al.[25] described an in vitro procedure, the *lymphocyte transformation test* (LTT). When lymphocytes from the blood of sensitized patients are incubated with food antigens, certain foods increase the activity of the lymphocytes, transforming them to a more blastic form, whereas other foods produce no change. In 1972, May and Alberto[26, 27] selected foods positive by the LTT and challenged patients with these foods. After harvesting the lymphocytes, they demonstrated these cells to be active and transformed even when not exposed to in vitro antigen. They postulated that ongoing in vivo proliferation of lymphocytes was induced by antigens absorbed in the challenge procedure. Transformation of lymphocytes, not subjected to food antigens in vitro, did not occur when the oral challenge was not performed. In 1976, Scheinmann et al.[28] repeated and confirmed these studies.

In 1980, Valverde et al.[29] studied 258 patients with idiopathic chronic urticaria and angioedema with the LTT for foods and additives. The LTT response index was positive in 238 patients: 44 positive to additives, 83 to food extracts, and 111 to both foods and additives (Table 31–3). The implicated additives and foods demonstrating a possible LTT response were eliminated from the diets of patients, with complete remission of symptoms in 61.6 per cent, partial remission in 22 per cent, and no change in 16.2 per cent (Table 31–4). These investigators concluded that the LTT was accurate in identification of foods responsible for patients' symptoms. Typically, patients with chronic idiopathic urticaria and angioedema have normal levels of total IgE. There is no evidence of IgG-mediated disease, biopsies of lesions demonstrating no vasculitis as observed in immune complex reactions, and no necrosis of the vessel walls or presence of nuclear dust. Neutrophils are not prominent in these biopsies, and immunofluorescent studies for the deposition of immunoglobins and complement are negative. Thus, there is no evidence of a type I IgE-mediated reaction or a type II or III IgG-mediated reaction. Nevertheless, the LTT is positive in these patients; that is, the lymphocytes are stimulated by the foods, and the elimination of these foods improves the condition of the patients.

The immunologic reaction implicated in producing the urticaria is type IV delayed hypersen-

Table 31–3. NUMBER OF PATIENTS REGISTERING A POSITIVE RESPONSE INDEX (RI) TO ADDITIVES, FOOD EXTRACTS, OR BOTH

	No. of Patients (n = 238)
Positive RI to additives	44 (18.4%)
Positive RI to food extracts	83 (35.2%)
Positive RI to both	111 (46.6%)

From Valverde et al.[29]

Table 31–4. RESPONSE TO SPECIAL RECOMMENDED DIET ON THE BASIS OF RESULTS OBTAINED IN VITRO

	No. of Patients (n = 258)
Total remission	159 (61.6%)
Partial remission	57 (22.0%)
No change*	42 (16.2%)

*This group included 20 patients who did not show any response to foods or additives.
From Valverde et al.[29]

sitivity. Valverde et al.[30] have performed similar experiments on patients with the allergic tension-fatigue syndrome, with total remission occurring in 86.3 per cent of the patients. These studies are not direct evidence of T cell activity but are deductive evidence. There is more direct evidence from studying enteropathy in patients with food-induced symptoms.

Ashkenazi et al.[31] studied cell-mediated immunity within the small intestinal mucosa in celiac disease utilizing a test for T cell activation by measurement of leukocyte inhibition factor (LIF), which decreases white cell migration. When the patient's T cells and the antigen are incubated together in an agar well, migration from the well (or lack of it) can be easily measured. This test obtained in a group of patients with celiac disease demonstrated that celiac disease symptoms resolved when specific foods producing an LIF positive response were eliminated from the patients' diets. In 1980, Minor et al.[32] measured LIF responses to milk-

from the diet and may last indefinitely. Therefore, treatment for IgE-mediated food sensitivity is elimination of the offending food.

The second type of food allergy is the cyclic form or the non–IgE-mediated delayed sensitivity, accounting for 60 to 80 per cent of the food sensitivity problems seen in clinical practice. These are probably IgG-mediated, representing an immune complex disease. Identification of this type of sensitivity depends primarily on history taking. Verification may be accomplished with a measurement of specific IgG or immune complexes using RAST, but it must be noted that a high level of IgG or immune complexes does not necessarily mean that the person is clinically sensitive to this particular food. The immune response could just be protective in nature. Following the in vitro testing, the foods that show a high IgG level should be tested with an oral challenge test.

Cyclic food allergy, unlike fixed food allergy, is exposure-dependent (see Chapter 33). Increased frequency of ingestion leads to increased sensitivity; that is, the more frequently the food is eaten, the higher the concentration of specific IgG and immune complexes, and the greater the symptom production. When exposure is present at nearly every meal, as occurs in such hidden foods as corn or milk, a condition of masked food allergy may occur in which a small amount of the food actually relieves symptoms for a short period of time. Treatment for this type of food sensitivity is elimination of the food. This elimination need not be indefinite but rather for only five to six months. At that time the food can be reintroduced into the diet but not consumed every day. Foods should be rotated so that exposure to any food is no more frequent than every four to five days. Infrequent exposure commonly ensures that the specific IgG to these foods will not become elevated and symptom-producing levels will not be reached. The cyclic pattern of delayed food sensitivity may be explained through an IgG immune complex mechanism (Fig. 31–1).

As shown in Figure 31–1, in stage I masked sensitization, the food is eaten frequently, and when a particularly large amount of food is ingested, the immune balance is shifted into antigen excess and pseudotolerance is produced. No immunoglobulin is produced, and the symptoms abate or are "masked." As the antigen level decreases, the level of optimal antibody (IgG) production in response to antigen exposure is again produced. Symptoms will recur. The response is delayed by the time it takes for that level of antigen to decrease to the level of optimal antibody production. If the antigen or the food is omitted for a period of four to five days, the food antigen is cleared from the body; however, there is still a high level of IgG being produced. If a large amount of food is

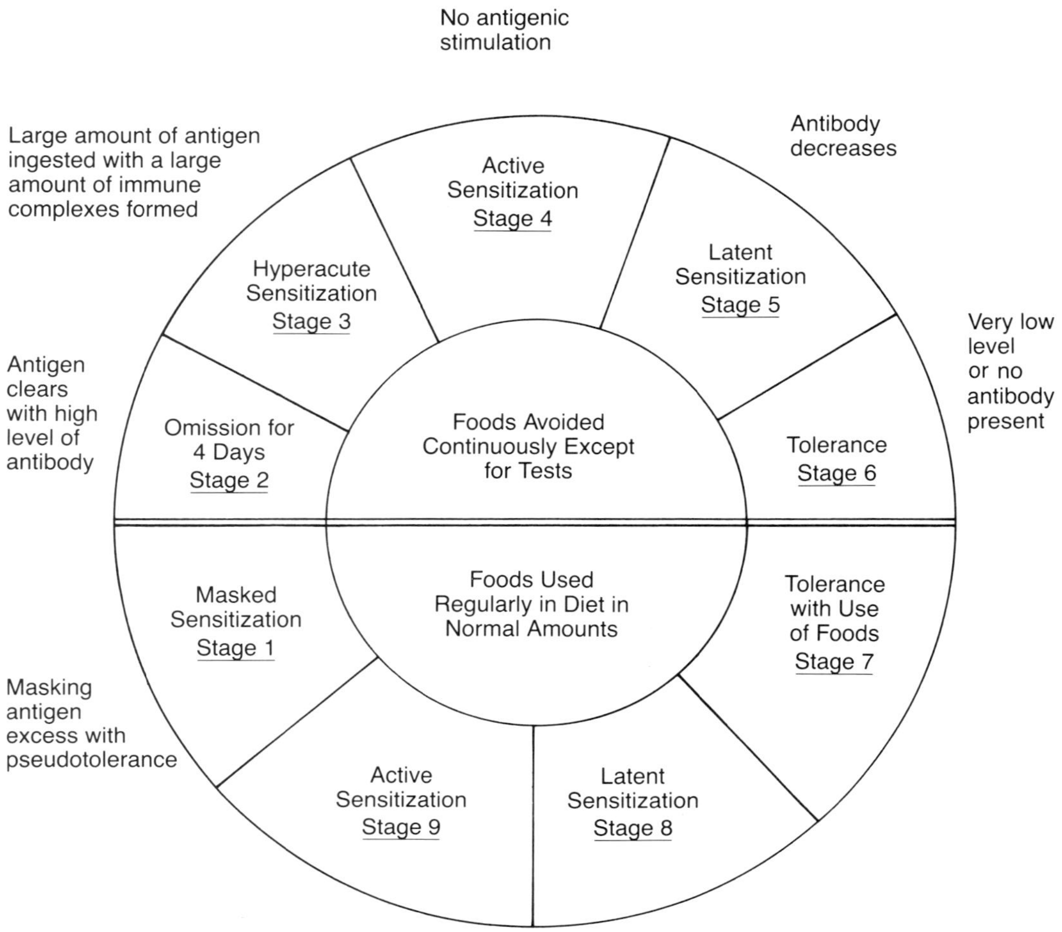

FIGURE 31–1. Increased immune complex disease with increased antigen exposure. (From Rinkel HJ, Randolph TG, Zeller M: Food Allergy. Springfield, IL, Charles C Thomas, 1951. Courtesy of Charles C Thomas, Publisher.)

then consumed, numerous immune complexes form and an exacerbation of symptoms is incited. This is the basis of the oral challenge test in which a person acquires exaggerated symptoms after a four- to five-day fast from that food.

If the patient continues to omit the food in question from the diet, the level of IgG gradually falls until the tolerance phase (stage IV) is attained. At this point there is a very low level of IgG, if any, to that food antigen. At this stage, if the food is reintroduced, there will be some elevation of IgG; but with limitation of the exposure interval, the level of IgG with symptom production will not be reached. In this tolerance phase, the food or foods in question should be rotated to prevent symptom recurrence to a particular food. If the allergic individual again ingests the food frequently, the immune system will be stimulated to produce IgG, and eventually the immune response will become elevated enough to again produce symptoms.

Clinically, there are several ways to test for food sensitivities. For IgE-mediated allergic reactions, the RAST is diagnostic but rarely necessary, since these food sensitivities are usually well known to the patient, producing immediate reactions. Two types of in vivo testing for the more delayed food sensitivities are available. The oral challenge test involves the elimination of a specific food for a period of four to five days followed by ingestion of that food in large amounts. If the patient has a delayed IgG type of sensitivity to this food, he or she will respond in an exaggerated symptomatic manner.

There are occasions, however, when certain foods cannot be eliminated or are very difficult to eliminate from the diet, for example, very common foods such as corn, soy, or wheat.

Other common foods may be difficult to eliminate for a period of four to five months and to rotate in the diet, particularly for a person who travels frequently and is dependent on restaurants. In these cases, provocation with neutralization may be utilized. These techniques for diagnosis of food allergy or hypersensitivity are discussed in more detail in subsequent chapters.

Neutralization

Three mechanisms (most likely working together) may explain the neutralization phenomenon. Two are immunologic, one is nonimmunologic, and more mechanisms may be involved that are still unknown.

In 1974, Jerne[33] proposed a hypothesis to explain the complex interactions that regulate antibody formation (Fig. 31–2), suggesting that the immune system is self-regulating and is composed of a network of idiotypes and anti-idiotypic antibodies. According to this hypothesis, an antigen elicits the production of an antibody (Ab_1) that creates a unique sequence of amino acids, the idiotype, in its antigen-binding region distinguishing it from other antibodies. The unique sequence displayed by idiotype 1 (Id_1) may also function as an immunogen in the same host, since this new array of amino acids is not recognized as self and stimulates the production of another antibody (Ab_2) that has anti-idiotypic specificity for Ab_1. At the same time it displays another unique idiotype, idiotype 2 (Id_2). Ab_2 suppresses the production of Ab_1. In a similar manner, Ab_2 will stimulate the production of Ab_3 and its own unique idiotype 3 (Id_3), displaying anti-anti-idiotypic antibody activity against Ab_2 and so on such that each idiotype that is expressed will stimulate the production of a corresonding anti-idiotypic antibody to suppress the production of the antibody (Ab) against which it was produced. It should be noted that the network can also involve T cells, whereby helper or suppressor T cells can suppress idiotypes identical to those displayed on antibody molecules. Perturbation of this network initiated by exposure to antigen evolves in interactions between idiotypes, anti-idiotypes, and anti-anti-idiotypes. They either turn on or turn off antibody formation to the activities of the various subsets of immunoregulatory T cells. With low doses of antigen exposure this regulatory system is shifted toward shutting off Ab_1 to the original immunogen, and the person moves into the low-dose tolerance phase.

The second immunologic mechanism involved with low-dose therapy is the T cell regulatory system. Figure 31–3 schematically represents proposed cellular interactions that might occur among the already recognized subsets of regulatory T cells. This mechanism involves the direct effect of antigen on T cells. Presentation of the immunogen to macrophages results in the activation of helper-effector T cells and helper-suppressor inducer cells, which cooperate with B cells to initiate antibody formation (pathway 1). At the same time, the helper-suppressor-inducer T cell population is activated to stimulate the regulator T cells, which influence the suppressor-effector T cells to exert their regulatory suppressor effect (pathway 2).

It is currently believed that the suppressive effects initiated by the suppressor-effector T cells are manifest at the level of the helper-effector T cells rather than by direct action of B cells. In situations in which the immunogen appears to bypass interaction with macrophages (e.g., high antigen dose), suppressor-effector T cells can be directly activated by antigen (pathway 3). These cells also exert their suppressive effects at the level of the helper-effector T cell. This pathway may explain the state of pseudotolerance that occurs in the presence of antigen excess.

The final pathway to consider, the contrasuppression circuit (pathway 4), is initiated by the activation of contrasuppressor-inducer T cells. It has a dual regulatory effect interfering with the suppressive activities of the suppressor-effector T cells as well as rendering the helper-effector T cells resistant to the activity of the suppressor-effector T cell.

With very high antigen stimulation, pathway 3 is dominant with suppression of antibody production, creating the pseudotolerance state. With less antigen administration but still high dose, the level of optimal antibody production is reached and pathway 4 predominates. With less antigen administered or low antigen dose, the suppressive effect through pathway 2 predominates and this is the stage of low-dose tolerance. Thus, with low-dose therapy the T cell regulatory mechanism shifts more toward the suppression of antibody production. This eliminates immune complex disease.

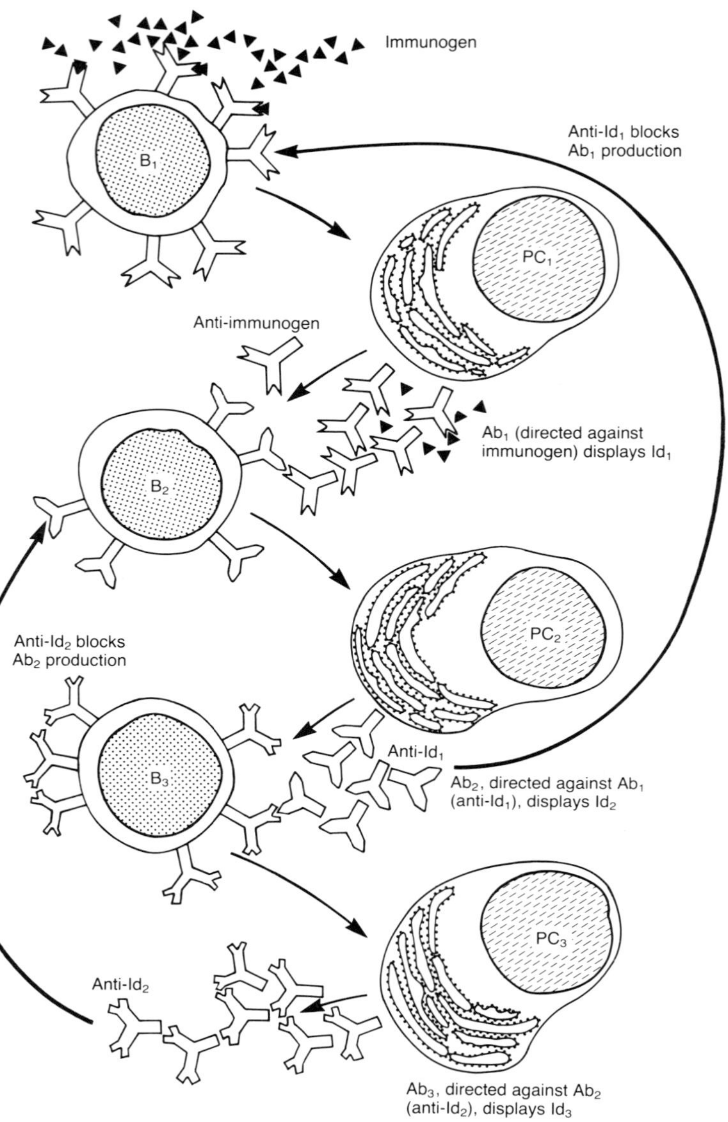

FIGURE 31–2. Schematic representation of idiotype–anti-idiotype regulation of antibody formation. (After Jerne.)

The third mechanism that affords protection to cells when exposed to low-dose antigen exposure is not immunologic but rather involves prostaglandin production. In 1979, Robert et al.[34, 35] reported on cytoprotection by prostaglandin. These investigators gave rats oral administration of caustic substances inducing extensive necrosis of the gastric mucosa. Pretreatment with exogenous prostaglandin either orally or subcutaneously prevented necrosis. They then produced endogenous prostaglandins by pretreating the rats orally with small amounts of the caustic material. This also prevented the necrosis when the caustic material was given. They called this phenomenon the cytoprotective effect. Pretreatment of the rats with indomethacin completely ablated the cytoprotective effect of the low-dose oral feeding. Thus, blocking endogenous prostaglandin production blocked the cytoprotective effect.

Based on these studies, Boris et al.[36] in 1983 studied this cytoprotective effect on antigen-induced asthma in humans. Bronchospasm was evaluated with pulmonary function testing in double-blind studies on 19 subjects with a history of wheezing to animal dander. The subjects were challenged with gradually increasing doses of inhaled animal dander until the dose that

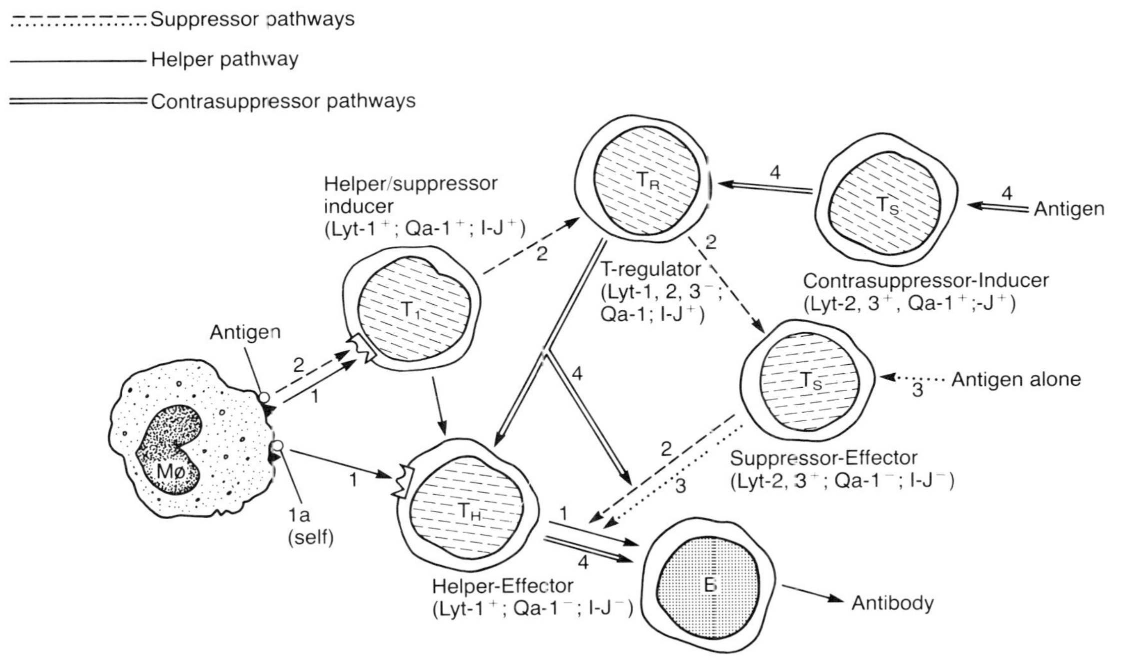

FIGURE 31–3. Schematic representation of T cell feedback regulatory circuits involved in the control of antibody formation. (After Gershon and Cantor.)

caused a 20 per cent increase in FEV_1 was achieved. Intradermal skin testing was then performed to ascertain the end point of the animal dander on each subject. The subjects were pretreated with subcutaneous injection of this endpoint dose and the inhalation provocation was repeated. There was significant prolongation of the FEV_1 up to 75 per cent when an identical inhalation challenge dose was administered. The subjects were then pretreated with indomethacin, the endpoint dose of antigen was administered by injection, and then rechallenge was performed by inhalation of the identical dose of animal dander as used previously. This pretreatment with indomethacin completely ablated the protection against bronchospasm that was produced by pretreatment with a low dose of injected antigen.

The conclusion is that low-dose therapy gives protection to the shock organ, and this is accomplished through prostaglandins. The cells of the shock organ, when exposed to a small amount of a noxious substance, produce prostaglandins that cause an increase in cyclic AMP and decrease in cyclic GMP intracellularly, leading to a reduced metabolism and reactivity of the cell. This is the same effect that is produced by the antiasthmatic medications theophylline and epinephrine. Small doses of immunogen initially protect the cells from the noxious effects of larger doses of the same immunogen.

That antigen dose that causes the shock organ to produce prostaglandins and thus increases cyclic AMP and decreases cyclic GMP, that causes the antibody feedback mechanism to shut off antibody production against that antigen, and that directly causes suppressor T cell activity to shut off antibody production is called the neutralizing dose. Therefore, small doses of immunogen initially protect the cells from the damaging effects of larger doses of the same immunogen.

REFERENCES

1. Coombs RR, Gell PG: Classification of Allergic Reactions Responsible for Clinical Hypersensitivity and Disease: Clinical Aspects of Immunology. Oxford, Blackwell Scientific Publications, 1975, p 761.
2. Danforth E, Moore RD: Intestinal absorption of insulin in the rat. Endocrinology 65:118, 1959.
3. Bernstein ID, Ovary Z: Absorption of antigens from the gastrointestinal tract. Int Arch Allergy Appl Immunol 33:521, 1986.
4. Korenblatt RE, Rothberg RM, Minden P, et al: Immune response of human adults after oral and parenteral exposure to bovine serum albumin. J Allergy 41:226, 1968.

5. Wilson SJ, Walzer M: Absorption of undigested protein in human being. Am J Dis Child 50:49, 1935.
6. Hoffman DR, Haddad ZH: Diagnosis of IgE mediated immediate hypersensitivity reaction to foods by radioimmunoassay. J Allergy Clin Immunol 54:165, 1974.
7. May CD, Brock SA: A modern clinical approach to food hypersensitivity. Allergy 33:166, 1978.
8. Chua YY, Brenmer K, Lakdawalla N, et al: In vivo and in vitro correlates of food allergy. J Allergy Clin Immunol 58:299, 1976.
9. Wraith DG, Merrett J, Roth A, et al: Recognition of food-allergic patients and their allergens by the RAST technique and clinical investigation clinic. Allergy 9:25, 1979.
10. Merrett TG, Merrett J: The RAST principle and the use of mixed allergen: RAST as a screening test for IgE-mediated allergies. Methods Enzymol 70:376, 1980.
11. Monro J, Brostoff J, Carini C, Zilki K: Food allergy in migraine: study of dietary inclusion and RAST. Lancet 2:1, 1980.
12. Paganelli R, Levinsky RJ: Solid phase radioimmunoassay for detection of circulating food protein antigens in human serum. J Immunol Methods 37:333, 1980.
13. Schwartz HR, Nerurkar LS, Spies JR, et al: Milk hypersensitivity: RAST studies using new antigens generated by pepsin hydrolysis of beta lacto globulin. Ann Allergy 45:242, 1980.
14. Freed D: Laboratory diagnosis of food intolerance. Clin Immunol Allergy 2:181, 1982.
15. Scudamore HH, Philips SF, Swedlund HA, Gleich GJ: Food allergy manifested by eosinophilia, elevated immunoglobin E level, and protein-losing enteropathy: the syndromes of allergic gastroenteropathy. J Allergy Clin Immunol 70:129, 1982.
16. Sampson HA, Alberto R: Comparison of results of skin test, RAST, and double-blind, placebo-controlled food challenges in children with atopic dermatii. J Allergy Clin Immunol 6:26, 1984.
17. Hattevig G, Kjellman B, Johansson SG, Bjorksten B: Clinical symptoms and IgE responses to common food proteins in atopic and healthy children. Clin Allergy 14:551, 1984.
18. Lippard VS, Scloss OM, Johnson PA: Immune reactions induced in infants by intestinal absorption of incompletely digested cow's milk protein. Am J Dis Child 51:562, 1936.
19. Heiner DD, Sears JW, Kniker WT: Multiple precipitans to cow's milk in chronic respiratory disease. Am J Dis Child 103:634, 1962.
20. Holland HN, Hong R, Davis NC, West CD: Significance of precipitating antibodies to milk proteins in the serum of infants and children. J Pediatr 61:181, 1962.
21. Mathews TS, Soothill JF: Complement activation after milk feeding in children with cow's milk allergy. Lancet 2:893, 1970.
22. Sandberg DH, Bernstein CW, McIntosh RM, et al: Severe steroid responsive nephrosis associated with hypersensitivity. Lancet 1:388, 1977.
23. Trevino RJ: Immunologic mechanisms in the production of food sensitivities. Laryngoscope 91:1913, 1981.
24. Paganelli R, Levinsky RJ, Atherton DJ: Detection of specific antigen within immune complexes: validation of the assay and its application to food antigen-antibody complexes formed in healthy and food allergic subjects. Clin Exp Immunol 46:44, 1981.
25. Garcia P, Rodriguez JC, Vinos J: A new rapid and more sensitive microcytotoxicity test. J Immunol Methods 1:103, 1971.
26. May CD, Alberto R: In vitro responses of leukocytes to food proteins in allergic and normal children: lymphocyte stimulation and histamine release. Clin Allergy 2:335, 1972.
27. May CD, Alberto R: In vivo stimulation of peripheral lymphocytes to proliferation after oral challenge of children allergic to foods. Int Arch Allergy Appl Immunol 43:525, 1972.
28. Scheinmann P, Gendrel D, Charlas J, et al: Value of lympho-blast transformation test in cow's milk protein intestinal intolerance. Clin Allergy 6:515, 1976.
29. Valverde E, Vich JM, Garcia-Colderon JV, Garcia-Colderon PA: In vitro stimulation of lymphocytes in patients with chronic urticaria induced by additives and foods. Clin Allergy 10:691, 1980.
30. Valverde E, Vich JM, Garcia-Colderon JV, Garcia-Colderon PA: In vitro response of lymphocytes in patients with allergic tension-fatigue syndrome. Ann Allergy 454:185, 1980.
31. Ashkenazi A, Idar O, Handzel ZT, et al: An in vitro immunologic assay for diagnosis of coeliac disease. Lancet 1:627, 1978.
32. Minor JD, Tolber SG, Frick OL: Leukocyte inhibition factors in delayed onset food allergy. J Allergy Clin Immunol 66:319, 1980.
33. Jerne NK: Towards a network theory of the immune system. Ann Immunol 125c:373, 1974.
34. Robert A, Nezamis JE, Lancaster C, Hanchar AJ: Cytoprotection by prostaglandins in rats: prevention of gastric necrosis produced by alcohol, HCl, NaOH, hypertonic NaCl and thermal injury. Gstroenterology 77:433, 1979.
35. Robert A: Cytoprotection by prostaglandins. Gastroenterology 77:761, 1979.
36. Boris M, Schiff M, Weindorf S: Injection of low dose antigen attenuates the response to subsequent bronchoprovocative challenge. Otolaryngol Head Neck Surg 98:536, 1988.

CHAPTER 32

Antigen Selection for Food Allergy Testing

Hueston C. King, M.D., F.A.C.S., F.A.C.A.

The selection of antigen for food testing and treatment presents a different problem. Foods are not tested in batteries like aeroallergens. One cannot select the air that is breathed, so the pertinent potentially allergenic contents must be tested. In food, however, there is great variability in exposure. Pertinent foods are influenced by individual tastes, by local availability, by ethnic preference, and most strongly by cost. The antigen selection, therefore, may be widely divergent from one physician's practice to another's.

Hidden Foods

Since sensitivity is a direct result of exposure, it is not surprising that the most common food offenders are those foods most frequently encountered. One does not become sensitive to a food that is not eaten. Food substances used in preparation of a wide variety of dishes are by far the most common offenders in producing food sensitivity. Leading the list in children is milk; in adults it is corn. It must be remembered that neither need be present in its gross form to produce symptoms. Corn syrup, corn sugar, corn starch, and corn meal are as effective as is plain corn in producing allergic reactions. To gather an idea of the extent to which hidden foods appear in the diet, it is only necessary to read the labels of a few cans in the grocery store. Unless the patient is a health food fanatic, hidden foods must be investigated. A reasonable starting group might include corn, milk, wheat, egg, soy, malt, tomato, pepper, cane sugar, and yeast. Others will be added.

Common Foods

Most people are "habit" eaters. There is surprisingly little variation between the basic foods consumed day after day. A selection of common foods including beef, potato, lettuce, chicken, pork, onion, garlic, lemon, orange, apple, and cabbage would allow adequate testing on a wide variety of patients. It must be borne in mind that food families tend to cross-react; therefore, cabbage will also identify kale and Brussels sprouts, for example and nearly all cereal grains cross-react so that a wide range of grains are identified by testing for wheat. Doris Rapp[1] has produced an excellent list of food families and their cross-reactivity.

Local Availability

Some years ago the local availability of hidden foods was of major importance. An area producing sugar beets could be expected to predominantly use beet sugar in its products, whereas one producing cane would use cane sugar. The development of rapid, inexpensive transportation has fairly well eliminated this consideration. Whatever form of sugar is most readily available and least expensive will be used in production of a nationally sold product. Local availability is still important and should be considered in such things as farm products and seafood. This is a place where the seasonal availability of a product and the patient's tastes become of great significance, and the history will provide the necessary clues.

Ethnic Preferences

Ingrained ethnic habits may have a pronounced effect on the patient's food sensitivities. Daughters learn to cook from mothers, and many individuals still marry within the same ethnic group. Tastes acquired in childhood tend to be carried on, even in selecting from a restaurant menu. An astute investigator would not neglect to look for sensitivity to chicken or rice in a Latin, or to milk and beef in a midwesterner of Scandinavian descent, but would be unlikely to test an Orthodox Jew for pork sensitivity. In food, far more than in inhalants, proper selection of the item to be tested is imperative.

TREATMENT TABLE SELECTION

Whereas the available number of antigens is almost without limit, such a selection for the testing table is not essential. Hidden foods are necessary. Probably 10 will be needed. Another 10 to 15 common foods may be selected by considering the list of the most widely consumed and varying it in accordance with the region and ethnic preferences. This will provide a good overall evaluation for by far the greatest majority of patients. Individual items not present may be identified by elimination and challenge, as long as the number is not prohibitive. If the patient is particularly concerned about a special food, the same consideration described for inhalants may be used. Purchase a single vial, test the patient, and add it to the testing table long enough to see whether it is significant in a reasonable number of patients. If so, add it on a permanent basis. Rarely should a treatment armamentarium contain over 40 food antigens. Treatment of food allergy is a much less predictable procedure than is treatment of inhalants, and the fewer items being treated, the better the chance for success.

Foods rarely consumed may be eliminated or rotated with more satisfactory results than treatment. In general, it is wise to limit the number of food antigens for therapy to those almost impossible to avoid if the patient wishes to enjoy a normal life.

SUMMARY

A reasonable list of antigens has been described for food therapy. The reasons for their selection and for varying their selection have also been discussed. The number of antigens needed for practical therapy is not prohibitive, and may be expanded without difficulty as needed. By following these considerations, the beginning practitioner should be able to provide a satisfactory range of allergy care.

REFERENCE

1. Doris J. Rapp, M.D.: The ECR Collection, P.O. Box 615, Los Altos, CA 94022.

CHAPTER 33

Diets in Food Allergy: Testing and Therapy

William B. Pierce, M.D.

The diagnostic concept for the identification of food allergy utilized by otolaryngic allergists originated from the astute observations of Drs. Carlton Lee,[1] Herbert Rinkel,[2] French Hansel,[3] and Theron G. Randolph.[4]

Although the scientific method has yet to elucidate the exact mediators of the multiplicity of symptoms produced by the ingestion of foods, these men recognized that allergic reactions went beyond the realm of allergic rhinitis, asthma, urticaria, and eczema to include an interrelationship with the production of symptoms such as headaches, fatigue, mental confusion, insomnia, fluid retention, chronic diarrhea, indigestion, compulsive eating and drinking, and possibly others. The original techniques developed by these individuals for the specific identification and treatment of food reactions have been refined and redefined, but the concept of fixed and cyclic food reactions remains the basis for the diagnostic and therapeutic approach to the identification of food allergens.

FOOD ALLERGY: BASIC FORMS

Dr. Herbert Rinkel's observations led him to conclude that reactions to an ingested food became manifest in several different modes. He noted that some individuals would have a reaction to a food every time it was ingested regardless of the amount. This was classified as a fixed reaction. In others, he noted that reactions to ingested foods depended on the amount and frequency of exposure. Some individuals could tolerate what had previously been a problem food if it was ingested only once a week. Others demonstrated an addiction to specific foods. If the addicted individual missed a meal that included the food to which he or she was allergic, symptoms would develop, so he or she would keep eating that food to prevent the development of symptoms. This process by which an individual would seek to avoid symptoms by repeated ingestion was defined as masking. Other patients were observed to develop a period of acute hypersensitivity if they had no contact with their allergic food for a four- to five-day period. If the food to which they were allergic was ingested at the end of this four- to five-day period, they would have a significant flare of their allergic symptoms. From these observations, Dr. Rinkel proposed the "cyclic concept of food allergy"[5] and developed the individual deliberate feeding test[6] plus a method of diet therapy that he called the rotary diversified diet.[7]

To establish a diagnosis of food allergy by the individual deliberate feeding test, a cause and effect relationship must be demonstrated between the ingestion of the given food and subsequent production of symptoms or accentuation of symptoms. In utilizing this technique, the clinician is primarily concerned with observing the effects produced by ingestion of the test food when the patient is in the hyperacute sensitization stage. One must have the cooperation of the patient, be an accurate observer, and have a thorough understanding of the clinical manifestations and mechanisms of food allergy.

CYCLIC FOOD SENSITIZATION

In the concept of cyclic food sensitization, the degree of sensitivity is related to the incidence of each specific food in the diet. It is important to keep in mind that frequency of ingestion tends to increase that sensitivity, whereas avoidance tends to produce tolerance. The patient is encountered in phase I (Fig. 33–1), with chronic symptoms, usually from a food eaten at least once every three days. The food is eliminated for four to 10 days and the patient gradually enters phase II (Fig. 33–2), with resultant improvement in symptoms possibly following a withdrawal state. When the patient is in the allergic hyperacute phase, challenge with an eliminated allergic food will produce symptoms.

With continued elimination, the patient will enter phase III (Fig. 33–3), and subsequently may show tolerance on rechallenge to allergic food. One must be careful not to assume this is a safe food and allow it back in the diet on a regular basis, since symptoms will eventually reappear. Then one becomes lost in the attempt to explain and determine the cause of the patient's symptoms. The patient has reentered the cycle and tolerance is lost. Therefore, a detailed and comprehensive food diary is essential before testing. One must become a student of the food diary, learning from it the frequency of ingestion

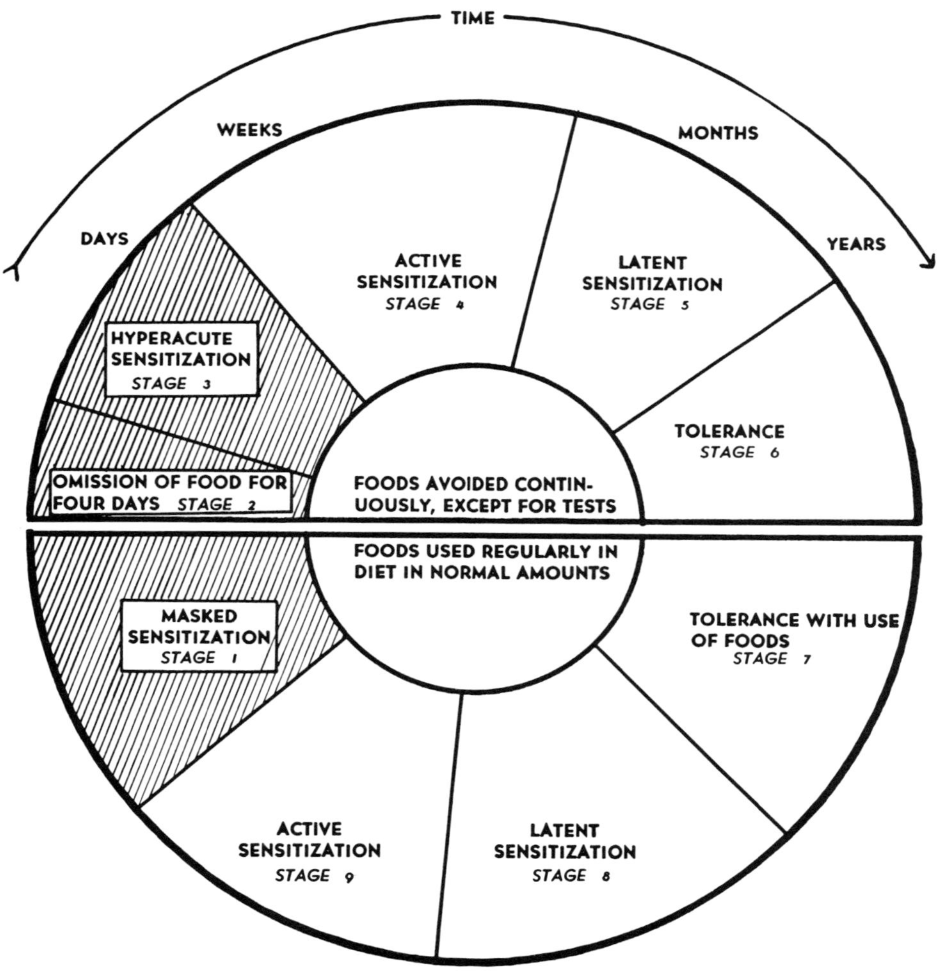

FIGURE 33–1. Phase I of the cyclic concept: masking, omission, and stage of hyperacute reaction. (From Rinkel HJ, Randolph TG, Zeller M: Food Allergy. Springfield, IL, Charles C Thomas, 1951. Courtesy of Charles C Thomas, Publisher.)

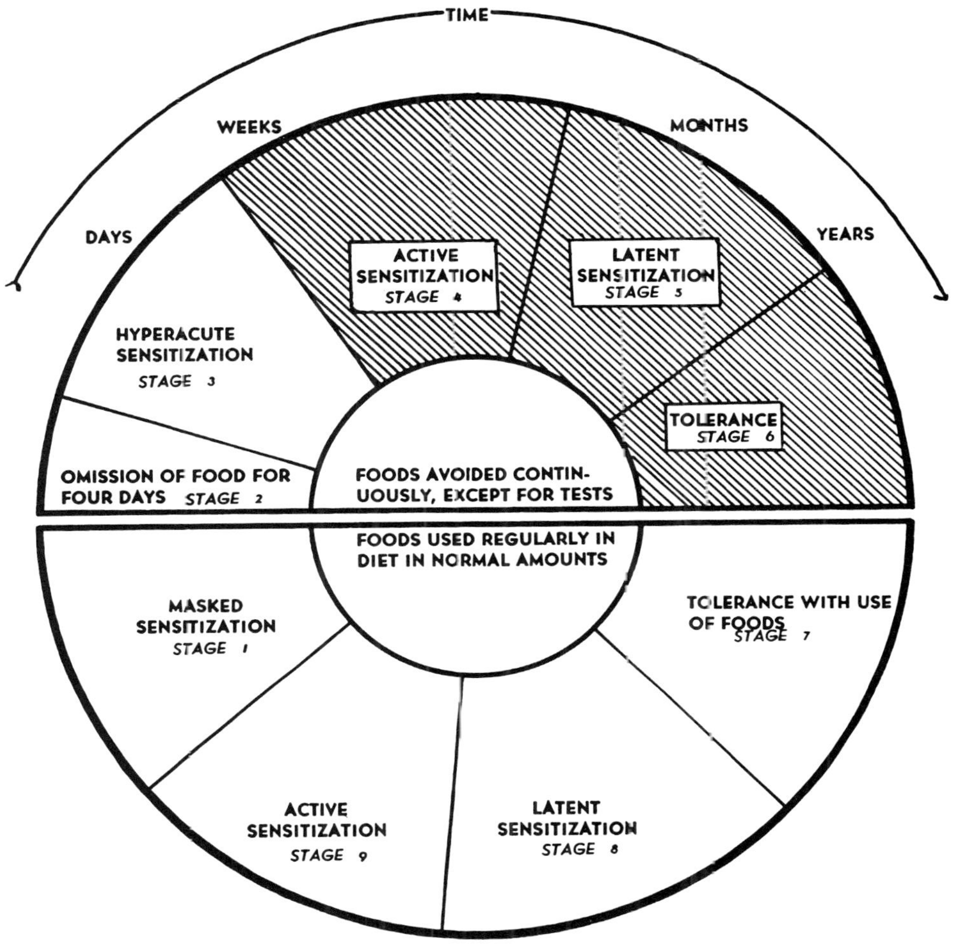

FIGURE 33–2. Phase II of the cyclic concept: active sensitization, latent sensitization, and tolerance with continued avoidance. (From Rinkel HJ, Randolph TG, Zeller M: Food Allergy. Springfield, IL, Charles C Thomas, 1951. Courtesy of Charles C Thomas, Publisher.)

of individual foods, the type of reactions the patient is experiencing, and the patient's general degree of sensitivity.

When analyzing a food diary, concentrate first on foods or liquids craved or eaten in binges, ones the patient suspects may be causing symptoms, and foods regularly in the diet. It is worthwhile making a list of those foods eaten once a week, those eaten twice a week, and those ingested more than once a day. In this manner you can develop an order of testing. Also, by separating foods eaten frequently from those eaten infrequently, we can identify which foods should or should not be tested.

HISTORICAL INDICATORS

Historical information that may indicate a possible food allergy includes

1. Symptoms beginning in infancy, such as eczema, frequent croup, colic, and diarrhea.
2. Perennial symptoms.
3. Symptoms that are worse after eating or are relieved by eating.
4. Food cravings and addictions.
5. Freedom of symptoms after a surgical or religious fast.
6. Fluid retention or frequent weight fluctuation.
7. Persistent symptoms in spite of adequate control of inhalant allergies.

FOOD TESTING

Individual food testing should be done in order of probability of sensitization (Table 33–1).

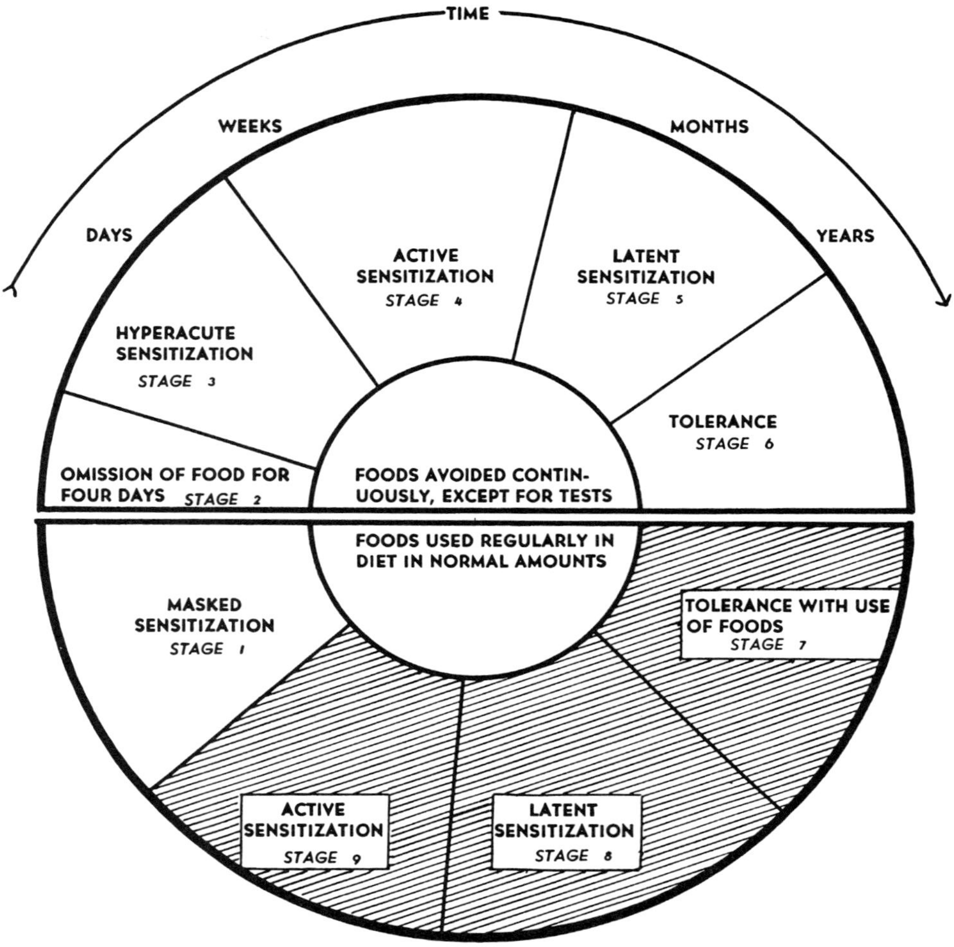

FIGURE 33–3. Phase III of the cyclic concept: period of tolerance after ingestion is resumed, followed by latent sensitivity, masking, and active sensitization with continued ingestion. (From Rinkel HJ, Randolph TG, Zeller M: Food Allergy. Springfield, IL, Charles C Thomas, 1951. Courtesy of Charles C Thomas, Publisher.)

Prior to testing an individual for food allergies by the individual deliberate feeding test, the following circumstances must prevail.[8]

1. Coexisting inhalant allergy should be diagnosed and treated.
2. The test food must have been in the patient's diet at least every other day for two weeks prior to its elimination.
3. The test should be postponed if the patient is ill or having an allergic flare.
4. Test foods should be chemically uncontaminated, individually prepared, and served in glass containers.
5. Shaving lotion and perfume are not to be worn on the test day.
6. Only one food can be tested at a time.
7. Give the patient detailed preinstructions regarding the food to be eliminated. This is especially important when testing for corn, soy, milk, and wheat, since they are common ingredients in processed food.
8. The test is performed on the fifth day following four days of complete elimination of the test food.
9. The patients are to fast from midnight and should not smoke for at least three hours before the beginning of the test.

Although the individual deliberate feeding test can be performed by the patient at home, it is best done in a physician's office under a controlled and quiet environment where the patient can be directly observed by the personnel administering the test.

Once the patient has arrived in the office and

Table 33–1. TEST FOOD

Wheat: ½ cup of pure Cream of Wheat prepared in distilled water
Corn: ½ cup of pure grits prepared in distilled water
Eggs: Two hard- or soft-boiled
Milk: 1 pint of plain cow's milk
White potato: One large or two small baked potatoes, plain
Oranges: Two medium or 8 oz of pure fresh orange juice
Peas: Can of dextrose-free June peas, unflavored
Beef: 4–6 oz of broiled beef, plain
Tomato: One large ripe, or one medium and one small ripe; pure tomato juice can also be used
Coffee: Two cups, black, of the patient's brand
Lettuce: One medium head, raw
Pork: Two chops fried in their own fat
Apples: Raw eating apple, patient's usual variety
Grapes: Raw if possible or pure grape juice; some patients are sensitive to purple grapes and not sensitive to green or white grapes
Cabbage: Portion of raw
Grapefruit: One whole, peeled or juiced
Chocolate: 1 teaspoon Hershey's Cocoa in water, sweeten with pure cane sugar

is comfortably seated, a baseline pulse, blood pressure, and respirations are taken.

Patients are supplied with a clipboard and paper for recording their symptoms.

Vital signs are repeated and recorded every 20 minutes of the two-hour test period, during which time the patient is observed for signs and symptoms. The test food should be eaten within a five-minute period. If a test food fails to produce definite symptoms at the end of 40 minutes, a 1/4 kicker portion is ingested.

Following ingestion of the test food, patients are observed for symptoms such as sniffing, sneezing, runny watery nose, scratching or itching of the nose, nasal stuffiness, throat clearing, coughing, chest tightness, wheezing, excessive gas, bloating, heartburn, nausea, abdominal cramps, vomiting, diarrhea, and borborygmus as well as fatigue; headache, pain or aching in any location; itching of the skin, lips, palate, or throat; development of hives or exacerbation of eczema; flushing of the face; or a sensation of chilling.

In general, early development of symptoms and a sustained reaction indicate a high degree of sensitization. A sustained, clinical reaction is considered diagnostically important. Some patients may develop delayed symptoms, usually within 10 to 14 hours following the test. The majority of these patients will have had some indication of a positive reaction within the first hour following ingestion of the test food. Either an increase or decrease in pulse rate may be observed. Also, the pulse may become irregular and thready. From a symptom standpoint, a symptom noted by the patient and the observer, such as throat clearing, rubbing of the nose, or facial grimacing, is more important than subjective symptom expressions such as "I think I have a tightness in my head" or "a muscle tightness in my throat." Patients with these kinds of subjective symptoms usually have no pulse change.

Subjective responses are not good indicators because the patient may have a preconceived idea that he or she is allergic to the test food and, if so, is more likely to express a symptom. It is also important not to preinstruct patients that they might receive a kicker dose if they do not react. They will often produce a symptom so they do not have to eat any more of the challenged food. If a patient reports that he or she feels better than usual following the ingestion of the test food, it is likely that the test food has been eaten in some form during the elimination. It is often advisable for the patient to keep a food diary during the four days of elimination.

WATER FAST

A more rigorous method of oral food challenge involves admission to an environmental care unit, followed by four days of fasting on spring or filtered water. The fast is followed by an individual food challenge in a quantity sufficient to satisfy hunger, usually four times in a day. The safe foods are subsequently rotated and reactive foods eliminated.

FOOD TEST CRITICISMS

Oral food challenge tests have been criticized in the following areas:

1. They are nonscientific and do not necessarily represent an immunologic response when positive.

2. Since food and eating occupy a predominant interplay in our psychological world, the imaginary physical reactions cannot be distinguished from true reactions without the scientific use of a double-blind food challenge.

3. There is an inherent bias on the part of physicians and patients relative to their symp-

toms as a result of ingestion of a specific food. At least 25 per cent of the reactions are either psychological or imaginary.

METHODS USED BY OTHER ALLERGISTS

General allergists consider the double-blind placebo-controlled oral challenge as the "gold standard" for the determination of food allergies. It is primarily utilized in a clinical research environment because it is somewhat impractical for office diagnosis.

The test food is administered in capsules or through a nasogastric tube. Test food selection is based on a strong history of possible food allergies and/or positive skin prick tests. Some physicians use a laxative to purge the intestinal tract prior to testing. One test method[9] performs two challenges each day, one placebo and one test food, utilizing up to 8 gm of dehydrated powdered food administered in size 0 capsules or in 100 ml of juice or broth over a one-hour period. Physicians or research nurse clinicians evaluate all possible reactions and symptoms. These are then recorded on symptom sheets. A single blind food challenge method has also been described.

ROTATION DIETS—BACKGROUND HISTORY

From the earliest concept of manipulation of diet to influence adverse reactions to foods, alteration of diet was employed for either diagnostic or therapeutic purposes or both. Historically, Dr. Rinkel first utilized the rotary diversified diet in 1934 for the purpose of maintaining tolerance to a problem food. Subsequently, he employed the diet to prevent the occurrence of new sensitizations and, finally, to preserve tolerance and to prevent the development of new food allergies in allergic individuals. It can also be utilized as a diagnostic tool to unmask hidden food allergies.

A. H. Rowe elimination diets[10] have been utilized for approximately 60 years in the diagnosis and control of food allergies by many allergists. Prior to 1926, Dr. Rowe advocated elimination of wheat, milk, eggs, and other suspicious skin-reacting foods. By 1926, he added fish, nuts, chocolate, coffee, condiments, and a few vegetables and fruits to this list. He subsequently devised three diets that were originally published in *JAMA* in 1928.[11] In several instances these diets did not totally eliminate the problem food and did not take into account the biologic grouping of foods. These diets have been modified from their original form and include a cereal-free elimination diet, a fruit- and cereal-free elimination diet, and a cereal elimination diet for infants.[10]

L.P. Gay of St. Louis presented an article in July 1941 in the *Journal of the Missouri Medical Association* entitled "Menu for Dietary Management of Allergic Disease."[12] He felt that wheat, milk, eggs, white potato, pork, tomato, citrus fruit, chocolate, and pineapple were the most common food offenders for most patients. Therefore, these foods were removed from the diet and substitutions were made. A menu for five successive days was worked out. On the sixth day, the patient started over with the first day but with a different group of foods. In essence, this represented a form of a rotary diversified diet.

Warren T. Vaughan laid the foundation of dietary management for allergic disease by the recognition of the biologics of food sensitization relating to their genetic classification.[13] Ellis expanded the listings further into the animal kingdom and clarified various cross-reactivities.[14]

Dr. Rinkel first employed his rotary diversified diet in 1934. However, an article on the subject was not published until 1948.[7] There have been few major changes to the basic diversified rotary diet concept since publication of *Food Allergy* by Randolph, Rinkel, and Zeller in 1951.[2] Refinements have included further diversification and greater than four-day intervals of rotation. At the time of the writings of these early clinicians, most children were breast fed, and early introduction of solid foods into their diet was not advocated. There had been little change in farming methods, and no herbicides or pesticides had been introduced into the food chain.

Modifying the diet today is much more difficult, particularly with the recognition of corn as a major allergen by Dr. Randolph,[15] because it has become a common ingredient in processed foods of today.

Many allergists feel that major eliminations in the average western diet must be accomplished before any biologic food source changes become meaningful. They advocate elimination of processed food as the first step and find in many instances that nothing else is required, since it reduces the intake of chemical additives, sugars, salt, and common denominators such as yeast, soy, and spices.

Any physician who embarks on the utilization of diet to help patients establish control of their food allergies must be prepared to do extensive reading and become familiar with the various diets, including their advantages and disadvantages. Do not totally transfer this responsibility to the patients by giving them an instruction sheet on food rotation or even a single food elimination list. The most successful treatment of an individual patient with a food allergy results from developing an approach that leads to the greatest compliance. Therefore, enough time has to be spent with the patient to determine his or her capability of compliance. Approach and counsel the patient as an individual, adapting for socioeconomic circumstances, life style, ethnic background, age, nutritional requirements, and occupation. It must be determined what dietary approach is realistic for each patient.

FOOD DIARY

Evaluation of a patient's food diary, coupled with an understanding of the cyclic nature of food sensitivity, will usually provide a definable starting point for nutritional management. The food diary will reflect the amount of food consumed per day, the number of foods eaten including their individual ingredients, the patient's eating habits, and any correlation to symptoms. The diary should be recorded for at least one week. By combining the patient's history with this information, examples of masking, food addiction, tolerance, withdrawal symptoms, and exaggerated reactions may become evident. Chronic symptoms such as headaches, insomnia and hyperactivity, abdominal discomfort, flatulence, diarrhea, arthralgia, laryngeal edema, rhinitis, eczema, asthma, and chronic urticaria may represent delayed food reactions.

You may notice during evaluation of food diaries that some patients consider this a very intimate piece of information. They have a personal, almost sensual relationship with their food. When you ask questions about their diary, they may react as though you were asking questions about their sex life. When patients react in this way, it is highly suspected that they have a food allergy. Other patients, after completing a food diary, will begin to suspect what their problem food may be. When elimination of one or more suspected foods is recommended on a trial basis, they may respond emotionally. People who consider eating purely a functional requirement usually have no food problems. These people will treat their food diaries as "matter-of-fact" information.

CYCLIC FOOD ALLERGY TREATMENT

Treatment of cyclic food allergy can best be accomplished by elimination. Whenever a patient is proved sensitive to a food, elimination is the treatment of choice. Omission of the food is required until tolerance develops, which may take anywhere from three to 18 months, depending on the inherent tolerance of the patient. It is reasonable to exclude that food from the diet for three months and then test it by a single challenge feeding. If no symptoms result, that food is rotated into the diet and consumed once a week for six weeks. If there are no resultant symptoms, the food can be added to the diet every four to five days. However, if a single feeding causes symptoms, it will be necessary to avoid that food for another three months and retest it. If the result is negative, the food is allowed once daily at four- to five-day intervals for six weeks to determine if sensitization recurs, since symptoms will not mask themselves at this interval. In the absence of symptoms after six weeks at this interval, the patient is instructed to reduce the interval from five to three days. The food is then used at this interval for three months and, if still tolerated, may possibly be reduced to a single use once every two days.

Tolerance will vary from individual to individual and will vary with different food groups. If the patient develops an increase in symptoms during the course of using the diet in this manner, the possibility of recurring allergy as the result of insidious and progressive sensitization must be considered. If this is true, the elimination must be repeated. The type of patient who can be treated satisfactorily by eliminating known allergens with a narrowed limited diet is considered to have a high inherent tolerance for foods.[2]

Those patients who tend to become sensitive or who are sensitive to any food that appears in their diet on a daily basis are considered to have a low inherent tolerance to foods and require a more stringent rotary diet.[2] We are then faced with providing the patient with a diversified diet consisting of foods to which he or she can develop and preserve tolerance, as well as preventing the development of new sensitizations while providing foods for a well-balanced diet.

FOOD ROTATION

Since the frequency of any food as a specific allergen is determined more by its frequency in the diet than its biochemical makeup, individuals with multiple food sensitivities need to eat as varied a diet as possible and limit the frequent ingestion of the same food. The basis of the nutritional regimen, therefore, is a "rotary diversified diet," which means that all food items in an individual's diet are rotated by food families[16] for a specified number of days, usually with a given food being ingested only once every four days. The diet should be diversified to include as many different kinds of compatible foods as possible. A four-day rotation is most commonly used. It represents the average transit time for food to pass through the gastrointestinal tract. If the food is eaten on Monday, it should not be eaten again until Friday. For example, if an apple is eaten on Monday, a pear or an apple could be eaten on Friday, since they are in the same biologic plant group. The same principle is applied with the food groups for meat, grains, vegetables, nuts, oils, and sweeteners as well as fruits. Rotation is best accomplished by limiting the number of foods per meal and increasing their quantity per serving.

The number of foods allowed per meal and the number of meals per day may be an individual decision based on the patient's food tolerance, individual sensitivity, and symptoms. Food families based on their biologic form and origin (Table 33–2) are also rotated. Once eaten, a member of a food family may not be repeated for another four days. With this timing, as previously mentioned, the patient enters a hypersensitivity stage so, on challenge, the food ingested will produce a reaction and sensitivities are unmasked. Allergenic foods determined in this way are eliminated for three months. If the patient does well, they are reintroduced at a minimum four-day rotation. Occasionally, a seven- to 10-day rotation is required to maintain tolerance.

The rotation diet emphasizes

1. Whole, less refined foods—will be higher in fiber and lower in simple carbohydrates; encourages consumption of complex carbohydrates.

2. Foods free of pesticides, antibiotics, steroids, hormones, food additives, preservatives, artificial sweeteners, and waxes.

3. Foods lower in salt and in hydrogenated fat.

THE CONCEPT OF MINIMAL ELIMINATION

Where a few specific foods are highly suspect, a single food elimination may be tried. The suspect food is eliminated completely from the diet for a minimum of four days and a maximum of ten days. The food is reintroduced during the four- to ten-day period, and observations are made over the next 24 hours for symptoms. This may be used when the patient feels well most of the time and has only a few suspected foods. The disadvantages of the single food elimination are

1. Detailed instructions must be given to the patient regarding those foods that occur as hidden ingredients, such as corn, soy, milk, and wheat. The patient must read labels and question waiters.

2. It may be hard to detect a reaction to that food if the patient has multiple food allergies and is reacting to other foods.

The water fast, such as is utilized in environmental units, may also be considered. In seriously debilitated, underweight patients, some physicians use an elemental diet, such as Vivonex or Ultrabalance. However, the patient may react to the food residue from which the essential amino acids are derived, usually soy.

Table 33–2. FOOD PROTEINS CLASSIFIED ACCORDING TO BIOLOGIC RELATIONSHIP

Animal Groups

1. Amphibians
   - frog
2. Bird (flesh and organs)
   - chicken
   - Cornish hen
   - duck
   - grouse
   - goose
   - guinea hen (fowl)
   - partridge
   - pheasant
   - pigeon
   - squab
   - turkey
3. Crustaceans
   - crab
   - crayfish
   - lobster
   - prawn
   - shrimp
4. Eggs (bird)
   - ovomucoid
   - ovovitellin
   - white
   - whole
   - yolk
5. Fish (representative families)
   - Acipenseridae
     - sturgeon (caviar)
   - Anguillidae
     - eel
   - Argentinidae
     - smelt
   - Carangidae
     - pompano
   - Centrarchidae
     - black bass
     - crappie
     - sunfish
   - Clupeidae
     - herring
     - sardine
     - shad
     - sprat
   - Cyprinidae
     - carp
   - Esocidae
     - muscallonge
     - pickerel
     - pike
   - Gadidae
     - cod
     - haddock
     - hake
     - pollock
     - scrod
   - Mugilidae
     - mullet
   - Percidae
     - perch
   - Pleuronectidaes
     - flounder
     - halibut
   - Salmonidae
     - grayling
     - salmon
     - trout
     - whitefish
   - Scienidae
     - croaker
     - drum
     - redfish
     - sea trout
     - weakfish
   - Scombridae
     - bonito
     - mackerel
     - tuna
   - Serranidae
     - grouper
     - rockfish
     - white bass
   - Siluridae
     - bullhead
     - catfish
   - Soleidae
     - sole
   - Sparidae
     - porgy
     - red snapper
   - Stolephoridae
     - anchovy
   - Xyphidae
     - swordfish
6. Red meats (flesh and internal organs)
   - a. *Bovidae*
     - Cow
       - beef
       - calf
       - steer
       - veal
     - Gelatin
     - Goat
     - Ox
     - Sheep
       - lamb
       - mutton
   - b. *Suidae* (pig)
     - bacon
     - boar
     - ham
     - hog
     - pig
     - pork
     - sausage
     - scrapple
     - sow
     - swine
7. Milk products (cow, goat)
   - butter
   - buttermilk
   - casein
   - cheese
   - cream
     - sour
     - whipped
   - ice cream
   - lactalbumin
   - milk
     - condensed
     - evaporated
     - homogenized
     - powdered
     - raw
     - skimmed
   - selected infant formulas
   - yogurt
8. Mollusks
   - abalone
   - clam
   - cockle
   - mussel
   - octopus
   - oyster
   - quahog
   - scallops
   - snail (escargot)
   - squid
9. Reptiles
   - alligator
   - crocodile
   - rattlesnake
   - terrapin
   - turtle

Plant Groups

10. Apple family
    - apple
      - cider
      - vinegar
    - crabapple
    - pear
    - quince
    - quince seed
11. Banana family
    - banana
    - plantain
12. Beech family
    - beechnut
    - chestnut
    - chinquapin
13. Birch family
    - filbert
    - hazelnut
    - wintergreen
14. Buckwheat family
    - buckwheat
    - rhubarb
    - sorrel
15. Cashew family
    - cashew
    - mango
    - pistachio
16. Citrus family
    - citron
    - grapefruit
    - kumquat
    - lemon
    - lime
    - orange
    - tangelo
    - tangerine
17. Cola nut family
    - chocolate (cocoa)
    - cola (kola) nut
18. Fungi
    - mushroom
    - truffle
    - yeast
      - baker's
      - brewer's
      - distiller's
      - Fleischman's
      - lactose-fermenting
      - lager beer
19. Ginger family
    - cardamom
    - East Indian arrowroot
    - ginger
    - turmeric
20. Goosefoot family
    - beet
    - lamb's quarters
    - spinach
    - Swiss chard
21. Gourd (melon) family
    - cantaloupe
    - casaba
    - Chinese watermelon
    - citrus melon
    - cucumber
    - gherkin
    - honeydew melon
    - Persian melon
    - pumpkin
    - summer squash
    - watermelon
    - winter squash
22. Grape family
    - champagne
    - grape
    - raisin
    - vinegar (white)
    - wine (grape)
23. Grass (cereal) family
    - bamboo
    - barley
    - corn (maize)
    - hominy
    - malt
    - millet
    - oat
    - popcorn
    - rice
    - rye
    - sorghum
    - sugar cane
    - wheat
      - bran
      - germ
      - gliadin
      - globulin
      - glutenin
      - leucosin
      - proteose
      - whole
24. Heath family
    - black huckleberry
    - blueberry
    - cranberry
    - wintergreen
25. Laurel family
    - avocado
    - bay leaf
    - cinnamon
    - sassafras

Table continued on following page

Table 33–2. FOOD PROTEINS CLASSIFIED ACCORDING TO BIOLOGIC RELATIONSHIP *Continued*

Plant Groups *Continued*

26. Lecythis family
    - Brazil nut
27. Lily family
    - aloe
    - asparagus
    - chives
    - garlic
    - leek
    - onion
    - sarsaparilla
    - shallot
28. Madder family
    - coffee
29. Mallow family
    - cottonseed
    - marshmallow
    - okra (gumbo)
30. Mint family
    - balm
    - basil
    - catnip
    - hoarhound
    - Japanese artichoke
    - lavender
    - marjoram
    - mint
    - oregano
    - peppermint
    - rosemary
    - sage
    - savory
    - spearmint
    - thyme
31. Morning glory family
    - sweet potato
    - yam
32. Mulberry family
    - breadfruit
    - breadnut
    - fig
    - hop
33. Mustard family
    - broccoli
    - Brussels sprouts
    - cabbage
    - cauliflower
    - collards
    - garden cress
    - horseradish
    - kale
    - kohlrabi
    - mustard
    - radish
    - rutabaga
    - turnip
    - watercress
34. Myrtle family
    - allspice
    - clove
    - guava
    - myrtle
    - pimento
35. Nightshade family
    - bell pepper
    - cayenne pepper
    - chili (paprika)
    - eggplant
    - ground cherry
    - melon pear
    - potato (white)
    - strawberry tomato
    - tobacco
    - tomato
    - tree tomato
36. Nutmeg family
    - mace
    - nutmeg
37. Olive family
    - jasmine
    - olive
38. Orchid family
    - vanilla
39. Palm family
    - cabbage palm
    - coconut
    - date
40. Papaya family
    - papain
    - papaya
41. Parsley family
    - anise
    - caraway
    - carrot
    - celeriac
    - celery
    - coriander
    - dill
    - fennel
    - parsley
    - parsnip
42. Pea (legume) family
    - acacia
    - alfalfa
    - black-eyed pea
    - broad bean
    - carob bean
    - chickpea
    - common bean
    - kidney
        - navy
        - pinto
        - string (green)
    - Jack bean
    - lentil
    - licorice
    - lima bean
    - mesquite
    - pea
    - peanut
    - soybean
    - tamarind
    - tragacanth
43. Pepper family
    - black pepper
44. Pine family
    - juniper
    - pine nut (Pignolia)
45. Pineapple family
    - pineapple
46. Plum family
    - almond
    - apricot
    - cherry
    - peach, nectarine
    - plum, prune
47. Poppy family
    - poppyseed
48. Rose family
    - black raspberry
    - blackberry
    - boysenberry
    - dewberry
    - loganberry
    - red raspberry
    - strawberry
49. Saxifrage family
    - currant
    - gooseberry
50. Sunflower (composite, aster) family
    - absinthe
    - artichoke
    - camomile
    - chicory
    - dandelion
    - endive
    - escarole
    - Jerusalem artichoke
    - lettuce
    - oyster plant
    - safflower
    - sunflower
    - tansy
    - tarragon
51. Tea family
    - tea
52. Walnut family
    - black walnut
    - butternut
    - English walnut
    - hickory nut
    - pecan

THE "CAVEMAN OR STONE AGE" ROTARY DIVERSIFIED DIET

For initial dietary manipulation, the caveman diet can be used in the office management of patients suspected of having a food factor as a disease element. It is an alternative to the fasting type program, as it eliminates the most common foods implicated in chronic illness.

Foods eliminated:[17]

1. Refined sugar.
2. Wheat and cereal grains.
3. Milk and all products containing milk.
4. Processed foods; also artificial colors, flavorings, preservatives, and additives.
5. Yeast, malt, mold foods, and mold-containing foods.

Foods allowed:

1. Meat.
2. Fish.
3. Fowl.
4. Fruits and vegetables—all fresh or fresh-frozen.
5. Seeds and nuts—raw or in the shell.

The foods allowed should be in their least chemically contaminated form or organically grown. This diet can also be used for diagnostic purposes, since the foods to be eliminated should be excluded from the diet for seven days and then can be reintroduced on a four-day rotational basis. This constitutes an individual deliberate feeding test. During the initial seven days of elimination, a determination must be made to see if presenting symptoms are modified. If a patient does not experience any improvement, it is then likely that one of the foods in the diet may be a causative factor and subsequently would have to be evaluated by avoidance and reexposure.

The food consumed while on this diet should be spaced so that the same food group or family is not used more often than once every fourth day. Before beginning the diet, some physicians will clear the gastrointestinal tract by use of laxatives such as Sal Hepatica, epsom salts, or unflavored Fleet Phosphc-Soda.

Again, instructional time must be spent with the patient so that he or she may acquire the appropriate foods, and they should be chosen to represent a variety of the food families. Keep in mind that foods in the same biologic family may cross-react. Sesame seed, sunflower, and olive oil may be used as oils for rotation, whereas soy, peanut, cottonseed, and corn should be avoided.

As with other rotational diets, if a food is found that causes a reaction after prolonged avoidance, it is eliminated from the diet for at least three months and then may be tested with a single feeding. If no reaction occurs, it could be reintroduced into the diet once a week for six weeks, and if all is well, it may be rotated on a four-day rotation regimen. However, if the test feeding is positive, three additional months of avoidance should be instituted followed by retesting. After two years of avoidance, if the food continues to cause a reaction, it can be considered a fixed reaction and will always have to be avoided.

ADDITIONAL INSTRUCTIONS

Foods that come in plastic bags should not be used. Foods are used plain, but they can be mixed together. The foods should be rinsed with spring water from glass bottles. Tap water may be utilized if it is filtered through an approved charcoal filter. No spices, herbs, or pepper are allowed, but sea salt can be utilized. In the cooking and preparation of the foods, they should be broiled, baked, or roasted plain. Electric cooking should be utilized, and items should be cooked in glass or stainless steel containers. Aluminum and cast iron should not be used. Fruits, vegetables, and fish can be steamed with a small amount of spring water in stainless steel containers. Foods should be cooked only with spring water. Gas stoves should not be used. Foods should be stored in the refrigerator in either glass or stainless steel containers. Toothpaste and tooth powders are eliminated. Baking soda may be utilized for brushing. Only unscented white tissues and white toilet paper should be used.

REFERENCES

1. Lee CH, Shephard EM, Scala LS: Allergic neutralization. Tri Sigma Press, St. Joseph, MO, 1987.
2. Rinkel HJ, Randolph TG, Zeller M: Food Allergy. Springfield, IL, Charles C Thomas, 1951.
3. Hansel FK: Clinical Allergy. St. Louis, CV Mosby, 1953.
4. Randolph TG: Human Ecology and Susceptibility to the Chemical Environment. Springfield, IL, Charles C Thomas, 1978.
5. Rinkel HJ: Food allergy. J Kansas Med Soc 37:177, 1936.
6. Rinkel HJ: Food allergy. II. The technique and clinical application of individual food tests. Ann Allergy 2:504, 1944.
7. Rinkel HJ: Food allergy. IV. The function and clinical applications of the rotary diversified diet. J Pediatr 32:266, 1948.
8. Williams RI: The Management of Clinical Allergy. Cheyenne, WY, Frontier Printing, 1983, pp 121–122.
9. Sampson HA: Immediate hypersensitivity reactions to food, emphasizing blinded food challenges in children with atopic dermatitis. 5th International Food Allergy Symposium, October, 1984.
10. Rowe AH, Rowe A Jr: Food Allergy. Springfield, IL, Charles C Thomas, 1972, pp 41–75.
11. Rowe AH: Food allergy: its manifestations, diagnosis, and treatment. JAMA 91:1623, 1928.
12. Gay LP: Menu for dietary management of allergic disease. J Missouri State Med Assoc 38:233, 1941.
13. Vaughan WT: Food allergies. A genetic classification with results of food testing. J Allergy 1:385, 1930.
14. Ellis RV: Rational grouping of food allergens. J Allergy 2:246, 1931
15. Randolph TG: Food allergy. Med Clin North Am 32:245, 1948.
16. American Academy of Allergy and Immunology Committee on Adverse Reactions to Foods: Adverse Reactions to Foods. U.S. Department of Health and Human Services, NIH Publication 84–2442, July 1984, pp 17–25.
17. Dickey LD, MacLennan SG: Clinical Ecology Office Procedures Manual. 6th ed. Denver, Clinical Ecology Organization, 1981, p 71.

CHAPTER 34

Diagnostic Provocation Testing and Neutralization Therapy for Food Allergy

William P. King, M.D.

DIAGNOSTIC TESTING BY PROVOCATION

Over a quarter century ago, Dr. Carlton Lee recognized an urgent need for a more practical food allergy test than the time-consuming and awkward food challenge technique. As an answer, he developed an intracutaneous provocation food test.[1] This test mimicked intracutaneously the classic deliberate challenge food test, but required less time and preparation and was much more convenient. In addition, he noted that he could neutralize the provoked symptoms with slightly weaker dose application, whereas still weaker doses would sometimes aggravate the symptoms.

Dr. Herbert J. Rinkel became interested in the work of Lee, and after collaboration developed a revised technique.[2] Because of Dr. Rinkel's untimely death, it fell upon the shoulders of one of his disciples, Dr. Dor Brown, to present this modality for the first time at the First International Congress of Food Allergy in Vichy, France, in June 1963. Rinkel originally had considered administration of this provocation injection test subcutaneously as well as intracutaneously. After the original paper was presented, both techniques were advanced and taught by his successors. A variant of these injection techniques utilizes sublingual administration of the tested food extracts.

Although some physicians continue to use the classic techniques of Rinkel, most utilize further refinements proposed by Lee and later by Dr. Joseph Miller, referred to generally as "definitive" intracutaneous provocative food testing.[3–5]

The original essence of these injection provocation tests was diagnosis by provocation of symptoms in minutia on quantitative injection of the test food extract, followed by a so-called neutralization of the produced symptoms by orderly subsequent injections of more dilute dilutions of the same food extract. Advocates of this technique claim the procedure provides more practical diagnostic and treatment modalities than is allowed with pure dietary management.

Principally because the claimed qualities of the test could not be readily explained immunologically, these procedures were not readily accepted by all allergists. After 20 years of favorable experience, however, they now are being enthusiastically embraced by a growing number of physicians. The 1983 Position Statement of the American Academy of Otolaryngic Allergy (AAOA) endorses the intracutaneous and subcutaneous versions of this provocative food test, although this organization has not as yet endorsed the sublingual variant as has the

American Academy of Environmental Medicine. In May 1984, the American Academy of Otolaryngology–Head and Neck Surgery (AAO–HNS) agreed in a statement by its Board of Directors that "intracutaneous and subcutaneous provocative food testing and neutralization therapy are accepted clinical procedures in the practice of this specialty."

Techniques in General

The advantages of these provocative/neutralization techniques are their ability to conveniently identify the foods to which the patients are allergic and to provide a neutralizing dose that may be utilized for practical treatment. The foods chosen for testing are deduced from a combination of knowledge of the most commonly offending foods and inspection of the patient's prepared diet/symptom diary. Patients should not be tested by these modalities for a fixed food allergy well established by history where treatment by strict elimination is required by the severe nature of the problem. It is the more common, nonfixed, delayed, hidden variety of food allergy for which these tests are designed. Seldom does adequate symptom control necessitate testing more than 30 foods, and frequently 15 or less will suffice.

While the test in experienced hands is very safe, some foods by nature are more allergenic than others and should be tested only with extreme care. Examples are cottonseed, fish, peanut, and shell fish. Also, brittle patients, that is, those with a history of asthma, angioedema, or other such notable symptoms, should be approached with greater caution, as when any in vivo test is utilized. Detailed recommendations follow.

All of these tests are performed single-blind, that is, the patient is not aware of which food is being tested. To achieve a priming for provocation, it is preferable that the patient eat the foods to be tested within the 24-hour period prior to testing. The patient, thus, needs to be provided a list of foods to be eaten in some form that includes, among others, the foods to be tested. The patient must be well-schooled in advance as to what to expect during the test procedure, and how to report on a provided clipboard any and all subjective symptoms, their time of appearance, severity, and degree of waxing and waning.

Any symptoms the patient may be having prior to testing are recorded to establish a baseline for comparison purposes. One must not confuse an already present symptom with a provoked symptom. It is not unusual for a patient to come in with a symptom, say headache, and have the symptom relieved on neutralization of a particular food. It is imperative that the tester be constantly present and acutely observant. For added guidance, the tester should record the patient's pulse before each test and every five minutes during the test, noting any sizable increase or decrease of rate or appearance of any arrhythmia.

Classic Intradermal and Subcutaneous Injection Provocative Test and Sublingual Test

All techniques utilize 1:5 dilutions of the extract concentrate, exactly as prepared for inhalant skin endpoint titration. Food extract concentrates, however, may be 1:10 wv in strength as well as 1.20 wv, depending on the provider.

One must be constantly cognizant of possible biphasic symptom provocation whereby administration of doses of allergen not only too strong but also too weak may initiate symptom production, with the symptom-relieving or "neutralizing" dose lying in-between. In the classic test versions, delivery of the test dilutions proceeds generally from stronger dilutions to weaker dilutions. Attempt at provocation of symptoms is initiated by injection of 0.05 ml intracutaneously or 0.1 ml subcutaneously of dilution #1. Ten to 20 minutes is allowed for observation. If no symptoms are provoked in the allotted time period, many physicians then proceed to inject a similar "kicker" dose of the #3 dilution, that is, a dilution 25 times weaker, assuring thereby no symptom provocation by delivery of a weaker biphasic dose. If again no symptoms result within 10 to 15 minutes, the test is considered negative.

If symptoms are provoked after the first injection of the #1 dilution, then the tester, without further delay, initiates identification of the "neutralizing" dose. It is advised to proceed weaker one dilution at a time until the best symptom-relieving dose is determined. This practice disallows inadvertent biphasic "weak dose" symptom aggravation. The time interval allowed between injections generally is 10 to 15 minutes, but may be accelerated when it is obvious that the last injection is of no benefit. If the patient should become worse after a weaker dilution is administered, one should immediately return to the next stronger dilution, although this is an infrequent occurrence if one proceeds one dilution at a time. Occasionally, symptoms may be relieved only partially, or temporarily for a few minutes. Generally, repeat injection of the same dilution results in lasting relief. In such an instance, the neutralizing dose recorded is the sum total volume required; that is, it may be a sum dose multiple up to four, since a multiple of five would equal the same dose as the preceding unsuccessful stronger dilution. When symptoms are provoked by the dilution #3 "kicker" dose, the skipped #2 dilution will be the neutralizing dose in the majority of cases.

In the sublingual modification, the test procedure is the same except the dilutions of the food extract are delivered as a sublingual drop held under the tongue for 30 seconds. This method is preferred by some physicians because they feel it is more convenient and less painful, especially for children. Critics, however, question whether sublingual absorption is as dependable as intracutaneous or subcutaneous administration.

Definitive Intracutaneous Provocative Food Test of Lee-Miller

Although there are slight variances of the "definitive" variety of intracutaneous provocative food test, the test typically is accomplished in the following fashion. Initial testing for each food is started with the administration of a 4 mm intracutaneous wheal of the selected allergen dilution. This size wheal results when 0.01 ml volume is administered in the average adult skin. In theory, this size dose is first used to identify by its whealing response a safe dilution to start true provocative testing with a larger 7 mm intracutaneous test wheal. The latter typically results when 0.05 ml volume is administered intracutaneously in the average adult skin. In more sensitive individuals, symptoms may be provoked after application of the smaller initial test dose, in which case the test is completed utilizing the smaller wheal instead of advancing to the larger wheal.

Patients with brittle histories, that is, a history of asthma, angioedema, or other serious varieties of symptoms, are usually started with a dilution no more concentrated than a #4. The same is true when any of the more allergenic foods are tested, whether the potential danger is inherent from the food itself or is suspected from the patient's history. Otherwise, the usual test starting dose generally is a #2 dilution.

Since the tester is guided by the whealing response, it is very important that a negative control first be established. Dilutions 1:5 of 50 per cent glycerin, as contained in extract concentrates, are utilized. The #1 dilution of the glycerin control usually produces a positive wheal owing to irritation from the high glycerin content. Varying with the individual, weaker dilutions may also produce positive whealing. A positive wheal may be defined as a wheal that exhibits a 2 mm average growth over a 10- to 15-minute period.

If the initial test wheal results in a negative response, that is, grows less than 2 mm in 10 to 15 minutes without symptom provocation, the next applied wheal may be of a dilution not more than 25 times stronger. Thus, if the initial negative 4 mm test wheal was a #4 dilution (commonly referred to as 1/4, because typically this size wheal results from 0.01 ml volume), the next wheal could be made from the #2 dilution (1/2). Likewise, if the 1/2 wheal is negative without provocation, the next application may be 5/1 (a 7 mm wheal from 0.05 ml of the #1 dilution).

If and when a positive wheal response greater than the negative control results, the next step depends on whether such a positive wheal is accompanied by provocation of symptoms. If the initial #4 dilution test wheal responded positively without symptom provocation after 20 minutes, the strongest dilution that resulted in a negative wheal would be determined. If, say, this proved to be the #5 dilution, then the next wheal applied would be a .05 cc 7 mm. wheal with the #5 dilution (a 5/5). Thus, testing initially with the smaller dose allows initiating testing with the larger dose at a safe dilution. The weakest dilution that produces a positive whealing response with the larger wheals is then identified. This dose represents the most likely neutralizing dose, and its application theoretically should help ensure against a later delayed reaction (Fig. 34–1).

Some physicians feel symptom provocation is a test variable and assume positive whealing response indicates test positivity. They utilize the strongest negative whealing dilution for specific allergen neutralization treatment even when no symptoms are provoked. Others, who demand provocation of symptoms for assurance of test positivity, retest after a few days' wait, starting with the first positive wheal strength. Such a repeat test disallows prevention of provoked symptoms by a prior inadvertent application of a neutralizing dose.

When provocation of symptoms occurs, one proceeds to identification of the "neutralizing" dose. This is accomplished by applying consecutively 1:5 weaker dilutions at approximately 10-minute intervals until the neutralizing dose is determined. Because neutralization generally does not occur on a dilution that produces a positive wheal, recognition of an obvious positive skin response allows a more rapid application of the next weaker dilution.

The "neutralizing" dose most often is the strongest, thus usually the first, negative dilution applied. Seldom is it the next weaker dilution, and rarely the third. Occasionally, neutralization is only partial or temporary, as previously explained when the classic techniques were reviewed, requiring a multiple of a particular dilution dose to afford complete neutralization. For example, if 5/3 results in a negative wheal and gives only partial symptom relief, and application of a 5/4 is of no help or perhaps makes the provoked symptoms worse, multiple applications, up to four, of 5/3 may produce the desired neutralization. As explained before, if one applied five 5/3 wheals, one would be back to the equivalent of 5/2, a previously unsuccessful dose. If three applications of 5/3 are required to achieve a good response, then the neutralizing dose is 0.15 ml (15X) of that dilution.

Remember, when decreasing the dose to dilutions weaker than the strongest negative while searching for the best neutralizing dose, provoked symptoms may actually flare. If such should occur, one should immediately return to the stronger negative dilution. It is because of this possibility that it is advised to limit negative "jumps" to 1.5 dilutions.

Once the provoked symptoms caused by a provocative test are neutralized, a new test for a different food may be begun. If, however, complete neutralization cannot be achieved, then further testing must be delayed until the provoked symptoms have completely disappeared, which may require anywhere from 30 minutes to hours.

Occasionally a patient may develop delayed symptoms after leaving the office, either later in the day, that night, or, infrequently, the following morning. This happens because it is not always possible to exactly balance the neutralizing dose.

For the occurrence of such delayed symptoms, the patient should be instructed to first

1. *Negative Skin Test and Provocation*
   1/4 → 10 min neg → 1/2 → 10 min neg → 5/1 pos → 20 min, no symptoms → strongest neg wheal (probably 5/2 or 5/3) and record.
2. *Positive Skin Test, Negative Provocation*
   1/4 → 10 min neg → 1/2 pos → 20 min, no symptoms → 5/2 pos → 20 min, no symptoms → 5/3 pos → 20 min, no symptoms → strongest neg wheal (probably 5/4 or 5/5) and record.
3. *Positive Skin Test, Positive Provocation*
   a. 1/4 → 10 min neg → 1/2 pos → 20 min, no symptoms → 1/3 neg, no symptoms → 5/3 with symptoms → STAT neutralizing dose (probably 5/4 or 5/5).
   or
   b. 1/4 → 10 min neg → 1/2 pos, with symptoms → STAT 1/3 = neutralizing dose.
   if not
   c. → STAT 1/3 → 10 min neg, no or partial neutralization → 1/4 neg = neutralizing dose.
   if not
   d. → 1/4 → 10 min or less, symptoms same or worse → STAT 1/3 → 10 min, no or partial neutralization → 1/3 → 10 min, partial neutralization → 1/3 → 10 min, full neutralization = 3/3 neutralizing dose.

FIGURE 34–1. Examples of provocation testing.

attempt to self-neutralize these symptoms by utilizing the masking phenomenon, as explained in Chapters 30 and 33. This is simply accomplished by eating a little of the foods tested at the previous session, trying one food at a time in small quantity at approximately 15-minute intervals until relief occurs. During the testing session if a particular food produced rather striking symptoms or was difficult to neutralize, that food is the one most likely causing the problem and should be the first taken.

Tri-alkali salts, composed of three parts sodium bicarbonate, two parts potassium bicarbonate, and one part calcium carbonate, may be used for nonspecific treatment of any food allergy symptoms, including delayed symptoms from provocative testing. The dose of the trisalts is one to two teaspoons in a glass of cool water for an adult, with the children's dose being reduced directly in proportion to body weight reduction. A convenient substitute is Alka-Seltzer Gold, composed of sodium bicarbonate and potassium bicarbonate, two tablets for an adult and one tablet for a child dissolved in a glass of cool water. Allergic reactions interfere with the natural buffering systems, producing intracellular edema and acidosis. The purpose of these alkali salts is to counteract this untoward response. Secondarily, they also act as a mild laxative to rid the gut of any retained guilty food.

Test Comparisons

Proponents of the classic form of provocation testing propose that starting with a maximal provoking dose disallows false negativity that may result from inadvertent administration of the neutralizing dose when an arbitrary weaker dilution is initially injected. Proponents of the definitive method take comfort in that they define the degree of a patient's sensitivity prior to the application of stronger doses. Also, in the definitive technique, wheal size provides an objective guide for dosing during both the provocation and neutralization phase of the test. Such an objective guide is not available in the classic techniques, in that whealing response is regarded of less significance in the intradermal variety and is unavailable in the subcutaneous and sublingual approaches.

Further, proponents of the definitive test refute the often taught premise that skin whealing is purely an IgE-mediated response. A recent study by Johnson and Rea, now being finalized for submission for publication, seems to illustrate this point well. In the study, the results of challenge food testing, definitive intracutaneous provocative testing, and modified radioallergosorbent test (RAST) on 159 consecutive food allergy patients hospitalized in an environmental control center are compared. There proves to be a high correlation of 96 per cent between oral challenge and the intracutaneous provocative test results, whereas the RAST correlates only 44 per cent and 42 per cent with the other two tests respectively. It would appear, thus, that food challenge and the definitive intracutaneous provocative test similarly diagnose all types of food allergies, unlike the RAST, which diagnoses only the IgE-mediated variety. It follows that allergenic skin response is not solely dependent on IgE mediation.

As was the case for inhalant immunotherapy when it was administered for over half a century prior to the discovery of IgE, a precise immunologic explanation for provocation/neutralization is not available. With current research, however, the answers appear to be rapidly evolving.[6–9]

Neutralization Therapy

The provocation/neutralization techniques were derived to provide a practical and convenient diagnostic and treatment modality for delayed food hypersensitivities. Patients with this variety of medical infirmity are especially unfortunate in that they usually manifest problems with multiple foods, most of which are difficult to avoid "staples" such as corn, wheat, egg, milk, soy, and yeast.[10–12] Their problems are compounded because these foods are persistent ingredients in most prepared and packaged foodstuffs, the new mainstay of the modern American diet.

More often the symptoms produced by this variety of food allergy are insidious while they compound because they are delayed, providing little recognition of cause and effect. All organ systems may be affected.[10–17]

Multiple systems are often concomitantly involved, with a resultant cornucopia of complaints incomprehensible to many physicians.

Table 34–1. TREATMENT PROGRAM

Injections	Sublingual Drops
b 1 week × 1 month	bid × 4 months
q week × 1 month	qd × 4 months
q o week (use 2-month intervals if sublingual drops not used)	qod × 4 months
	b 1 week × 4 months
	prn ×

Even when the responsible foods are diagnosed by challenge diets, one is left with only avoidance for definitive treatment. Because of inevitable multiple exposures to these staple-hidden causative foods, such an approach often is doomed to failure. Herein lies the great advantage of the provocation/neutralization allergy techniques. They provide not only an added method of diagnosis, but an additional means of practical treatment. Although an admitted compromise with total avoidance, neutralization treatment allows most patients at least a limited intake of their allergenic staple foods, improving thereby patient compliance and quality of life.

Fixed food allergies and food sensitivities that provoke severe symptoms should be treated by strict elimination rather than by neutralization. Likewise, easily avoided foods, such as coffee, chocolate, and other such nonhidden foods, are better treated by avoidance when the patient will comply.

More often, neutralization treatment is combined with some variety of a rotary diet,[10, 11] which furnishes a general blunting of the various food sensitivities by decreasing the frequency of their intake. The rotary diet also helps identify other allergenic foods in the diet by accomplishing, in essence, challenge food testing on each food as it is rotated. This is accomplished because the intake of each ingested foodstuff is repeated only at several-day intervals, allowing a better recognition of cause and effect symptom response. Details of the rotary diversified diet are discussed in Chapter 33.

Whatever initial treatment routine is adopted, it should never be prescribed in a cookbook fashion. The patient needs to be carefully followed, with changes in treatment routine accomplished as indicated by clinical response. It is not unusual to have to occasionally recheck the patient's neutralization endpoints. The need for such a recheck is often heralded by a decrease in symptom relief after initial success. Endpoints, however, usually stabilize with prolonged treatment. Another possibility to be kept in mind as a cause for renewed symptom production is the development of new food allergies to previously nonallergic foods now substituted for nontolerated foods on a regular basis.

Neutralization treatment involves administration of the exact neutralizing dose of each positive responding food at intervals dictated by clinical need and response. The neutralizing dose is administered subcutaneously from a multifood allergen vial. Initial treatment injection may be given anywhere from once a day to twice a week. Strictness of a companion rotary diet varies with severity of the individual problem. With increasing tolerance, the patient should be able to stop treatment injections and control symptoms by only diet manipulation.

Although not as yet an approved technique of the AAOA or AAO–HNS, sublingual drop therapy is utilized by many physicians in place of or in combination with neutralization injections. Sublingual drops contain in a given amount of volume, usually in one drop, the same dose of allergen administered in a neutralization injection. Drops are typically given initially from once to four times a day, and their frequency decreases according to the patient's response and need. One of the claimed advantages of combining sublingual drop treatment with subcutaneous injection is the attainment of symptom relief with fewer bothersome injections. A typical starting schedule for such a neutralization program is presented in Table 34–1.

Food injections, as with inhalant immunotherapy injections, may be self-administered or given in the office per the desire of the individual physician. Food neutralization injections, in the experience of the author, are far less likely to result in untoward reactions than are routine inhalant immunotherapy injections. As with any immunotherapy regimen, it is advised to always give the first injection from a new vial mixture in the office in the event of human error, so that appropriate treatment for any provoked symptoms may be promptly accomplished. While local reaction from a properly prepared neutralization vial is unusual, systemic reaction is a rarity. One must always be alert for the exception, however, and office personnel and the patient must both be prepared for appropriate response.

Table 34–2. MULTIPLE FOOD TREATMENT MATERIAL PREPARATION

Multiple Food Injection Vial

A. 0.25 ml volume per dose
 20-dose vial = 5.00 ml volume

B. With only a few foods, may be prepared from endpoint dilutions.

Food	*Neutralizing Dose*	*20-Dose Volume*
Milk	5/3	1.00 ml of #3
Corn	5/2	1.00 ml of #2
Wheat	1/4	0.20 ml of #4
Egg	1/5	0.20 ml of #5
		2.40 ml total volume
		2.60 ml added diluent
		5.00 ml = 20-dose vial

C. With many foods, may need to be prepared from stronger dilutions.

Food	*Neutralizing Dose*	*20-Dose Volume*	*Stronger Dilution*
Milk	5/3	1.00 ml of #3	0.20 ml of #2
Corn	5/2	1.00 ml of #2	0.20 ml of #1
Wheat	1/4	0.20 ml of #4	0.20 ml of #4
Egg	1/5	0.20 ml of #5	0.20 ml of #5
Yeast	5/2	1.00 ml of #2	0.20 ml of #1
Soy	5/3	1.00 ml of #3	0.20 ml of #2
Beef	5/2	1.00 ml of #2	0.20 ml of #1
Orange	5/2	1.00 ml of #2	0.20 ml of #1
Lettuce	5/2	1.00 ml of #2	0.20 ml of #1
Tomato	5/4	1.00 ml of #4	0.20 ml of #3
		8.40 ml total volume	2.00 ml
			3.00 ml diluent
			5.00 ml = 20-dose injection

Sublingual Drop Multiple Food Bottles

A. Dropper bottle: Meridian Bio-Medical, Inc., 1700 Royston Lane, Round Rock, TX 78664
 Bottle (#4) ¼ ox.
 Caps for above
 Tips for above

B. 1. Make up so that one drop = one neutralizing dose.
 2. 100 of such doses in the above bottle = 6 ml total volume.
 3. 100 doses requires 5 times more food allergen than the 20-dose injection vial.
 4. With multiple foods, you may need to drop back two dilutions stronger *(where you can)* to make up.

Food	*Rx Dose*	*100-Dose Volume*	*Stronge Dilution*
Milk	5/3	5.00 ml of #3	0.20 ml of #1
Corn	5/2	5.00 ml of #2	0.20 ml of concentrate
Wheat	1/4	1.00 ml of #4	0.20 ml of #3
Egg	1/5	1.00 ml of #5	0.20 ml of #4
Yeast	5/2	5.00 ml of #2	0.20 ml of concentrate
Soy	5/3	5.00 ml of #3	0.20 ml of #1
Beef	5/2	5.00 ml of #2	0.20 ml of concentrate
Orange	5/2	5.00 ml of #2	0.20 ml of concentrate
Lettuce	5/2	5.00 ml of #2	0.20 ml of concentrate
Tomato	5/4	5.00 ml of #4	0.20 ml of #2
		42.00 ml total volume	2.00 ml
			4.00 ml diluent
			6.00 ml = 100-dose drops

Multiple food injection and sublingual treatment vial preparation instructions are provided in Table 34–2.

REFERENCES

1. Lee CH: A new test for detection of food allergies, pollen and mold incompatibilities. Buchanan Co Med Bull 25:9, 1961.
2. Rinkel RJ, Lee CH, Brown DW, et al: The diagnosis of food allergy. Arch Otolaryngol 79:71, 1964.
3. Lee CH, Williams RT, Binkely EL: Provocative testing and treatment. Arch Otolaryngol 90:87, 1969.
4. Missal SC: Food allergy in ear, nose and throat disease. Otolaryngol Clin North Am 4:479, 1971.
5. Miller JB: Food allergy, provocative testing and injection therapy. Springfield, IL, Charles C Thomas, 1972, pp 33–115.
6. Sobotka AK, Dembo M, Goldstein B, Lichtenstein LM: Antigen specific desensitization of human basophils. Ann Immunol 122:511, 1979.
7. Mendoza GR, Kiminobu M: Subthreshold and suboptimal desensitization of human basophils. Int Arch Allergy Appl Immunol 65:101, 1982.
8. Scadding GK, Brostoff J: Low dose sublingual therapy in patients with allergic rhinitis due to house dust mite. Clin Allergy 16:483, 1986.
9. Boris M, Schiff M, Weindorf S: Injection of low-dose antigen attenuates the response to subsequent bronchoprovocative challenge. Otolaryngol Head Neck Surg 98:536, 1988.
10. Rinkel JH, Randolph TG, Zeller M: Food Allergy. Springfield, IL, Charles C Thomas, 1951, pp 5–147.
11. Rinkel JH The management of clinical allergy. Part IV. Food and mold allergy. Arch Otolaryngol 77:302, 1963.
12. Brenemen JC: Basics of Food Allergy. Springfield, IL, Charles C Thomas, 1978, pp 156–163.
13. Brenemen JC: Basics of Food Allergy. Springfield, IL, Charles C Thomas, 1978, pp 8–9, 14–15.
14. Speer F: Food Allergy. 2nd ed. Boston, John Wright PSG, Inc, 1983, pp 1–2.
15. Rowe AH: Food allergy, its manifestations, diagnosis and treatment. JAMA 91:1623, 1928.
16. Rinkel HJ: The management of clinical allergy. Part I. General considerations. Arch Otolaryngol 76:491, 1962.
17. Gordon VH, Liu HY, Gerrard JW, et al: *In* Gerrard JW: Food Allergy, New Perspectives. Springfield, IL, Charles C Thomas, 1980 (Chapters 2–4).

CHAPTER 35

In Vitro Evaluation of Food Allergy: Current Status

Hueston C. King, M.D., F.A.C.S., F.A.C.A.

With the refinement of "in vitro" testing technologies available today, the evaluation of inhalant allergy has become a predictable science. Essentially all inhalant problems appear to be IgE-mediated, Gell and Coombs type I reactions. The evaluation of food allergy, unfortunately, is not so simple. Foods have been shown to utilize all four Gell and Coombs pathways with no definable pattern, and at times a single food may become involved in two or more pathways in the same patient. The variety alone creates major identification problems. To compound the difficulty, the foods utilizing different pathways may exhibit major differences in character.[1]

The most easily recognized allergenic foods are those whose reactions are caused by IgE (Gell and Coombs type I). These are humorally mediated, rapid in onset, and potentially anaphylactic in nature. They may be identified by skin testing or by IgE RAST with a high degree of accuracy. Such study is rarely necessary, however, as the prompt onset of symptoms allows the victim to make a cause and effect identification of the offender. The availability of definitive identification is of value, however, and may be employed for confirmation. It has been estimated that between 20 and 30 per cent of allergenic foods are mediated by IgE. (The difficulty in making a more reliable estimate of the percentage lies not in identifying the IgE-mediated foods, but in estimating the larger number of non–IgE-mediated foods for which no such definitive test is available.)

Gell and Coombs type II food allergies produce their reactions by means of a direct cytotoxic action on the target cells without the formation of immune complexes. Antibodies become adherent to the surface of the target cells through a variety of mechanisms and, when exposed to more antigen in the presence of complement, react to destroy the cell involved. This is actually an extension of the body's normal mechanism for removing offending substances from the system; only correct identification of offenders has been altered. No test is currently in use that reliably defines the foods involved. It may well be that the cytotoxic test of Black and the Bryans identifies foods reacting through this mechanism, but such has never been proved. (The test described has been in use since 1926, and is discussed later. Despite its persistence in the armamentarium of food allergy evaluation, the test has never been reproducible and remains in the limbo "of potential value".) Because of the unavailability of a reliable test for the involved foods, no estimate of the importance of type II food allergy is available. Even the supporters of the cytotoxic test have been unwilling to categorize it as being specific to type II foods.

Gell and Coombs type III reactions are defined as those resulting from immune complexes. Immune complexes result from the reaction of an antigen and antibody, stimulated by complement. These structures circulate through the bloodstream and have an affinity for small blood vessels. Immune complexes tend to accumulate in a given area and attach to the vessels of an organ. In quantity they are toxic to the vessels, producing a vasculitis that allows fluid to leak from the circulation into the tissue of the organ. While the pathologic process of this type of reaction remains constant, the variety of organs involved allows a wide range of symptoms to be produced; for example, if the target organ is the skin, the result may be a rash, whereas if the target organ is the lungs, the result may be asthma.

Both types II and III reactions may be prompt, or delayed for as much as three or four days. They are also cumulative and dose-related; that is, a small amount of the offending food may produce no symptoms, whereas a large amount will. Also, an offending food eaten once in several days may not produce symptoms, but the same food eaten two or three times in succession may precipitate a problem. This only serves to underscore the difficulties of identifying such offending foods by clinical means and emphasizes the need for a reliable in vitro test.

Techniques are available to assay the level of specific food immune complexes in the serum; however, to date, such assays are in limited supply. More readily available are food-specific IgG assays, both those utilizing individual subgroups (IgG_2, IgG_3, or IgG_4) or the entire IgG complex. Since IgG is the predecessor of the immune complex, such assays provide a much simpler and less expensive form of evaluation.[2] The difficulty in evaluating the significance of IgG levels in the serum stems from several causes. First, everyone forms IgG antibodies after eating a food. At what point the level of IgG antibodies becomes pathologic has not yet been established. Some of the original investigators have estimated that the upper levels of class III and class IV antibodies appear to occur just before the formation of immune complexes by reaction with complement. They have attempted to produce a positive identification by elimination and challenge of foods reaching this level. The results indicate that this indeed is so, but the investigators are the first to stress that double-blind studies are still lacking and may be impossible to carry out owing to the dose and frequency requirements present in producing such food reactions.[3] This difficulty, of course, is compounded enormously when food identification is attempted by elimination and challenge without some form of screening.

Although serum assays may be made in a reliable manner, the significance of various levels of IgG and/or immune complexes is not yet established. The immune complexes actually responsible for symptoms are bound to the tissue, and only the unbound portion free in the serum may be assayed. It also remains to be established what relationship the time of ingestion of the food bears to the serum IgG level. All of these parameters are being studied.

It should be apparent the food-specific IgG assay does not possess the level of reliability of the IgE assay; at least not today. Bearing in mind the practical impossibility of accurately evaluating non–IgE-mediated food by clinical methods, the IgG assay appears to have a useful place. It cannot be considered a definitive test, but in the patient with a widely diversified diet, it may provide a useful starting point for further testing by elimination and challenge.

Gell and Coombs type IV food allergy (cell-mediated) has been shown to exist. Clinical tests for this type of allergy are not available; hence, the prevalence of this type of problem, as for types II and III, is not known.

It has been commented upon by investigators in both in vitro and in vivo food allergy studies that results of testing by various methods rarely give uniform responses. This does not necessarily indicate invalid results on the part of any one test. So many aspects of the immune system are affected by foods that a study limited to one or two aspects may well miss others, whereas a different approach may identify these only. In addition, the immune system is subject to shock due to various forms of stress, especially in the selective absorption ability of the intestinal tract. This allows the production of apparently allergic symptoms in the absence of true allergy, as incompletely broken down foods are absorbed through the incompetent defenses of the shocked intestinal mucosa. Attempts at identification of offending foods by in vivo methods will often include these foods, adding to the confusion.

It quickly becomes apparent that the diagnosis

of food allergy by any means is far from easy. Clinical approaches become an exercise in frustration due to the number of variables possible. In vitro tests would provide a much more viable solution even if several were needed to complete the identifications. Inroads are being made into this area, but, to date, the results are incomplete. It appears that some time will be necessary before the evolution of the far more complex field of food allergy will approach the reliability of aeroallergen identification.

REFERENCES

1. Breneman JC: Basics of Food Allergy. 2nd ed. Springfield, IL, Charles C Thomas, 1984.
2. Dockhorn RJ: In Vitro Immunologic Techniques in the Diagnosis of Adverse Reactions to Foods. Lecture, V International Food Allergy Symposium, American College of Allergists, Atlanta, Georgia, October 1984.
3. Dockhorn RJ, Frick OL: Delayed Onset Food Reactions. Lecture, VI International Food Allergy Symposium, American College of Allergists, Boston, Massachusetts, November 1987.

Addendum: For Historical Interest
The Cytotoxic Test

Hueston C. King, M.D., F.A.C.S., F.A.C.A.

Since the first recognition of the nature of allergy, the number of possible offenders has made the allergist's task appear overwhelming. People must function within their environment, and any contact is potentially capable of producing an adverse reaction. Many offenders may be present simultaneously, supplementing each other's actions, and any organ system of the body may react independently to any individual offender. Foods and inhalants may interact. Without some means of identifying the individual allergens, care of any sort would seem to be impossible.

The urgent need for a simple, practical means of identifying individual allergens may be responsible for the persistence and recurring episodes of popularity of such diagnostic technologies as the cytotoxic test. The test has never gained general acceptance by the allergy community. It has been misused by commercial franchises in recent years, becoming the incentive for condemnation.

The basic attraction of the cytotoxic test has been that it is performed on living cells outside the body: an in vivo test performed on an in vitro basis with the accompanying convenience of in vitro testing. Although in its early days the test was applied to both foods and inhalants, today it is reserved for foods. Much better methods for studying inhalant sensitivity are available. In the absence of a detailed knowledge of the immunologic mechanisms of food sensitivity, such a test might be the closest thing possible to the difficult approach of elimination and challenge. Rarely has a simplistic approach turned out to be as successful as could be hoped for, and the cytotoxic test is no exception.

The evolution of the test shows a series of swings from enthusiasm to deprecation. Whereas it is discussed in most of the literature as a single test, few laboratories have performed it in a manner identical to another laboratory, and even within the same laboratory the technique inherently allows variability of interpretation. Even today it would be impossible to describe the accepted method of performing the test, as it differs from one laboratory to another. A look at the test's history may give a clearer picture of both the approach and the problems.

The original test was described by Arthur P. Black[1] in 1955.

During the 1960s the Bryans[2] improved upon Black's original format, using Siliclad glassware to reduce the Hageman factor, plus accurately measured amounts of antigen and other controls. Their technique, as reported in 1971, is reproduced here for history and potential research value.

TECHNIQUE OF THE IN VITRO TEST

Step 1: Preparation of the Glassware

All glassware, especially the slides and coverslips, must be thoroughly cleaned and treated with Silicad, a silicone product. We have found that plain glass is toxic to the leucocytes because of activation of the Hageman factor. Three rings of petrolatum are placed on each slide. These are made with a syringe and a 25 gauge needle which has been cut short, by extruding the petrolatum on the slide over a pattern. Clemis and Interlandi have made mechanical ring-makers. The outer circumference of each ring should be exactly the size of the glass coverslip that will be used later to seal the serum and cell suspension.

Step 2: Preparation of the Food Extracts

Food extracts have been obtained usually from the suppliers of allergy products (Hollister-Stier, Stemen Laboratory). However, for the coffee test regular perculated [*sic*] coffee is used. The obtaining of food extracts is an area open for exhaustive investigation, and in time improved extracts may be developed. However, the extracts now available do work well.

The amounts are critical. Approximately 10 mg. of powdered extract is weighed with an analytical balance. Exactly 1 ml. of pyrogen-free distilled water is added to each milligram of powdered extract. This is mixed and allowed to stand overnight—not longer, because bacteria and fungi may multiply and interfere with the test. After 24 hours the supernatant fluid is removed, and this solution is diluted 1:4 in most cases. It is by varying this dilution that the sensitivity of the test is adjusted. Three drops of the solution are put on the clean silicated slides within the ring of petrolatum. While drying, they are covered to protect them from dust.

When one is starting with a different antigen, it is well to try several dilutions: 1:2, 1:4, 1:8, and 1:16, for example. Filtering the solution has lessened the error of supersaturation of some foods, especially yeast, which without filtering had to be diluted 1:1000. Supplies of slides are made up in advance, allowed to dry, and stored in slide boxes.

Step 3: Preparation of the Serum-Cell Suspension

Ten cubic centimeters of fresh venous blood is taken and put into a test tube with 0.8 cc. of sodium citrate. After mixing, the citrated blood* is put into special tubes about 4 inches long and ¼ inch in diameter with constricted middle portions. These are centrifuged slowly for one and one-half hours. The buffy coat containing the white cells and platelets forms over the packed erythrocytes in the constricted part of the tube. The constriction thickens the buffy coat so that it can be easily removed with a pipette. It is then mixed with some of the serum.

In order to compensate for the drying of the food extracts on the slides and the drying of the serum itself, one drop of sterile distilled water is added to four drops of serum; this improves cellular motility.

Enough serum is added to the cells to form a suspension of scattered cells convenient for microscopic examination. A sample of this suspension is put on a slide in a petrolatum ring without food antigen and sealed with a coverslip. This is used as a control by which one can determine the need for adjusting the concentration of cells and check the normal viability of the cells periodically. It is desirable to have approximately 15 to 20 neutrophils per high power field.

In order to obtain uniformity, enough of the suspension is made for about 50 tests, but it is necessary to remix it frequently because the cells settle rapidly. The amount put in the ring of petrolatum should just fill it after the coverslip is lightly pressed down. The coverslips are put on as soon as possible to minimize uneven settling and drying of the suspension. They should be placed carefully on the petrolatum rings to avoid air bubbles. Nine to 12 tests should be prepared and sealed before the procedure is repeated with remixing of the suspension. Drying and undue settling of the cells are thus avoided. It is important to remember that variations in the quantities of cells, and especially the presence of air bubbles and drying due to a break in the petrolatum seal, will vary markedly the degree of reaction.

*This by itself has proved destructive of the test. We have to use blood transfusion citrate, which is better balanced, containing dextrose and potassium citrate as well as sodium citrate.

Reading the Results

We have found that the most convenient microscope objective to use in routine observation of the test is the apochromatic 60 high dry lens or its equivalent. Phase-contrast microscopy reveals more intracellular detail, such as vacuoles, movements, and degree of density of the granules, but although interesting at present these details do not add to the facility in the routine reading of the test.

If a reaction does not occur within two hours, the test is considered to be negative. Longer periods have been used and sometimes reactions have progressed, but most were stationary. Reactions are not missed when the tests are read at two hours. If the technique is performed correctly—with no bubbles allowed and tight sealing—normal cells will remain active into the third day. Reading the tests does require some judgment, mainly because not all cells are of the same age and hence vary in viability. Therefore, not all cells are affected to the same degree, and an overall estimate of degree of reaction must be made.

The Bryan technique quickly became the standard of the profession, although not all laboratories confirmed its results.[3, 4] Individual laboratories made their own variations upon it. Since the shock organ consisted of living cells, these variations may have had a strong effect upon the reproducibility of the test. Black was greatly concerned about the maintenance of a stable temperature. Few other studies mention the temperature. The stability of the pH is similarly unstated. Varying amounts of serum and/or distilled water may be added to the cell suspension to improve reading.

The incubation time of the suspension prior to reading varies from one laboratory to another. All of these variations and others have been developed to improve the readability of an intrinsically subjective study; however, in the presence of such variations, comparison of results between laboratories becomes virtually impossible.

Probably the most important variation in testing technique is the length of time between the patient's consuming the suspect food and the drawing of blood for performing the cytotoxic test. Recommendations have been made from 12 hours to eight days.[5] Some investigators do not specify the time of abstinence from the food to be tested.[3, 4] Recent studies suggest that much of the variation in reproducibility of the test may be due to the time of abstinence, and that invalidating the cytotoxic test on the basis of variability over hours or days may be comparable to invalidating a glucose tolerance test because the results differed over different time intervals. This has not yet been clarified, and may be difficult to do in the presence of other variables.

The wide range of testing techniques in performing the cytotoxic test is not the only oddity of the study. From its inception, and even with its precursor, the leukopenic index, investigators have reported a disparity of findings. Most have reported a leukopenia appearing after consumption of a positive food; however, other careful observers have consistently reported a leukocytosis.[6, 7] Zeller[8] reported four possible reactions: (1) none; (2) leukocytosis; (3) leucopenia; (4) variable.

It can be no surprise that a test subject to the wide range of variations in use and a diversity of positive findings has not achieved uniform acceptance. Added to this is the subjective nature of the interpretation: all reliability depends upon the astuteness of the technologist doing the reading. Not only the actual number of cells present must be determined, but also their health and activity. The most reliable technologist has been described as one expert in performing sperm counts and analysis, also an inexact study. When a subjective test is read by different technologists, variations may be expected. Even the same technologists may interpret findings differently on different days.

Despite all the problems, the tests continue to show a tantalizing validity. All who have studied it in person admit to observing a response on the part of the white blood cells on exposure to a positive food. What is lacking is a means of quantifying the response, and this seems little closer than it was over a quarter century ago.

Very recently specific assays for IgG_4 and food immune complexes have become available. A strong correlation between these and the best controlled forms of the cytotoxic food test seems to be present. It seems a fair possibility that these reproducible tests will clarify some of the obscure mechanism behind the cytotoxic response. If this indeed proves to be the case, the inherent validity of the test may be confirmed, in principle at least. It will also be made obsolete by a superior form of testing.

REFERENCES

1. Black AP: A new diagnostic method in allergic disease. Pediatrics 17:716, 1956.
2. Bryan WTK, Bryan MP: Cytotoxic reactions in the diagnosis of food allergy. Otolaryngol Clin North Am 4:523, 1971.
3. Lieberman P, Crawford I, et al: Controlled study of the cytotoxic food test. JAMA 231:728, 1975.
4. Benson TE, Arkins JA: Cytotoxic testing for food allergy; evaluation of reproducibility and correlation. J Allergy Clin Immunol 58:471, 1976.
5. Hughes EC, Gottschalk GH, et al: Effect of time of blood sampling on in vitro tests for food sensitivities. Ear Nose Throat J 61:34, 1982.
6. Ulett GA: Cytotoxic testing and leucocyte increase as an index of food sensitivity. Ann Allergy 33:23, 1974.
7. Updegraff TR: Food allergy and cytotoxic test. Ear Nose Throat J 56:48, 1977.
8. Zeller M: The leucopenic index in intractable asthma. Illinois Med 69:54, 1936.

Additional Suggested References

Leary HL Jr, Halsey JF: An assay to measure antigen-specific immune complexes in food allergy patients. J Allergy Clin Immunol 74:190, 1984.

Necessary PC, Leary HL Jr, Dockhorn RJ, Halsey JF: Allergen-specific immune complexes in food sensitive patients. Ann Allergy 52:232, 1984.

Halsey JF, Necessary PC, Leary HL Jr, Dockhorn RJ: Food antigen-specific immune complexes in food sensitive patients. Unpublished data.

Delire M, Cambiaso C, Masson P: Circulating immune complexes in infants fed on cow's milk. Nature 272:632, 1978.

Paganelli R, Levinsky R, Atherton D: Detection of specific antigen within circulating immune complexes: validation of the assay and its application to food antigen-antibody complexes formed in healthy and food-allergic subjects. Clin Exp Immunol 46:44, 1981.

Brostoff J, Carini C, Wraith D, Johns P: Production of IgE complexes by allergen challenge in atopic patients and the effect of sodium cromoglycate. Lancet 1:1268, 1979.

Inganas M, Johansson SGO, Dannaeus A: A method for estimation of circulating immune complexes after oral challenge with ovalbumin. Clin Allergy 10:293, 1980.

SECTION FOUR

ENVIRONMENTAL SENSITIVITY

CHAPTER 36

Introduction to Chemical-Environmental Allergy

John H. Boyles, Jr., M.D.

In 1951, Theron Randolph, M.D., discovered that our increasing pollution of the environment with chemicals was a major source of chronic illness. Sensitivity to a multitude of seemingly common and harmless substances in use in our homes, offices, and workplaces is not to be confused with damage caused by toxic chemicals, which are known to cause exposure problems in the majority of individuals. This poorly understood problem hinges on individual susceptibility and individual adaptation to our modern environment.

Individual susceptibility is not concerned with the middle of the distribution curve, but with the far end. Whereas acute and chronic toxicity studies of new chemicals in animals are indispensable as preliminary screening processes, they will do nothing to predict problems in those individuals who have an individual susceptibility to small doses of common chemical substances. Certainly, toxicology studies in animals will protect the majority of humans from obvious serious chemical reactions but will do little to address the situation confronting humans in their daily lives. Exposure to excitants—poisons, irritants, and various other manmade chemicals usually regarded as harmless in the doses encountered—may induce acute or chronic clinical effects, depending principally on dosage and host susceptibility. On one extreme are the acute, immediate reactions from massive exposures. These are readily apparent and generally harmful to all. We are largely protected from such acute effects by a general knowledge of their harmfulness. At the other extreme are the chronic symptoms traceable to the long-term, subtle impingement of frequently encountered chemicals to which an ever-increasing minority are apparently becoming susceptible. Unfortunately, we are neither adequately protected from these chronic effects nor generally aware of the potentially noxious nature of such chemical exposures.

The immunologic mechanisms of chemical sensitivity or allergy have in the past been as mystifying as those involved in food allergy. Recent refinements of RAST testing and RAST inhibition tests have shown that many chemical sensitivities are IgE-mediated, and specific tests are becoming available that can accurately diagnose chemical allergy by "in vitro" techniques. This type of diagnostic testing is desperately needed in our modern society to remove those individuals susceptible to low-dose chemical exposure before they are physically and mentally harmed.

Since it has been estimated that as many as 3000 new compounds are introduced annually, the widespread presence of hazardous chemicals in our environment has made the problems of chemical susceptibility critical to our survival. In addition, recent research has shown that chronic exposure to levels previously thought to be safe is now incriminated with not only an increase in chemical allergy but also an increase in carcinogenesis. With the discovery that the chemical excitant may trigger a maladaptive response in virtually any of the four smooth muscle systems (cardiovascular, respiratory, gastrointestinal, and genitourinary) or the skin has come the realization of the gravity of chemical sensitivity. This problem is particularly important in the diseases of the ear, nose, and throat and must be understood by otolaryngologists if they are to properly diagnose and treat the chronic disorders found in these organ systems.

Virtually all the symptoms found in chronic food and inhalant allergy can be encountered in those patients with chemical sensitivity.

Head/neural	Headache including migraine, nonspecific dizziness and fainting, neuralgias and neuritis, convulsive seizures, and throbbing or stabbing pain.
Ears	Loss of hearing, recurrent infection, Meniere's syndrome, hyperacusis, fluctuating tinnitus and vertigo.
Nose	Postnasal discharge, itching, sneezing, sinus pain, rhinorrhea, recurrent sinusitis.
Mouth and throat	Canker sores, mouth breathing, itching, chronic pharyngitis, excessive salivation, hoarseness, coated tongue, dysphagia.
Respiratory	Chest congestion, chronic cough, wheezing, shortness of breath, hyperventilation.

In the chemical or food allergic patient these symptoms will be chronic, intermittent, and usually unresponsive to antihistamines, steroids, and traditional immunotherapy. Many other organ systems are affected by chronic chemical sensitivity and the physician should be familiar with the clinical picture. There may be other common clinical characteristics. Drug sensitivity often occurs in these patients. Usually one or more drugs bother the patient, and often five or more different drugs cannot be tolerated. Some patients develop difficulty with all oral medications because of sensitivities to pharmaceutical dyes, stabilizers, adhesives, preservatives, and other chemicals that are common additives to most medications. Some patients are already aware that certain volatile chemicals, such as perfumes, aerosols, air fresheners, and exhaust fumes, produce severe symptoms. They are frequently intolerant to synthetic clothing, bedding, and building materials. Women often find that their symptoms become worse after each pregnancy. Patients will often feel sluggish or have a lack of energy after eating. This may be due to the chemical contamination of the food rather than a specific food allergy or combination of both. Bloating is also a frequent symptom and lasts for one to two hours after eating. Many patients discover intolerance to their local water supply. Weakness may be a prime complaint in adult patients, while hyperactivity is frequently found in children. History taking may be facilitated by having the patient fill out various forms or questionnaires (Fig. 36–1).

CHEMICAL SOURCES

Since the mid-19th century, chemistry has revolutionized modern life. The United States alone produces over 500 billion pounds of chemicals per year, and over 35,000 different compounds are in common use in the United States with approximately 3000 new chemicals discovered and entered into the environment each year. Despite the Toxic Substances Control Act of 1976, few of these chemicals are adequately tested before being introduced into the marketplace. Since these substances have become an integral part of our current existence, they are usually not suspected as being the cause of chronic illness and are not usually avoided deliberately. In addition, there is an element of addiction to some of these chemicals and some victims do not wish to avoid such exposure. Thus, understanding of this program has been obstructed by both the constant nature of the chemical exposure and the self-perpetuation of the process. Many chemicals in use today are combustion products or derivatives of gas, oil, and coal. Because of the complexity of this problem and the sheer numbers involved, clinical testing is usually confined to the major basic chemicals, although new testing procedures may soon be available so that specific chemical sensitivity may be accurately diagnosed.

Name ____ Date ______________

Yes	No	1. Do you dislike the taste of your tap water or do you feel that it causes symptoms?
Yes	No	2. Do you react to wood-burning stoves, fireplaces, or kerosene space heaters?
Yes	No	3. Do you react when entering fabric shops, carpet stores, grocery stores, or department stores?
Yes	No	4. Do you react or dislike the odor of perfume, soap, detergents, colognes, or other solvents, such as fingernail polish remover, paint remover, model airplane glue, etc.?
Yes	No	5. Do you dislike or react to disinfectants, insecticides, sprays, ammonia, or moth balls?
Yes	No	6. Do you react to or dislike the odor of Christmas trees or other indoor evergreen decorations, odor from sanding or woodworking, odor of a cedar closet, or pine-scented household deodorants, shampoos, or turpentine-based paints?
Yes	No	7. Do you react to or dislike the odor of exhaust fumes, jet airplane exhausts, oil, or gas fumes or diesel fumes from trucks and buses?
Yes	No	8. Do you feel that you react to your working environment, either continuously or depending upon the area of the workplace that you are in?
Yes	No	9. Do you have hobbies that involve exposure to smells odors, chemicals, paints, ceramics, or dusty, moldy, chemically contaminated areas?
Yes	No	10. Do you have a tendency to have unpleasant feelings or reactions to all medicines taken by mouth regardless of what condition they are given for?
Yes	No	11. Do you take large amounts of over-the-counter medications, such as vitamins, headache pills, sinus pills, etc.?
Yes	No	12. Do you react to other people's use of tobacco (cigarettes, pipes, cigars)?
Yes	No	13. Do you react to all types of fresh fruit and vegetables and improve if the substances are cooked or peeled?
Yes	No	14. Do you react to foods that are commercially prepared while not reacting to the same foods that are eaten fresh or prepared at home?
Yes	No	15. Do you have difficulty eating in restaurants, but are able to eat the same foods when prepared at home?
Yes	No	16. Do you feel that you perform or feel better in natural lighting compared to fluorescent lighting?
Yes	No	17. Do you react to newsprint or other printed material?

FIGURE 36–1. Chemical allergy questionnaire.

Chemical excitants are encountered in the three major components of our environment—air, food, and water. The concept of total body load is the sum of all excitants found in these three categories, in addition to allergic organic inhalants and foods. The total load principle seems simple until one perceives the amount and scope of chemical pollution that has crept into our environment. Chemicals causing individual susceptibility are found in

1. Domiciliary air pollution.
2. Drugs and anesthetics.
3. Ambient air pollution.
4. Food additives and contaminants.
5. Water additives and contaminants.

Some of the common classes are (1) formaldehyde and its derivatives, (2) natural gas, (3) pesticides, (4) volatile solvents, (5) rubber and plastics, (6) combustion products and fuel, (7) paints and varnishes, (8) miscellaneous.

Air

Contamination of the air may be found in the ambient air as well as in the air within homes and buildings. Our concern with energy preservation has resulted in closed circulation systems in many of our buildings, and the "closed building syndrome" is now being recognized as a common occurrence resulting in many various complaints, absenteeism, and, in some cases, widespread illness for a large majority of inhabitants. When chemical susceptibility was first described by Randolph in 1951, the most common indoor pollutant was natural gas because of its widespread use not only in heating but also in powering appliances. Since electricity has been used to energize appliances, natural gas is no longer a large problem. In today's world, the most common indoor air pollutant is formaldehyde and its derivatives, which are commonly used in construction (Table 36–1). Phenol and its by-products (Table 36–2) are also found in ever-increasing amounts, as are derivatives of ethanol (Table 36–3). Much work needs to be done in educating architectural and structural building companies in the design and construction of safe housing and buildings. This type of construction is readily available if care is taken in selecting safe building materials.

The problems with outdoor air contamination are becoming increasingly severe. The air in cities with a population of 50,000 or more has an outside pollution greater than 50 times that

Table 36–1. SOURCES OF FORMALDEHYDE
Used to make other chemicals
Tanning agents
Fertilizers
Pesticides
Additives to concrete, plaster, and waterproof materials
Antiperspirants
Shampoo
Hair spray and hair products
Detergent soaps
Mouthwash
Dentifrices
Germicidal products
Air deodorizer
Disinfectants
Dyes and dyed fabrics
Stripping agents
Embalming fluids
Adhesives
Waxes
Polishes
Fabrics—permapress
Flame retardant
Synthesis of some vitamins, esp. A and E
Paper products—wetproof quality
Photo chemicals
Wood veneer
Wallboard
Nail polish
Antifreeze
Carpet
Cellophane
Cleaning solutions
Contraceptive creams
Cosmetics
Dry cleaning chemicals
Enamels and latex paints
Exhaust fumes
Fabric softener
Facial tissue
Foam insulation
Plastic
Plywood
Newsprint
Tampons
Toothpaste
Wallpaper
Wax paper

Formaldehyde is an industrial chemical manufactured from methanol, natural gas, and some of the lower petroleum hydrocarbons found widely in urea formaldehyde foam insulation used in homes and mobile homes.

of sea air on good days; amounts range from 2000 to 4000 on bad days. Problems such as acid rain are now attracting widespread attention, but much needs to be done to correct this problem.

Foods

Contamination of our food supply with various chemicals is now widespread and complete. It is estimated that over 95 per cent of commercial foods contain pesticides. It is literally impossible to find organically grown foods in most areas of the country. It is estimated that the average individual ingests one gallon of food additives yearly. Foods may be contaminated in the growing process with pesticides, herbicides, and nitrates as well as in the collection process. Commercial preparation involves many chemical processes using dyes, preservatives, and stabilizers. Commercially grown meats are contaminated with hormones; antibiotics are used in both the growing animals and in preparation for storage. Plastics, phenols, and other gases and

Table 36–2. SOURCES OF PHENOL—CARBOLIC ACID OR HYDROXYBENZENE
Epoxy
Synthesis of aspirin and some drugs
Manufacture of explosives
Herbicides, pesticides, and germicides
Thermal insulation panes
Laminated boards
Nylon
Polyurethane
Detergents
Perfume
Gasoline additives
Dyes
Photo solution
Preservatives in medications and allergy shots
Acne medications
Baking powder
"Bakelite"
Caulking agents
Disinfectants—Lysol, Pine Sol, etc.
Enamel paint
Fiberglass
Flame retardant finishes
Food additives
Inks (fountain pen, printers)
Stamp pad
Insulation (thermal and acoustical)
Jute or hemp fiber preservative (carpet backing, area rugs, rope, twine)
Laundry starches
Matches
Mildew proofing
Paint
Plastics
Plywood
Preservatives in cosmetics
Preservatives in hair care products
Sealants
Shaving creams and lotions
Shoe polishes
Soundproofing
Solvent
"Spandex" (girdles, support hose, etc.)
Tin can inner linings
Water color paints
Wood preservatives

Table 36–3. SOURCES OF ETHANOL

Shellac
Oil
Rubbing alcohol
Ether
Rubber
Perfumes
Deodorant
Soaps
Detergents
Shampoo
Aftershave
Moth balls
Hair spray
Insect spray
Asphalt
Paint
Varnish
Glue
Gasoline
Exhaust fumes
Crude petroleum and its derivatives

Ethanol is made from ethylene gas by the oil companies and is used widely in its products. Ethanol is also made from grain.

chemicals are used in packaging in bulk storage. Preparation of food, particularly in restaurants, involves gas, preservatives, and artificial coloring.

Water

Perhaps the most difficult problem to correct is the contamination of our water supply. Chlorination is used for bacterial control but often acts as a catalyst, turning chemicals into other chemicals that are more toxic and harmful to humans and animals. Many of the contaminants that are secondary to agricultural methods do not break down naturally and cannot even be removed by distillation. The same is held true for industrial wastes, many of which are poisonous. It has been said that there is no longer any pure water left on earth.

The modern otolaryngologist should be able to recognize chemical sensitivity and be able to diagnose, treat, and prevent further damage to patients who have this difficult and serious problem.

REFERENCES

1. Dickey LD (ed): Clinical Ecology. Springfield, IL, Charles C Thomas, 1976.
2. Golos N, Goblitz FG, Leighton FS: Coping With Your Allergies. New York, Simon & Schuster, 1979.
3. Randolph TG, Moss RW: An Alternative Approach to Allergies. New York, Lippincott & Cromwell, 1980.
4. Randolph TG: Adaptation to specific environmental exposures enhanced by individual susceptibility. *In* Dickey LD (ed): Clinical Ecology. Springfield, IL, Charles C Thomas, 1976.
5. Randolph TG: Human Ecology and Susceptibility to the Chemical Environment. Springfield, IL, Charles C Thomas 1962.
6. State of California Department of Consumer Affairs: Clean Your Room! A Compendium on Indoor Pollution. Sacramento, Department of Consumer Affairs, 1982.
7. Zamm AV: Why Your House May Endanger Your Health. New York, Simon & Schuster, 1980.

CHAPTER 37

Therapy of Chemical and Environmental Factors in Allergic Disease

John H. Boyles, Jr., M.D.
Joseph P. Keenan, M.D., F.A.C.S.

The philosophy of treatment in chemical sensitivity is to avoid triggering symptoms in the first place, rather than to suppress them with long-term medications once they have happened. As a result, the main method of therapy consists of avoidance of offending substances. Frequently, this is not practical. The sensitivities may be so pervasive that it is impossible to avoid all of the allergens to which a person is sensitive.[1]

Consequently, the goal becomes to minimize the exposure to the offending allergens by environmental modification and a rotation diet of chemically uncontaminated foods, thereby reducing the allergic load. Neutralization of adverse reactions may at times be accomplished by alkaline salts or milk of magnesia. On occasion, the technique of neutralization by sublingual drops has been recommended in more severe cases, which have otherwise been difficult or impossible to benefit. Research into the mechanism of action is in progress.

THE ATMOSPHERIC ENVIRONMENT

The allergic patient often reacts to several outdoor as well as indoor contaminants including pollen, dust, mold, chemicals, and animals. Taking advantage of certain features of these different allergens can minimize the patient's exposure.

Pollens can be controlled by limiting vegetation around the home. Trees, especially, should be kept to a minimum. They create pollen problems as well as mold problems in the susceptible individual. In considering landscaping, the patient should be advised to plant flowering trees that have a low airborne pollen count, such as chestnut, willow, or locust. Suggest that these be planted a distance from the house. It must be kept in mind that pollens can be blown hundreds of miles and may affect an unsuspecting allergic patient. Also, a severely allergic patient might need to wear a face mask.

Trees near the house will create shade and increase moisture in the soil and create mildew problems on the house. Large exposures to mold should also be avoided. Raking of leaves, mowing the lawn, and weeding the garden should be jobs undertaken by nonallergic members of the family, or hired help should do them. If these tasks are unavoidable, the allergic patient must wear a face mask while performing them. Other sources of mold created by excess moisture around the house should be dealt with by the placement of drains. A person with mold allergies should not have a wood-burning stove. Storing wood near the house and bringing the moldy wood into the house greatly increases the mold exposure.

Since chemical exposure to pesticides, fungicides, fertilizers, fossil fuels, and other manmade substances can severely aggravate the allergic person, avoidance of these is strongly recommended. In general, the new fad of having the lawn sprayed with various chemicals is contraindicated for sensitive individuals. Residual molecules of these sprayed chemicals are carried by the wind and can affect people living several hundred yards away. Some states have imposed restrictions on the application of these chemicals. The allergic patient should not allow these chemicals to be sprayed on his or her lawn and should remain indoors with the windows closed if neighbors are using such substances. Gasoline-powered tools such as hedge trimmers, weed eaters, and chain saws should be replaced with electric-powered tools if possible.

Some patients will have to change their residence from a chemically or smog-infested area to one in which the outdoor air is less contaminated with chemical substances. Patients must be advised to live for brief periods of time in all four seasons of the year before they change locations from one area of the country to another, or even from one side of a city to another.

In general, having clean air to breathe in the home is the goal. Cigarette smoking should be totally prohibited in the home of the allergic patient.

Smoke-generating devices such as wood-burning stoves, coal or kerosene heating devices, and fireplaces aggravate allergic symptoms. Indoor storage of strong chemicals used for cleaning or hobbies must be avoided. The home and work environments need proper ventilation of such chemicals, and the use of masks is recommended. Animal and animal products such as fur coats, hair carpet pads, stuffed animals, and down comforters or jackets should be avoided.

Depending on the environment, the workplace may need to be modified. For example, in the office and in the car, air cleaners can be installed as well as air conditioning. Care should be taken in the use of air conditioning to prevent mold generation in the moist pads over which the air flows. No smoking should prevail at the workplace and break area. It should be a right of the workers to have a pollution-free eating and break area. Encourage patients to become clean air advocates.

At home and work, other measures can be taken to improve the total home environment. The number of measures initiated by the patient will be related to the severity of symptoms and the amount of exposure needed to aggravate them. One major problem that must be faced is the financial constraints incurred when the patient carries out these measures. The patient needs to know that, sometimes, insurance will pay for the air cleaners and other devices that are necessary for the health of the patient. Tax benefits may also be possible if certain modifications to the environment are recommended by a physician as part of treatment. However, in our current tax environment, the patient should get advice from a tax consultant.

Another measure that can greatly reduce the dust levels in a home is the installation of a central vacuum system that is vented to the outside. The system removes dust, animal dander, and other debris, collects it, and exhausts it to the outside rather than recirculating the dust in the air.

By keeping windows shut in the summer and using an air conditioner, the pollen count will remain low. With all air circulating devices, special attention and care must be given to routine cleaning to prevent the growth of mold. For the patient with inhalant allergies, air cleaners both in the home and in the car may be recommended. Inhalant allergens, by definition, are carried by the air; therefore, anything that is done to reduce the concentration of allergens and pollutants will bring about significant improvement in the environmentally or chemically sensitive patient. It is best to avoid the use of plants in the interior decorating schemes of the house. The soil harbors molds, some plants emit harmful pollen, and leaves can collect dust that will aggravate the sensitive patient.

Petrochemically sensitive individuals should eliminate gas stoves and heaters. The small amounts of gas emitted from these appliances can be enough to provoke symptoms. Also, the use of pesticides, strong cleaning agents, and aerosol personal items should be minimized. When the patient has a choice, the use of hard floor surfaces is preferable to carpeted areas. Carpeting, no matter how thoroughly cleaned, acts as a dust collector. When it is walked upon or stirred up by cleaning, the airborne particles that have been previously entrapped in the carpet can aggravate patients with dust, dander, or molds or outgas the chemicals from which it and the pad are constructed, contributing to the patient's allergic load. Hobbies that require the use of chemicals, such as furniture refinishing, painting, dried vegetation as in flower arranging, and others, are undesirable. Major appliances should be vented to the outside to reduce air pollution, including the clothes dryer, oven, and stove. Humidity should also be vented outside from the bathroom and mildew prevented or carefully removed. Reduction in basement humidity would require a dehumidifier, and any mold present should be removed by professional fogging if necessary.

Indoor air pollution is a much more common source of trouble to most chemically allergic patients and, in cases of the working place, more difficult to manage. In the past, the most common source of indoor air pollution was natural gas used in the furnace or in appliances; however, in the modern home and office, formaldehyde has now become the number one source of trouble. Natural gas is now in the number two ranking, followed by pesticides. The major source of formaldehyde contamination is particle board, followed by carpeting and carpet padding. Particle board is found mainly in cabinets, furniture, and subflooring.

Epidermals are a significant source of sensitization of the allergic patient.[2] Animals should be eliminated from the home environment if there is evidence of sensitivity. The major problems in our culture are created by cats and dogs and other fur-bearing animals such as rabbits and, to a lesser extent, birds. Because the degree of sensitization and provocation of symptoms is directly related to the length of exposure, it is best to minimize this exposure even in patients without positive tests. If it is impossible to convince a patient to get rid of a dog that has been a family pet for years, have him isolate himself from the pet as much as possible. The allergic patient cannot be in charge of grooming or feeding the pet, and the animal needs to be kept outside of the house. If the animal is allowed in the house, the patient's bedroom must remain "off limits." Once the dander (especially cat) is present in the house, it will take months to completely eliminate it. Of course, barns and other buildings where animals are kept are no places for the allergic person. Hobbies involving animals are poor choices. If exposure to animals is a necessity, use long-sleeved coveralls and a mask. Having no pets is often a problem when children are involved. Fish and snakes are two extremely hypoallergenic pets that would be acceptable for the highly allergic child. Oftentimes, there can be an accidental exposure to the allergenic animal. It is possible for a highly allergic child who is sensitive to cats to have a provocation of symptoms at school even though no cat is present at school. Through a careful investigation, it is discovered that the allergic child is sitting next to a student who has cats at home. The student has brought in enough cat dander on his clothes to provoke symptoms in the allergic child. Without a thorough investigation, it might have been assumed that a food or building contaminant may have caused the symptoms rather than the cat dander.

ALLERGEN-FREE ZONE

The patient should be counseled in the importance of having an allergen-free zone in the home. Often, the bedroom is a good location because the patient will usually spend six to eight hours a day sleeping here. This room should be kept free of mold, dust, pollen, animals, and chemicals. This will give the allergic patient a safe place to recuperate. Certain measures need to be taken to make this environment as ideal as possible. This room should have no carpeting. Hardwood or tile floors prevent the build-up of dust, mold, and dander. The furnishings should be sparse, but what is present should be constructed of wood or metal. No bookcases, knickknack shelves, or other pieces of furniture that are dust collectors should be in the room. Upholstered furniture is similar to carpeting. It will hold allergens in the room, so it should be avoided. A water bed is desirable, but a mattress and box spring covered in allergen-proof encasings are acceptable. Pillows need to be covered also. Even with allergen-proof encasings, the pillows should not be feather or down. Polyester and Dacron are acceptable materials in patients not sensitive to them; for patients sensitive to these materials, covered down pillows kept very clean may, on occasion, be preferable. Wool, down comforters, chenille bedspreads, and heavy quilts are undesirable bedding choices. Cotton sheets and blankets are the most hypoallergenic but must be washed frequently in hot water to kill mites. Many patients can tolerate acrylic blankets as well. Windows need to be decorated with lightweight curtains that can be laundered frequently or blinds that are easily washed. Heavy drapes are tremendous dust collectors and, therefore, are unacceptable. Wallpaper can harbor molds, and oftentimes, patients are allergic to the material or paste used. Vinyl wallpaper is especially bad because of outgassing of the plastic. Painted walls are preferred with the patient not moving in until all odor is gone. Plants and animals are not allowed. Windows and doors need to be kept closed at all times. The use of an air conditioner and air cleaner will help keep the room allergen free. Depending on the climate, a humidifier or dehumidifier may be required. The use of a hygrometer to measure humidity in the room is helpful. The humidity needs to be maintained between 40 and 60 per cent. A variation from this will determine if the humidity control devices will be necessary.

Clothes worn outside are restricted from the bedroom and must be deposited directly into the laundry area. Cosmetics, including perfumes, hair sprays, and deodorants, cannot be used in the bedroom, and, of course, the bedroom must be cleaned frequently. Basically, anything that can be done to keep the room allergen free should be initiated. If the allergic person is a child, caution should be taken in allowing toys, books, bikes, and the like in the bedroom. Having toys located outside this area is best. Stuffed animals, in particular, act as dust collectors and may contain allergenic fillings. However, there are nonallergenic, washable ones now available. One or two of these as bedmates is acceptable as long as they are washed and dried weekly.

NEW HOUSE CONSTRUCTION

If the patient is fortunate enough to be in the process of building a new house, there are several factors concerning the construction and orientation of the house that should be considered. Geographical location is important in determining the exposure that a patient will receive from different allergens. Even given the same general geographical location, taking advantage of specific topography can greatly decrease the patient's exposure. The surroundings where the house is being planned should be carefully evaluated, whether it is inner city, country, valley, or hilltown. Air quality and wind patterns need to be considered in scouting out a suitable homesite. Once the general location is selected, the soil and surrounding vegetation should be examined. An ecologically oriented architect would be of tremendous assistance.

The house, itself, needs a well thought out plan to eliminate materials and techniques of construction that may be harmful to an allergic patient. The foundation of the house is best made with poured concrete with deep footings back-filled with gravel to reduce mold problems. No pesticide treatment should be allowed. These often outgas for years. Rooms below ground level or a cellar will increase mold exposure. To reduce chemical contamination within the house, hard materials are preferred in construction. Plywood outgasses less than particle board. Plaster walls are ideal, but sheet rock may be more cost effective; be careful to explore chemical treatments done to various sheet rock material before purchasing.

Insulating material requires some research and often may be placed outside the moisture barrier. A few years ago, the public was made aware of the health problems associated with urea formaldehyde insulation. Make sure the house is not "too tight." Air flow patterns are important to maintain fresh as well as clean air within the home. Many problems have recently arisen in homes and offices that are superinsulated. The air quality has reached critical levels, and families and employees have been experiencing health problems. In terms of heating and cooling, there has been some debate about the best approach. Baseboard hot water with an ancillary air conditioning system with air cleaners has been one choice versus heat pump systems, in which both hot and cold air are circulated as needed. In either case, the important factor to consider is a proper design to incorporate air cleaners when heating or cooling. The system needs to function effectively with the windows and doors closed. Therefore, exhaust fans that pull in outside air in the summer are prohibited. Gas heating systems and appliances should not be used. If attics and basements are unavoidable, good ventilation is a must. Radon levels need to be taken in the basement to avoid health problems associated with it. Hardwood floors or ceramic tile are the best materials to use with special grouting to prevent mold formation. Minimize the use of carpet. Although it is a cheap floor covering, it is very allergenic. Over time, hard floors are just as economical. They need to be replaced or resurfaced far less frequently than carpeting does.

The garage location is important for the allergic patient. Ideally, it should be a separate building connected to the house by a walkway. The outgassing of petrochemicals, exhaust fumes, and other types of chemical-based substances is very high in a garage. Besides cars, lawnmowers, chain saws, paints and paint thinners, fertilizers, pesticides, outdoor tools, and many other things are stored in a garage. These will present problems to the allergic patient. When the garage is located under the house or beside the house, these contaminants enter the house and create an air quality problem.

DIETARY CONTROL

Chemicals play an increasing role in contamination of our food supplies.[3] Spray residues are often found in fruits such as apples, cherries, peaches, pears, strawberries, raspberries, pineapples, grapes, oranges, grapefruits, and lemons. Vegetables sprayed include almost everything grown above ground. Most of these sprays are oil-soluble and permeate the food to which they are applied. Washing, peeling, soaking in water or vinegar, or even cooking will not remove all of the chemicals. Root vegetables are apt to be free of spray residue unless contaminated in transit, storage, and markets. Sprays also may contaminate forage plants and animal feeds. Therefore, lamb, beef, pork, and fowl may concentrate oil-soluble insecticides and herbicides in their fats and affect the highly sensitive patient. Hormones and antibiotics often contaminate both fowl and red meat animals. Foods often contaminated by fumigant residues include dates, figs, nuts, raisins, prunes, dried fruits, and cereal grains. Sulfur and its derivatives are used as fungal disinfectants, preservatives, and antibrowning agents in all stages of food processing. Coal tar dyes are commonly used to artificially color many foods. Gas finds its way into a wide variety of foods. Bananas and oranges are often artificially ripened by exposure to ethylene gas. Apples and pears are sometimes stored in the presence of ethylene. Coffee is usually roasted over an open flame, absorbing some of the combusted products. Cane and beet sugars are usually clarified through bone charred filters reactivated in gas-fired kilns. Residues are apparently passed along through the next batch of syrup filtered through. Honey, if it can be tolerated, is the preferred sweetener for the sensitive patient.

Containers often contaminate the food they are supposed to protect. Odorous plastic bags and cartons are used in most vegetable markets to package produce. In general, plastic tends to contaminate foods in direct proportion to the odor emitted by the material. If the material is odorous or if scraping, rubbing, or filing the surface of the plastic causes odor emission, there is increased reason to suspect it. Usually, the softer the plastic, the more unstable it is, and thus more likely to outgas in the surrounding air or closely contained food.

Foods are frequently contaminated by the gold and brown lining of metal cans. This lining, phenolic resin, prevents metal from bleaching the contents of the can but also contaminates them chemically. Paraffin wax is often used to dress up and preserve many fruits and vegetables.

Chemically treated water may induce symptoms in chemically susceptible patients who avoid other major sources of chemical additives and contaminants. Food may ordinarily be washed with tap water but may be contaminated if allowed to stand or cook in tap water. Some vegetables are contaminated by washing with detergents. Chemically softened water should not be used for cooking or drinking purposes.

SUMMARY

Despite the controversy surrounding the subject of food and chemical allergy, such reactions are an established fact. No matter how narrowly physicians limit their practice to a particular subspecialty, they will find it impossible to successfully diagnose and treat all their patients unless they have a comprehensive knowledge of the subjects of food and chemical allergy. Without this knowledge, they will be forced to treat their patients symptomatically with drugs. Unfortunately, many will ultimately decompensate and become therapeutic failures.

When counseling the patient in terms of environmental modifications, it should be stressed that avoidance of the offending allergens is the best approach. Financial constraints are definitely a consideration when making suggestions to patients. It may become necessary to limit some of the modifications to fit the patient's income. Compliance is vital, and a key point to remember is that a patient will not make changes in the environment unless he or she is effectively taught and made to see the benefits of these changes. Take adequate time with patients to emphasize their importance.

REFERENCES

1. Boyles JH Jr: Chemical sensitivity. Diagnosis and treatment. Otolaryngo Clin North Am 18:787, 1985.
2. Matthews KP: Aerobiology and inhalant allergens. Part II: *In* Middleton E (ed): Allergy Principles and Practice. St. Louis, CV Mosby, 1987, pp 1190–1201.
3. Saifer P, Saifer M: Clinical detection of sensitivity to preservatives and chemicals. *In* Brostoff J (ed): Food Allergy and Intolerance. London, Baillière Tindall, 1987, pp 416–420.

CHAPTER 38

Diagnostic and Therapeutic Techniques for Chemical-Environmental Allergy and Hypersensitivity

William P. King, M.D.

The fixed variety of chemical allergy, as exhibited by those individuals acutely allergic to monosodium glutamate or metabisulfate food additives, is diagnosed principally by astute history taking and, if necessary, carefully titrated direct oral challenge. In this section, however, we are addressing testing techniques for the more insidious environmental chemical allergy or hypersensitivity.

The portals of entry of this type of chemical problem are more often either vapor inhalation or oral intake. Skin absorption is also a possible source. As such, testing techniques, other than patch testing for contact allergies, are largely limited to some variety of blinded inhalant challenge or provocation/neutralization.

INHALATION CHALLENGE

Although various ingenious techniques for blind inhalation challenge have been devised, the most accepted method involves the use of a so-called chemical test booth. Whether a reaction to volatile chemicals is truly allergic, that is, involves some variety of immune response, or represents merely a hyperacute toxic reaction is moot, since treatment largely is limited to exposure avoidance.

The chemical test booth is constructed interiorly solely of aluminum and glass, neither of which emits outgassing contaminants. The walls and all contents of the room must be cleaned with bottled water and baking soda at regular intervals, dependent on the frequency of use of the booth, to ensure against any accumulation of surface contamination. Prior to a test, the booth must be ensured free of any contaminant residue in the air by replacing the air in the booth through a fan exhaust system. Baseline pretest existing symptoms and vital signs are recorded. The patient is seated within the booth on a non-outgassing stool in clear sight of the testing individual. A wide-mouthed jar containing 100 ml of a standard chemical solution (Table 38–1) poured over cotton balls is placed on a glass shelf in front of the patient. Suggested is a 1 pint jar with a 3-inch mouth containing 35 cotton balls. The jar is opened on signal. The patient is then carefully monitored by the testing individual for any untoward response, by both constant visual observation and direct communication through a two-way sound system. In addition, the pulse is monitored by utilizing a

Table 38–1. VOLATILE CHEMICALS FOR BOOTH TESTING

Formaldehyde	
Conc. =	37% formaldehyde
Test =	1:50 dilution (using saline)
Phenol	
Conc. =	87% phenol
Test =	4:1000 dilution
Chlorine	
Conc. =	5% sodium hypochlorite (Clorox)
Test =	concentrate undiluted
Alcohol	
Conc. =	91% isopropyl alcohol
Test =	concentrate undiluted
Insecticide	
Conc. =	nonaerosol insecticide (example: Raid and/or Hot Shot)
Test =	concentrate undiluted

pulse meter at five-minute intervals throughout the 20-minute test period.

The test is discontinued immediately if significant symptom provocation is obvious. Seldom is treatment other than brief oxygen inhalation or alkali salt administration required. Further testing, of course, cannot be accomplished as long as symptoms from a previous test are sustained.

It is important that the patient be thoroughly familiarized with the test procedure before beginning, to avoid anxiety or other interfering psychological manifestations. Normal saline placebos along with repeat blinded testing of questionable responses should be generously used to ensure accuracy, especially when only subjective symptoms result. This consideration is especially important when one considers the sobering thought that the primary treatment of positive responders is avoidance of the provoking chemical, a requirement that may be very inconvenient economically or socially when place of employment or home environment is involved in chronic exposure.

The five most common chemical families involved are phenols, chlorines, aldehydes, insecticides, and hydrocarbons. Typically tested for each group, respectively, is phenol, Clorox, formaldehyde, an insecticide, and isopropyl alcohol vapor. Also, often very informative is inhalation exposure to some kind of burning hydrocarbon gas; since this cannot practically be delivered in a blinded manner, simple inhalation of fumes over a lit gas stove or such suffices. The ambient air vapor concentration emitted from the test materials is not more than that typically well tolerated in everyday normal situations, so that only the hypersensitive will react. Also, when the blinded test materials are utilized, an identifying odor should not be perceptible, allowing efficacious use of placebos. Other vaporizing chemicals may be appropriately substituted as advised by the personal history.

ORAL CHALLENGE

Again, here we speak of testing techniques for the hidden, chronic variety of chemical allergy or hypersensitivity, rather than direct oral challenge of food additives that may be the cause of acute anaphylaxis.

The most common variety of oral challenge is sublingual provocation/neutralization. The technique used by the proponents of this modality has been previously described in Chapter 34. Most often this route of provocative/neutralization testing is chosen, rather than the intracutaneous or subcutaneous testing administration endorsed by the American Academy of Otolaryngic Allergy (AAOA) and the American Academy of Otolaryngology–Head and Neck Surgery (AAO–HNS), because the character of the testing material makes the latter approach ill-advised. The utilized concentrates for the chemicals commonly tested by the sublingual technique are listed in Table 38–2. Typically, testing is begun with the #1 dilution unless there is a suggestive history of notable sensitivity to the tested material. Because a temporary stinging occurs when the #1 formaldehyde dilution is delivered, some suggest starting this test with the #2 dilution.

Table 38–2. CONCENTRATES FOR CHEMICAL PROVOCATION/NEUTRALIZATION TESTS

Substance	Concentrate
Petrochemical ethanol	100% synthetic ethyl alcohol
Phenol	Buffered saline with 0.47% phenol
*Formaldehyde	37% formaldehyde
Red and yellow food dye	1:10 dilution of commerical food dye in saline
Tobacco smoke	Tobacco smoke mix, commercial extract
Glycerin	100% glycerin
Grain alcohol	190 proof
Chlorine	Clorox

*For formaldehyde, the maximal strength suggested for use sublingually is the #2 dilution, and intracutaneously the #3 dilution.

INTRACUTANEOUS CHALLENGE

The intracutaneous provocative/neutralization technique is used by a number of physicians for a few chemicals, specifically synthetic petrochemical ethanol, phenol, and formaldehyde. The concentrates utilized for this approach are the same as noted for sublingual testing. When intracutaneously testing for formaldehyde sensitivity, it is advised to utilize no stronger dilution than the #3.

HEMATOLOGIC TESTS

Although not related to allergy per se, hematologic tests for heavy metal poisoning, such as lead, mercury, cadmium, and arsenic, are well known. In addition, there are many sophisticated tests for toxicity levels to other specific industrial chemicals. Recently, there have been made available screening blood tests for minute levels, in the nanograms per milliliter range, of chlorinated phenols, chlorinated pesticides, and aromatic and halogenated volatile chemicals, plus a urine test for phenoxy acid herbicides.* Whereas the reported test levels of these chemicals are often well below so-called toxic levels, in some hypersensitive individuals it appears that even such low levels may be a hidden cause of chronic ill effects. Although of interest, these modalities concern diagnosis of hypersensitivity or toxicity more than true allergic phenomenon.

*Center for Bio-Organic Studies, University of New Orleans, New Orleans, LA 70148; Envirol-Health Systems, Inc., 990 North Bowser Road/Suite 800, Richardson, TX 75081.

THERAPY FOR CHEMICAL SENSITIVITY

Neutralization for Chemical Allergies

The most effective treatment for chemical allergies or hypersensitivities, as with any other such infirmity, is avoidance of the offending material. Total abstinence from such exposure in many cases, however, is impossible. In these instances, when a causative chemical can be tested by one of the provocation/neutralization techniques, treatment with a neutralizing dose may offer significant relief. Regardless of the test route of administration, sublingual or intracutaneous, treatment is usually administered sublingually in consideration of the character of all the test materials. The exception is phenol, which may also be delivered subcutaneously. The subcutaneous route is especially typical for patients receiving immunotherapy with allergens diluted with phenolated saline (0.4 per cent) phenol). In such instance, the neutralizing dose of phenol is administered subcutaneously 30 minutes prior to the therapeutic allergy injection.

The determination and preparation of the neutralizing dose is identical to that already described in Chapter 34. Frequency of administration varies with the individual frequency and severity of exposure. Initiation of sublingual therapy is generally at the one to three times a day level, with modification thereafter according to response and need.

SECTION FIVE

ADDITIONAL ALLERGY MANAGEMENT STRATEGIES

SECTION FIVE

ADDITIONAL ALLERGY MANAGEMENT STRATEGIES

CHAPTER 39

Surgery and the Allergic Patient

Helen F. Krause, M.D., F.A.C.S.

Patients with allergic diseases sometimes need surgery. It may be in the field of the allergic target organ, such as the nose or the throat, and directly related to the allergy, as in nasal polyposis; or it may be unrelated, such as correction of a deviated nasal septum. Even when surgery is at a distant site, the allergy still plays a role in the surgical management.

IS SURGERY NECESSARY?

In the practice of otolaryngology, we are again and again faced with several complex questions: In a patient with nasal obstruction, are the symptoms caused by a deviated nasal septum or by allergic edema? Is chronic or recurrent sinusitis simply infection, or is there an allergic basis that must be controlled? Does the chronic sore throat result from infection or from allergic postnasal drainage? Is the otitis media with effusion anatomic, infectious, or allergic in origin? Is the laryngeal edema caused by infection, voice misuse, or allergy? And, are these pathologic problems reversible without surgical intervention? Finally, what precautions should be taken in such patients? Again, we must never lose sight of the total patient, medically or surgically.

Of course, not every otorhinolaryngologic problem can be cured with a scalpel, nor can all be dispatched with a needle. But expertise in both surgery and allergy management places the otolaryngic allergist in a unique position to balance the multiple aspects of disease in the head and neck.

It may be impossible to determine by examination alone whether a problem is functional, that is, allergic or infectious; whether it is structural, due to deformities; or whether it is a combination of these. For instance, mucosal responses to prolonged structural obstruction can mimic allergic rhinitis; thus, nasal cytologic studies may be of considerable help in such cases.

ALLERGIC MANAGEMENT

In known allergic patients undergoing any type of elective surgery, not just rhinologic surgery, the allergic symptoms should be under the best possible management to ensure the safest anesthetic and postoperative care. In this way morbidity and surgical risk are decreased and the healing potential is improved. This is especially true in head and neck surgery and in endoscopy, be it intranasal, pulmonary, or gastrointestinal.

Allergy may, of course, be seasonal or perennial. If it is seasonal, the significant inhalant allergy season should be avoided if possible; otherwise the surgeon should be prepared to administer proper medications. In both seasonal and perennial allergy, the patient should be treated with medication and other measures, such as immunotherapy, long enough preoperatively to have comfortably clear mucous membranes. Patients with asthma should be wheeze free, perhaps requiring preoperative bronchodilators. Supplemental corticosteroids may be necessary in steroid-dependent asthmatics or in patients who have used them in the recent past. In allergy of the upper and lower respiratory tracts, steroids may be required during the surgery as well as postoperatively for the best result. Antihistamines and decongestants may also be of benefit, especially postoperatively. The hospital room should be smoke free, and specific allergy care, especially immunotherapy and diet management, should be continued. In some cases, plants and flowers may have to be eliminated from the patient's room. Increased humidification is sometimes of benefit.

UPPER AIRWAY OBSTRUCTION

There are many causes of upper airway obstruction seen in an otolaryngology practice, some structural, some functional (primarily allergic), or a combination of both (Table 39–1). A patient may present with obstruction due to mucosal, bony, or cartilaginous changes in the nose or due to thick nasal secretions or space-occupying lesions. Mucosal edema of the turbinates and septum may result from allergy, respiratory infections, hormonal changes, or vasomotor rhinitis. The turbinates may enlarge owing to mucosal hyperplasia secondary to chronic allergic edema, or because of bony hypertrophy from compensatory changes associated with septal deviations or perforations. Nasal choanal or sinus polyps may be related to allergy, infection, cystic fibrosis, or the aspirin sensitivity syndrome, or they may be idiopathic. Adhesions or stenosis sometimes result from trauma or previous surgery. Chronic upper airway obstruction may also originate in the nasopharynx due to adenoid enlargement, postoperative stenosis, tumor masses, or congenital deformities. In the mouth and pharynx, obstruction may be a consequence of massive tonsil hypertrophy, tumor involvement, ranulas, or congenital abnormalities. The history and physical are the keys that the surgeon-allergist must use.

Table 39–1. SITES OF UPPER AIRWAY OBSTRUCTION

Nose	Nasopharynx
Allergic rhinitis	Adenoid hypertrophy
Deviated nasal septum with or without external deformity	Tumors
Polyps	**Pharynx**
Nasal	Tonsil hypertrophy
Choanal	Macroglossia (pseudomacroglossia)
Turbinate abnormalities	Tongue cysts and ranulas
Hyperplasia	Palate abnormalities
Hypertrophic	
Polypoid	
Microrhino dysplasia	
Choanal atresia	
Foreign bodies	
Miscellaneous	
Tumors	
Stenosis	
Adhesions	
Chronic infection	
Neurogenic changes	

Table 39–2. AIRWAY EVALUATION IN 200 ORTHODONTIC PATIENTS

Referral Origin	Study 1	Study 2	Total
Orthodontists	74	63	137
General dentists	2	1	3
Pediatrician or family practitioner	18	26	44
Other otorhinolaryngologists	2	1	3
Patient self-referral	3	8	11
Speech pathologists	1	1	2

Obstruction, which may be diagnosed at any age, must be corrected to allow normal airway function and facial growth. The association of airway obstruction with the development of facial deformities has received considerable attention in recent years.[1–12] In 1983, the author completed an evaluation of 200 children between the ages of 4 and 16 years having malocclusion, and some also having facial deformities, selected at random from those referred because of upper aiway obstruction. Over 70 per cent were referred by dentists, especially orthodontists (Table 39–2).

The protocol (Table 39–3) involved (1) evaluation of the nasal anatomy, including both tissue edema and structural deformities; (2) assessment of the size of the adenoids and tonsils, with estimation of the degree of obstruction; (3) evaluation of patients with significant allergic history; and (4) diagnosis of structural deformities of the middle third of the face. Of these 200 children, 58.5 per cent were found to have allergies, alone or with some other factor associated; 38 per cent had hypertrophic lymphoid tissue; and 21 per cent had structural deformities, often a deviated septum. Ten per cent had microrhino dysplasia—a growth defect of the middle third of the face resulting in very narrow nasal fossae.[1] Allergies were diagnosed by his-

Table 39–3. MEDICAL FACTORS RELATED TO AIRWAY OBSTRUCTION

	Study 1	Study 2	Total	%
Nasal septal deformities (with or without related external deformities)	18	24	42	21
Hypertrophic or chronically infected lymphoid tissue (tonsils and/or adenoids)	41	35	76	38
Allergic diathesis	52	65	117	58.5
Growth abnormalities (microrhino dysplasia) (mid-facial dysplasia)	9	11	20	10

tory, skin endpoint titration or modified RAST testing, diet diaries, and diet elimination and challenge.

Of these children, 56, or 28 per cent, required tonsillectomies and/or adenoidectomies, most often because of chronic recurrent infections, rarely because of obstruction alone. Twenty-four, or 12 per cent, required nasal surgery, one having nasal polyps (Table 39–4). Some patients did not need previously anticipated adenoidectomy once control of the allergies was achieved (see Fig. 8–16). Thirteen children in the study had prior adenotonsillectomies but still had airway obstruction, most often due to allergic edema of the nasal mucosa.

Management of the airway was of significant importance in allowing proper orthodontic procedures, including tolerance of appliances, prevention of relapse after completion of orthodontic treatment, and prevention of further development of the classic long face syndrome (Fig. 39–1). Surgery alone would not have solved these problems. Dana is a case in point (Fig. 39–2). She had, at age 12, a typical long face syndrome with grotesque malocclusion. Allergy evaluation was completed and treatment started, followed by correction of her marked septal deformity. Within nine months (Fig. 39–3) her malocclusion was well under way to being corrected, and although stigmata of the long face syndrome do remain, she is a much healthier and happier child.

OTHER PROBLEMS

Problems requiring surgical care may arise from allergic upper airway disease. Nasal polyposis has most often been considered a result of allergy, although other causes are possible. In 1983 English[13] reviewed studies of the incidence of allergy in patients with nasal polyps (see Table 8–2). Allergies were diagnosed by history or by skin testing, with incidences ranging from 10 to 64 per cent. A number of patients included in this review had aspirin sensitivity with asthma—possibly skewing the figure lower, since only approximately 10 to 20 per cent with this syndrome have true atopy. Patients having aspirin sensitivity without asthma may also develop polyps. Asthma may develop years later. Also, studies of allergy based on history alone, not testing, may have resulted in some allergic patients being excluded from the statistics, for many patients are unaware of a chronic low-grade allergy.

Table 39–4. PATIENTS REQUIRING SURGERY

	Nasal Surgery	Tonsillectomy and/or Adenoidectomy
Study 1	12	33
Study 2	12	23
Total	24	56

Nasal polyps are mucosal in derivation, with an unclear pathogenesis. Management should include treatment of infection and allergies when present. Allergy control, including immunotherapy, intranasal steroids, and cromolyn, is rarely effective alone in the case of multiple, large polyps, although systemic steroids or direct injection into the polyps may be of benefit (see Chapters 23 and 25). When the disease is extensive and conservative measures are not sufficient, surgery is necessary in the attempt to attain normal anatomy. If the patient is atopic, the polyps are certain to recur unless the underlying allergy is treated.

Polypoid disease extending to the paranasal sinuses must be treated in conjunction with the intranasal disease. Infectious sinusitis with or without polyps may be related to allergy because of the chronic obstruction; or there may be true allergic involvement of the sinus mucosa. As with polyps alone, allergy control, bacteriologic studies, and proper antibiotic management are mandatory prior to surgical intervention. If obstruction is related to a deviated septum or to turbinate abnormalities, the problem should be

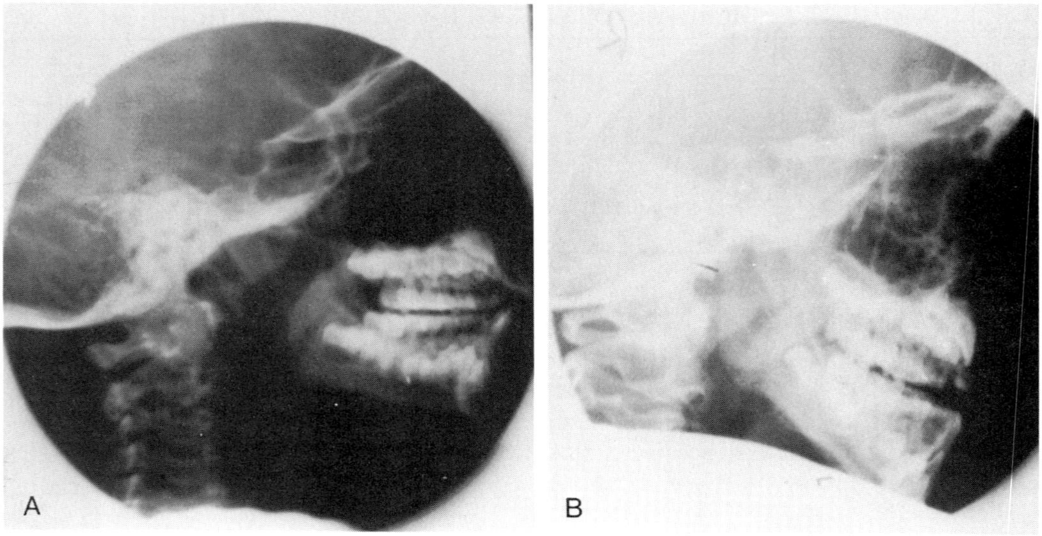

FIGURE 39–1. *A,* Normal facial structure, age 7. *B,* Abnormal characteristics of long face syndrome in a 7-year-old child.

corrected at the same time as the sinus surgery to prevent recurrences and provide an optimally functioning airway. Allergy management should *precede* the surgery, except in life-threatening situations such as those posed by ocular or intracranial complications.

There is no evidence that nasal or sinus surgery increases the potential for development of asthma. In fact, after sinus surgery, patients with asthma often show significant improvement and their medications can be decreased or stopped.[14–16] Elimination of the sinus disease improves the upper airway, often reduces the need for supportive care (especially medications), and decreases bronchial reactivity in many patients, as discussed by Dr. William Friedman et al.[14] in describing the sinobronchial syndrome (nasopulmonary reflex, Fig. 39–4).

Allergy may be involved in hyperplasia or inflammation of pharyngeal wall lymphoid tissue. Allergic management may reduce the inflammatory reaction as well as the size of the tonsils and adenoids, so that surgery is not needed. In such patients, thick postnasal drainage is often a clue that the inflammation is not infectious but allergic (see Fig. 8–18). Not all patients with allergies and chronic tonsil and adenoid disease adequately improve with allergy management alone; some still require adenoidectomy and/or tonsillectomy (Fig. 39–5). These are not obsolete procedures.

TECHNIQUES

Allergy should also be considered as a factor in the evaluation of laryngeal edema and even of vocal cord polyps. Laryngeal edema may occur either with a slow onset or as an acute episode. Sometimes appearing postoperatively after general endotracheal anesthesia for nonotolaryngologic procedures, it must be recognized and treated appropriately. Whereas edema may be merely due to the intubation, the possibility of allergy and increased mucosal reactivity must be kept in mind.

The relationship of chronic otitis media with effusion to allergy is still unclear, but allergy should certainly be considered. In some cases, allergy therapy may eliminate the need for repeated myringotomies with ventilation tube insertion. Both inhalant and food allergy may directly or indirectly cause eustachian tube and middle ear disease.[17–20]

Sinus surgery in allergic patients may entail antral surgery, ethmoidectomies, and sphenoidectomies. The use of good radiographic studies is essential. In addition to the standard radiographs and tomograms, computed axial tomography (CAT) scan is often invaluable, especially in difficult cases. Both sagittal (axial) and coronal views are helpful (Figs. 39–6 and 39–7). Magnetic resonance imaging (MRI) enhances such an evaluation if availability and cost are not

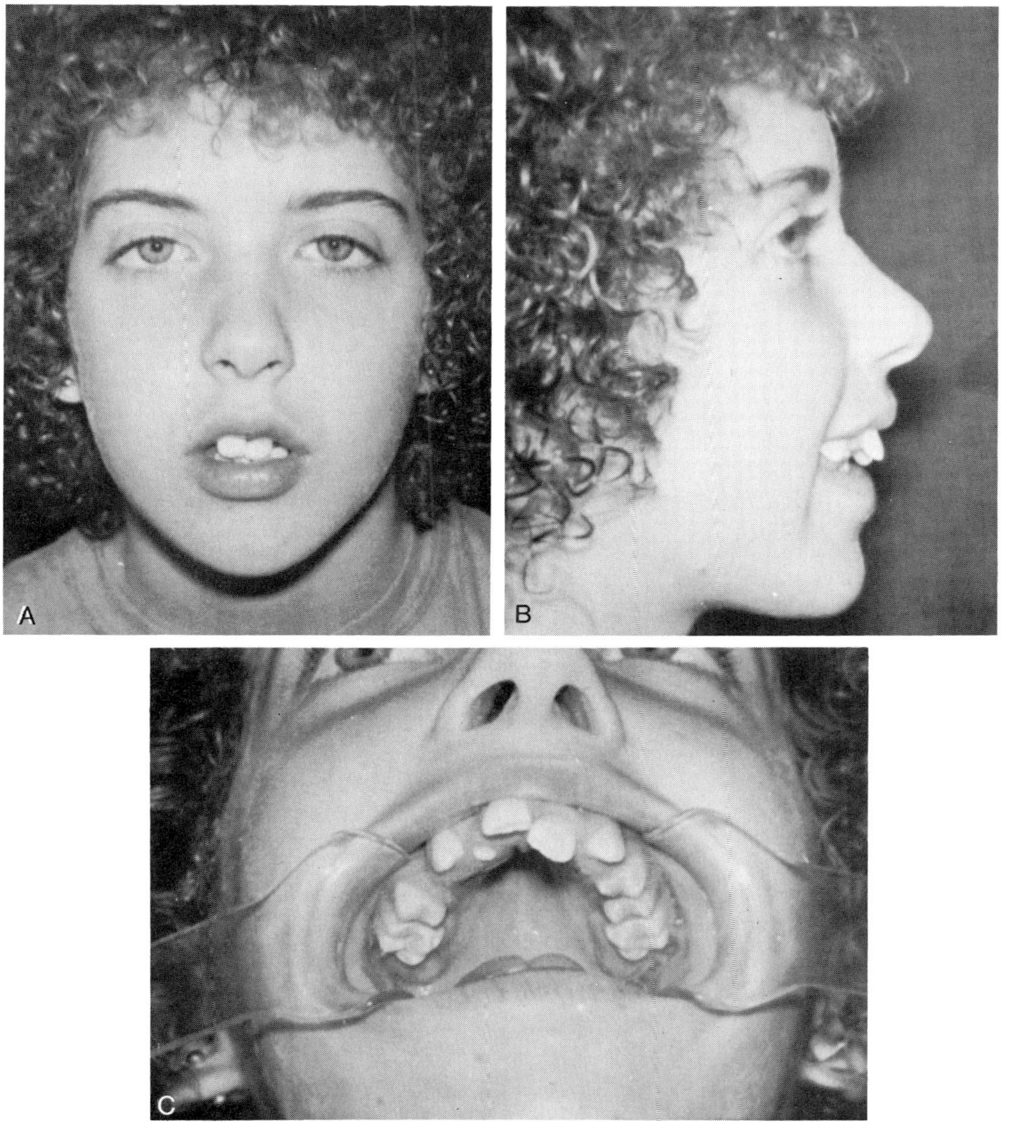

FIGURE 39–2. Twelve-year-old girl with long face syndrome and severe malocclusion prior to therapy.

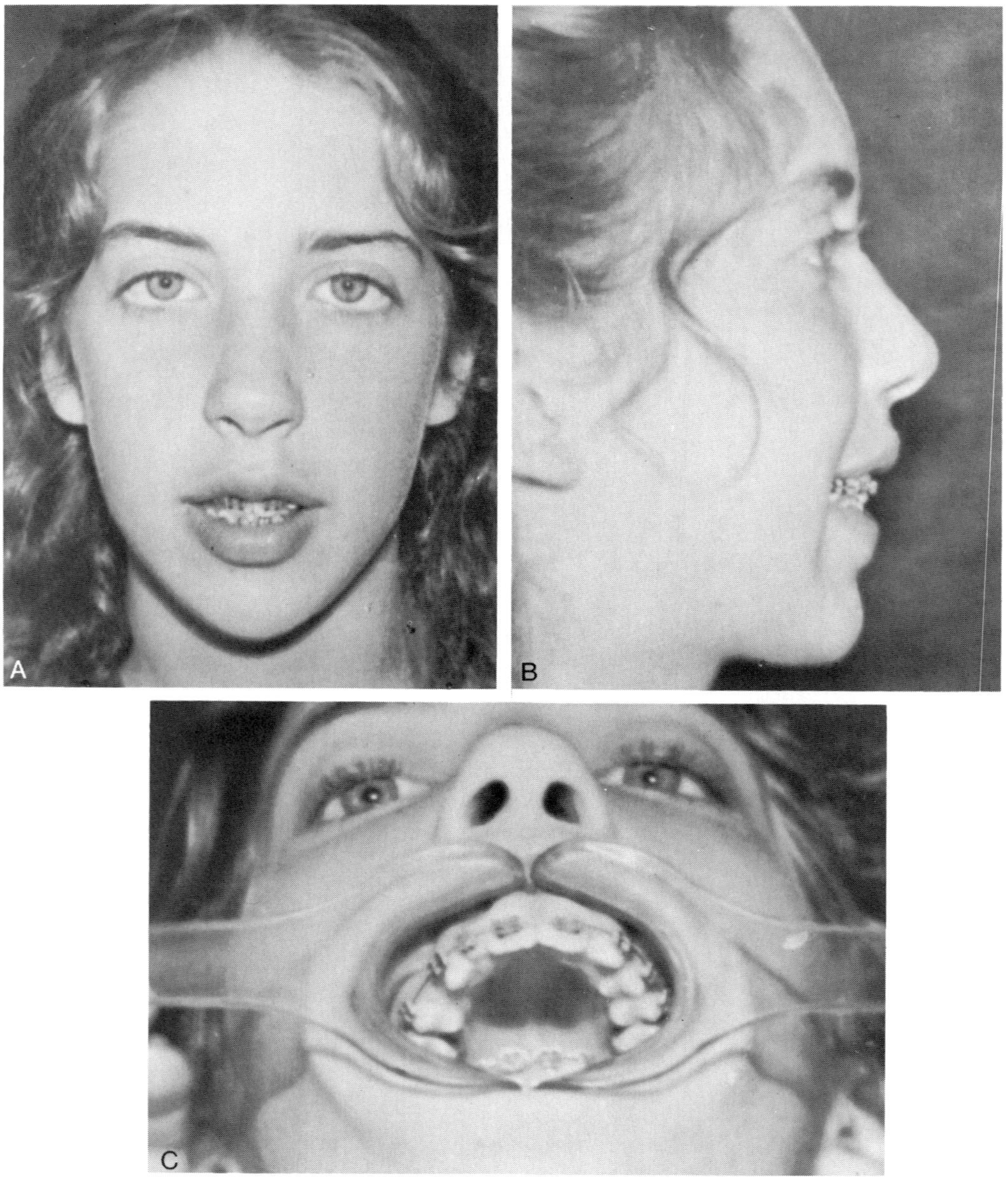

FIGURE 39–3. Child in Figure 39–2 nine months after nasal septal correction and commencement of allergy immunotherapy.

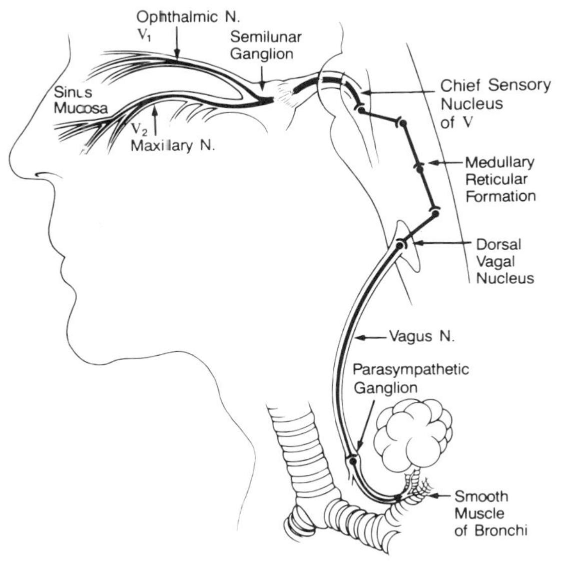

FIGURE 39–4. A proposed mechanism for the nasopulmonary reflex. (From Friedman WH, et al. Laryngoscope 96:473, 1986.)

restrictive. The ability of these new radiologic techniques to identify bony abnormalities or obstruction ensures more complete and safe removal of disease.

General or local anesthetics may be chosen according to the same guidelines used for comparable procedures in nonallergic patients. Very often the combination of local anesthetics and vasoconstrictive agents is helpful in tissues hypersensitive to mechanical as well as antigenic stimuli.

Intranasal endoscopy has increased the efficacy of paranasal sinus surgery, allowing complete elimination of disease with decreased morbidity. Antral surgery may also be approached transnasally via the medial wall of the maxillary sinus. A microscope or fiberoptic headlight and magnifying loupes are valuable if endoscopic surgery is not used. Some otolaryngologists still prefer the sublabial Caldwell-Luc approach. Rarely is an external exenteration any longer necessary, but complete removal of the disease is imperative.

Surgery on large, obstructing turbinates was extensively performed 30 years ago, at times resulting in atrophic rhinitis, but finally falling into disfavor. However, if conservative management fails to clear an obstruction, some type of turbinate surgery may be useful.[21–23] If mucosal involvement is predominant, a number of techniques have been recommended, including intraturbinate steroid injection, electrocautery, and

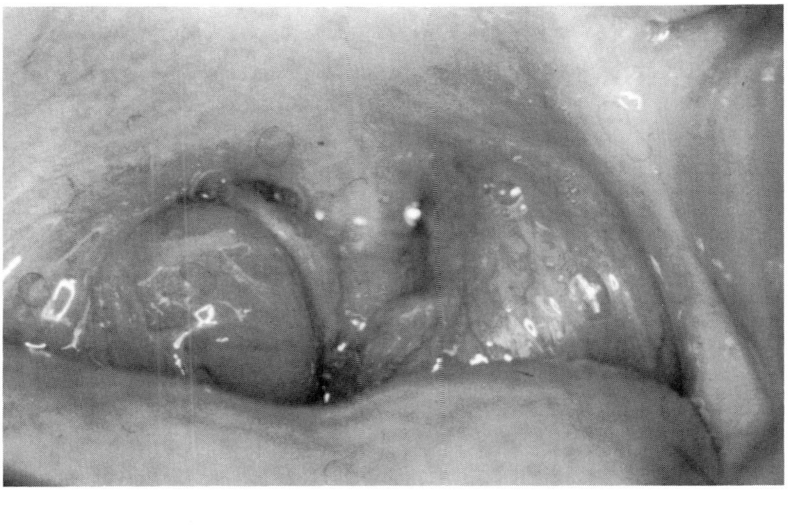

FIGURE 39–5. Massively enlarged, obstructing tonsils.

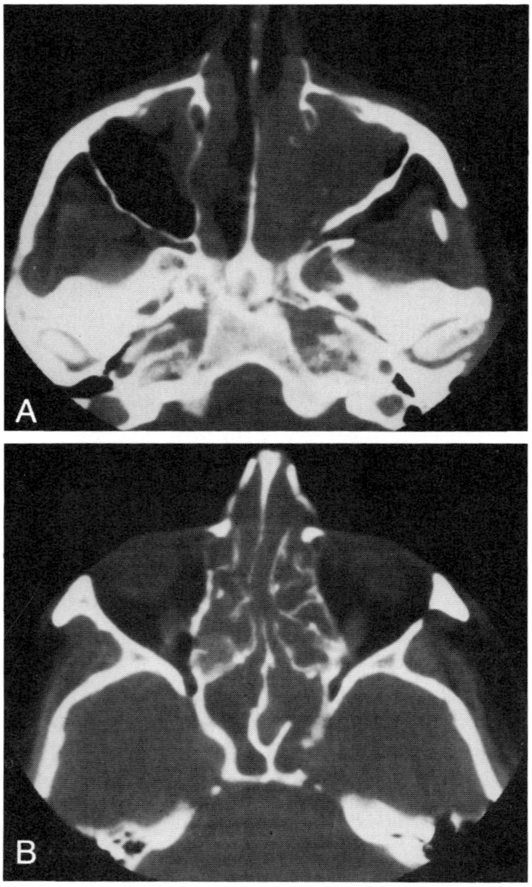

FIGURE 39–6. Sagittal (axial) views of paranasal sinuses with involvement of, *A*, maxillary sinuses and nasal fossa, and *B*, ethmoid and sphenoid sinuses. (Courtesy of S. Pawar, M.D., North Hills Passavant Hospital.)

cryosurgery. Laser surgery, a more recent technique, may be effective but carries special dangers; for instance, if bone is hit, the light flash may be blinding. It is not useful for bony hypertrophy. These procedures result in less obstruction and, often, decreased secretions. However, if the underlying allergic disease is not corrected, the turbinate disease will probably recur. If there is true bony hypertrophy, outfracture may help; but partial turbinectomy or submucous resection of the inferior or middle turbinates may still be necessary. Partial inferior turbinectomy with sinus surgery will leave a functional, unobstructed airway that can be maintained with good nasal hygiene and allergic management.

Vidian neurectomy has been used, especially in India and Japan, to reduce the secretory rhinopathy in allergic rhinitis. It has only infrequently been used in the United States for that purpose.

COMPLICATIONS

A number of complications may occur during or after surgery in allergic patients. We may see "twitchy" mucosa in the nose with excessive and prolonged rhinorrhea and sneezing after stimulation. There may be excessive intraoperative bleeding and edema in the pharynx and especially in the nose, resulting in postoperative bleeding and subsequent thickening and uncontrolled scarring. Healing may be prolonged, with tenderness, discomfort, and sensitivity. This must be particularly kept in mind prior to facial plastic procedures. Adhesions or stenosis may form, and there may be slow resolution of ecchymosis, with tissue staining and hyperplastic or metaplastic tissue changes. Tape sensitivity as well as drug allergies must be considered. Iodine reactions sometimes occur following use of Betadine as a preoperative preparation as well as in intravenous radiographic studies. The possibility of a reaction to suture material must also be anticipated. Research is still needed to identify which allergic patients are at greater risk for such complications.

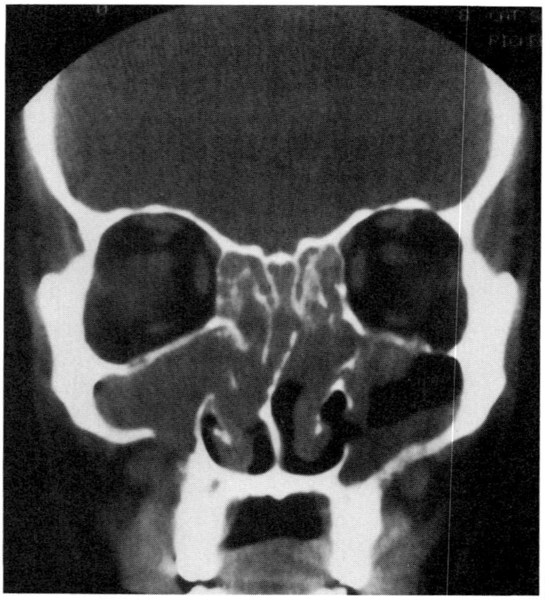

FIGURE 39–7. Coronal view of paranasal sinus with involvement of both maxillary sinuses and ethmoids. (Courtesy of S. Pawar, M.D., North Hills Passavant Hospital.)

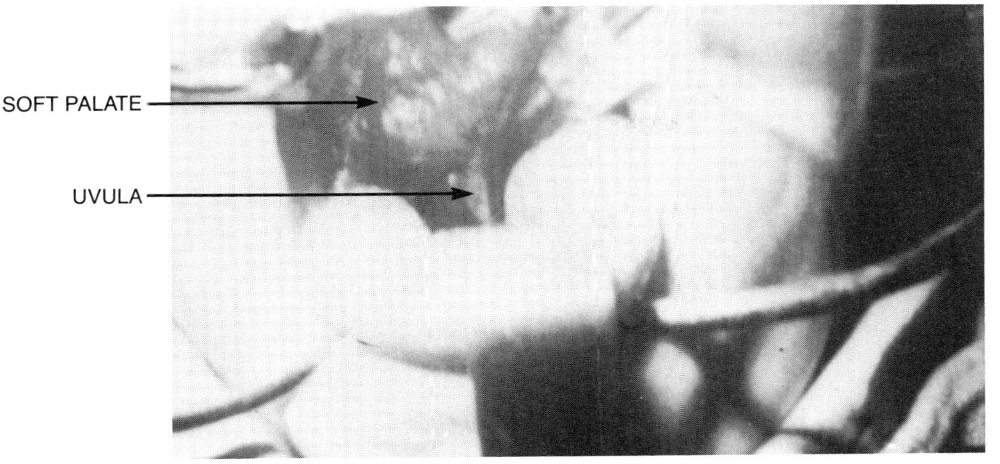

FIGURE 39–8. Markedly edematous palate early in tonsillectomy procedure in highly allergic 8-year-old girl.

A possible complication of adenotonsillectomy in the allergic child is rapidly developing palate and uvula edema during surgical manipulation. Intravenous steroids usually resolve the problem. The 8-year-old child in Figure 39–8 with multiple allergies under good control still developed marked soft palate edema with minimal, gentle manipulation. Ten minutes after intravenous steroid injection, the problem was resolving (Fig. 39–9). We must always be cognizant of the potential effect of allergy on other surgical procedures.

If surgery must be done in allergic patients, especially in emergency situations, medications such as steroids, antibiotics, antihistamines, and decongestants should be used judiciously. Surgical techniques should be done rapidly (although all tissues must be handled gently), preferably under local anesthesia using vasoconstrictors. Nasal packing should be inserted and removed carefully, and dressings should be firm and never hastily removed. Teflon splints may prevent adhesions.

Immunotherapy must be continued after surgery. Because many patients ignore this and neglect the allergy care, they must be reminded that they have a chronic disease.

It is wise to remember that allergy management cannot cure everything, and that surgery cannot cure everything. But the two disciplines often complement one another to a remarkable extent, increasing the chances for cures. For this reason, it is imperative that otolaryngologists become conversant with the symptoms and

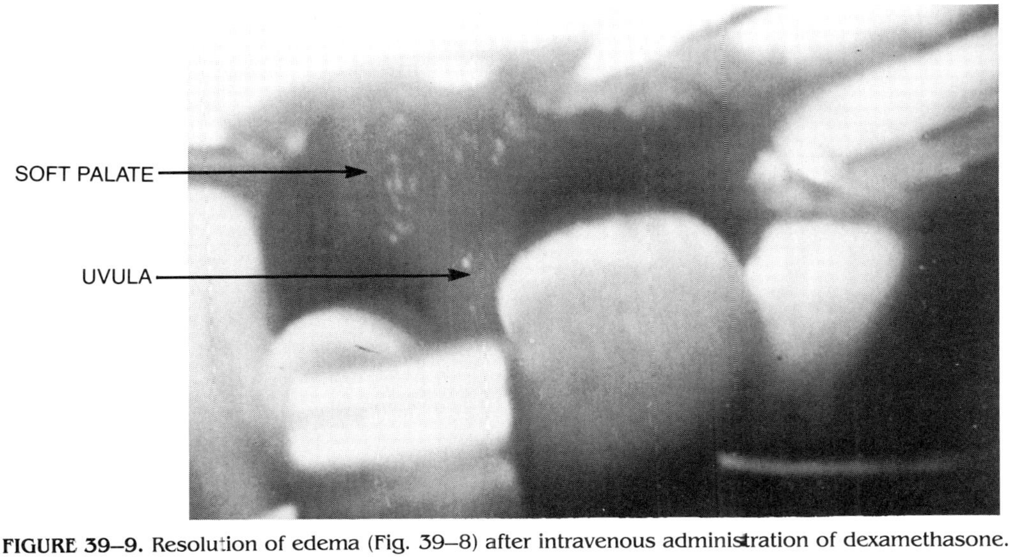

FIGURE 39–9. Resolution of edema (Fig. 39–8) after intravenous administration of dexamethasone.

management of allergic diseases in order to be the most successful surgeons.

REFERENCES

1. Ricketts RM: The interdependence of the nasal and oral capsules. *In* McNamara JA (ed): Naso-Respiratory Function and Craniofacial Growth. Monograph 9, Ann Arbor, University of Michigan, 1979, pp 165–198.
2. Hannuksela A: The effects of moderate and severe atopy on the facial skeleton. Eur J Orthod 2:187, 1981.
3. Rubin RM: The effects of nasal airway obstruction. J Pedodontics 78:504, 1983.
4. Ramadan MF: Effect of experimental nasal obstruction on growth of alveolar arch. Arch Otolaryngol 110:568, 1984.
5. Tankel JW, Cheesman AD: Symptom relief by adenoidentomy and relationship to adenoid and post-nasal airway size. J Laryngol Otol 100:637, 1986.
6. Subelny JD: Workshop on tonsillectomy and adenoidectomy. Ann Otol Rhinol Laryngol 84[Suppl 19]:250, 1974.
7. McNamara JA: Factors affecting the growth of the midface. *In* McNamara JA (ed): Naso-Respiratory Function and Craniofacial Growth. Monograph 6. Ann Arbor, University of Michigan, 1976.
8. Marks MD: Stigmata of Respiratory Tract Allergies. Kalamazoo, MI, Scope Publications, 1976.
9. Shapiro G, Shapiro P: Nasal airway obstruction and facial development. Clin Rev Allergy 2:225, 1984.
10. Warren DW: A quantitative technique for assessing nasal airway impairment. Am J Orthod 86:306, 1984.
11. Principato JJ, Kerrigan JP, Wolf P: Pediatric nasal resistance and lower anterior vertical face height. Otolaryngol Head Neck Surg 95:226, 1986.
12. Krause HF: Upper airway obstruction as a cause of dental and facial deformities. Primary ENT 3:2, 1987.
13. English GM: Nasal polyposis. *In* Otolaryngology. Philadelphia, Harper & Row, 1983.
14. Friedman WH, Katsantonis GP, Rosenblum BN, et al: Sphenoethmoidectomy: the case for ethmoid marsupialization. Laryngoscope 96:473, 1986.
15. Dixon HS: Microscopic sinus surgery, transnasal ethmoidectomy and sphenoidectomy. Laryngoscope 93:440, 1983.
16. Friedman WH, Katsantonis GP, Slavin RG, et al: Sphenoethmoidectomy: its role in the asthma patient. Otolaryngol Head Neck Surg 90:171, 1982.
17. Jordan RE: Deafness due to allergy. Laryngoscope 60:152, 1950.
18. Jordan RE: Role of allergy in otology. Arch Otolaryngol 55:363, 1952.
19. Shambaugh G Jr: Serous otitis media: are tubes the answer? Am J Otol 7:63, 1983.
20. Bernstein JM: The possible role of food "sensitivity" in the otitis-prone child. Manuscript presented at the American Academy of Otolaryngology—Head and Neck Symposium, Chicago, September 1987.
21. Fanous N: Anterior turbinectomy—new surgical approach to turbinate hypertrophy: a review of 220 cases. Arch Otolaryngol Head Neck Surg 112:850, 1986.
22. Fukutake T, Yamashita T, Tomoda K, Kumazawa T: Laser surgery for allergic rhinitis. Arch Otolaryngol Head Neck Surg 112:1280, 1986.
23. Ophiar D, Gross-Isseroff R, Lancet D, Marshah G: Changes in olfactory acuity induced by total inferior turbinectomy. Arch Otolaryngol Head Neck Surg 112:195, 1986.

CHAPTER 40

Aspirin, Rhinosinusitis, and Asthma

Helen F. Krause, M.D., F.A.C.S.

Aspirin sensitivity participates in a disease syndrome that appears to be neither allergenic nor immunologic in causation. It is so essentially interwoven with the practice of otolaryngology and otolaryngic allergy that we should be familiar with the current state of knowledge. The syndrome was described originally as a triad of chronic, progressive rhinosinusitis usually with nasal polyps, intrinsic asthma, and significant sensitivity to aspirin and certain other drugs.[1, 2] At times, in the natural history of the disease there may not be a clear-cut description of such an aspirin sensitivity. Also, in any individual, all three expressions may not be clinically apparent at the same time. The rhinosinusitis is often interminably progressive, despite careful avoidance of aspirin and other related drugs.

The pharmacopeia of antiquity suggests that willow bark teas and poltices were basic analgesics and antipyretics. These were used by the very earliest medicine men and women and down through the ages to the present time. Willow extracts are currently offered for sale in health food stores. Naturally occurring salicylates were extensively used until acetylsalicylic acid was developed in 1853, in Germany, by Gebhardt. Aspirin as we recognize it today was formulated by the Bayer Company in Germany, which began to produce it commercially in 1899. Reports of reactions followed very soon, as early as 1902. Reactions to preparations probably due to willow use itself date from ancient history to the present medical literature.

Abnormal responses to aspirin have been called allergy,[2] sensitivity,[3] intolerance,[4–7] and idiosyncrasy.[8, 9] This reflects the mystery of the mechanism that produces the abnormal reaction. Other drugs and chemicals have been recognized as causing the same patterns of disease as aspirin in susceptible individuals, especially many of the nonsteroidal anti-inflammatory drugs listed in Table 40–1.[3, 9, 10] Certain dyes, especially FD&C yellow No. 5 (tartrazine), and possibly some red dyes may also produce such reactions.[11–19] A few other drugs have been implicated that show variable results when challenged (Table 40–1).

Aspirin-related disease has been described not as a single entity but as several clinical syndromes. The pattern of nasal polyposis, asthma, and aspirin sensitivity was first described as a conglomerate of symptoms in 1937 by Drs. Prickman and Bucksten in the United States, and even earlier, in the 1920s, in the French literature. However, it was left to Drs. Samter and Beers in 1967 and 1968 to bring the triad to attention as a significant clinical entity. They also suggested that the aspirin sensitivity phase might be delayed, and that even without aspirin ingestion, the syndrome once started persists and the disease progresses. This description has proved to be accurate with later observations. In addition, occasionally the asthma does not become evident until after the other symptoms have been long recognized.

Samter described the asthma as "different"

Table 40–1. INCIDENCE OF "CROSS-SENSITIVITY" TO CHEMICALS

Chemical	Incidence
Nonsteroidal anti-inflammatory agents	
Indomethacin, naproxen, tolmetin, ibuprofen, mefenamic acid, sulindac, zomepirac, phenylbutazone	50–100%
Benoxaprofen	0%
Other drugs	
Sodium salicylate	rare
Acetaminophen	rare
Food dyes and preservatives	
Tartrazine	10%
Other azo and non-azo dyes	rare
Sodium benzoate, parabens	rare

After Lumry, Curd, and Stevenson.[49]

from other severe asthmas. It responded well to bronchodilators and was extremely sensitive to corticosteroids. He also described angioedema and urticaria associated with aspirin sensitivity, but later felt that this was a separate syndrome. Mathison and Stevenson[3] and others redefined this disease as two often interrelated syndromes stimulated by challenge testing to aspirin, one "naso-ocular" and the other "bronchospastic." The elements may appear concurrently or alone. In addition, they and others described urticaria and/or angioedema as another syndrome related to aspirin and certain drug sensitivities.[3, 9, 11, 20–23] The respiratory and cutaneous expressions rarely occur in the same patient.

The typical development of the respiratory syndrome (Table 40–2) is at first an intermittent rhinitis evidenced by a profuse, watery rhinorrhea, often sudden, without warning and most embarrassing, sometimes resembling a type of vasomotor rhinitis. The rhinorrhea usually persists and is followed by a gradual onset of nasal obstruction. The obstruction is also intermittent at first, responding well to decongestants. Often these symptoms are thought to be allergic rhinitis, and many patients undergo allergy testing; occasionally it is positive.[24] Symptoms become more persistent and less responsive to local vasoconstrictors and oral decongestants. Nasal polyps usually then develop along with hyperplastic rhinitis, followed by progressive hyperplastic sinus disease and very often secondary infection. In most cases there is bilateral involvement and usually frustrating progression even in the absence of aspirin, NSAIDs, or tartrazine, and even despite restriction of the naturally occurring salicylates in the diet. Simple nasal polypectomy is usually a failure, with the polyps recurring very quickly—within days or weeks.

Table 40–2. DEVELOPMENTAL PATTERNS OF ASPIRIN SENSITIVITY

Nasal symptoms and pathologic changes
Rhinorrhea—intermittent
Congestion—intermittent, then persistent
Polyp development
Paranasal sinus involvement
Pulmonary symptoms
Bronchoconstriction
Urticaria-angioedema
Shock

The asthma may appear concurrently with or occasionally prior to the rhinosinusitis, but the more common pattern described is the later development of the bronchospastic component. In a patient with rhinosinusitis even with a negative pulmonary history, baseline pulmonary function tests should be obtained, especially if surgery is contemplated. The response to aspirin ingestion may be dose-related and may be variable. Symptoms may be overwhelming, or at times not remarkable. And finally, in some patients after a number of years, the disease may appear to slow or stop its progression as mysteriously as it started.

The usual patient may be of either sex, in the mid years, often with a history of symptoms starting in the 20s or 30s. Its occurrence in childhood has been reported in studies by Rachelefsky[25] and Tan and Collins-Williams,[26] but is far less frequent. There are also reports by Lockey[5] and Delaney[27] and others of familial occurrence. The author recently has seen three patients with strong family histories. Some patients do have atopic histories, as mentioned before; others have only the history of aspirin sensitivity. Reports of atopy by skin or in vitro testing indicate that the frequency is extremely variable and there are indications that atopy, especially allergic rhinitis, may have been present early in the medical history, but is no longer active when tested. In an ongoing research project, the author is reviewing a large number of patients with documented or presumptive aspirin sensitivity, many with asthma, for the history of allergy, active or past, and other parameters. Polyps, pathologically, cannot be differentiated from those of allergic rhinitis, or from others for that matter, even with electron microscopy studies.[28, 29]

CLINICAL PRESENTATION

In a clinical practice, patients most often present with nasal, ocular, and/or pulmonary symptoms. Sometimes the history is diagnostic of an aspirin reaction, but it is often negative. The patient usually describes a facial flush, especially macular in location, the rhinorrhea (mentioned before), and nasal congestion. Cough and anosmia are very prominent symptoms. Loss of smell is almost constant, improving usually with steroid treatment, but recurring very quickly. If there is bronchospasm or asthma, we see recurrent wheezing and shortness of breath. There may be other associated symptoms to consider. A 1983 study proved proctocolitis was associated with the classic triad by challenge testing.[30] Hillerdal and Lindholm describe an adverse response in the larynx.[31]

The nasal examination often shows the mucosa to be bluish, thickened, and boggy with obstructive edema; the mucus may be profuse and watery or very tenacious and thick. If infection is present, it will be mucopurulent. Polyps are often present, but may not be seen early in the disease. They are usually multiple and may be flattened and discolored by the pressure of other polyps or the turbinates. If they have been present for a long period, there may be bony changes with widening of the nasal dorsum and even bone destruction (Fig. 40–1).

Laboratory studies may reveal elevation of the eosinophils in the serum and in nasal secretions as seen on a cytogram. Sinus radiographs and CT scans may demonstrate thickened mucous membranes, polypoid changes, complete opacification, or an air-fluid level if infection is present, all dependent on the duration of the disease (Figs. 40–2 and 40–3). The glucose tolerance test may be abnormal for some undetermined reason. The bleeding time may be prolonged to twice normal, especially in patients who have received recent aspirin. Total IgE by PRIST is usually normal or low. Allergy testing should be done if the history warrants. In vitro tests with proper control are often necessary

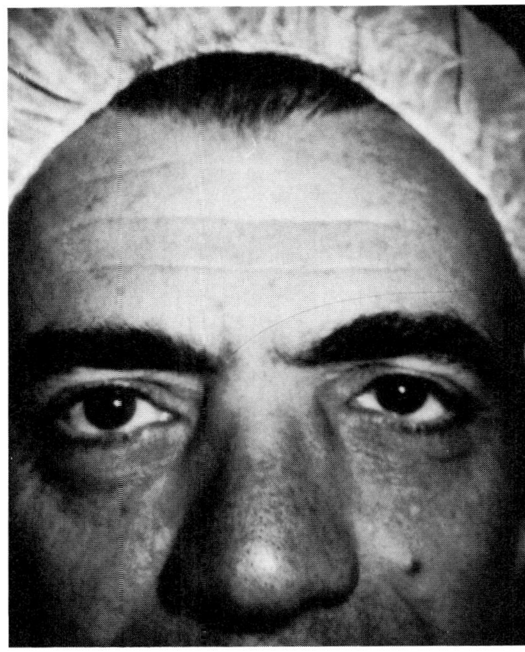

FIGURE 40–1. Destruction of the lateral (nasal) processes of the maxilla and widening of the dorsum in a 47-year-old man with a seven-year history of rhinosinusitis, nasal polyps, asthma, and reactions to asthma.

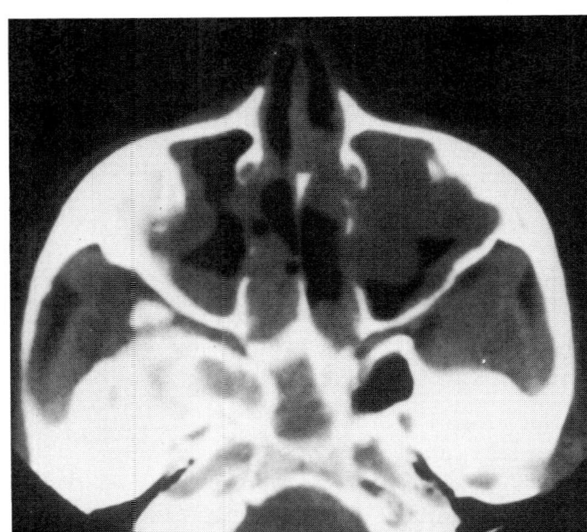

FIGURE 40–2. Sagittal view of CT scan with involvement of both maxillary antra, extending into the nasal fossae, in a 37-year-old woman with known aspirin sensitivity.

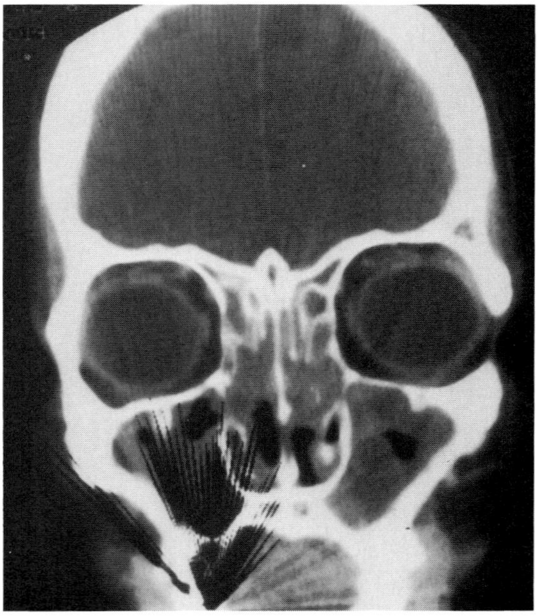

FIGURE 40–3. Coronal view (of Figure 40–3) illustrating involvement of the ethmoid and maxillary sinuses.

because the long-term use of drugs to control the respiratory symptoms negates the use of reliable skin tests. If positive, the patient should be appropriately treated with immunotherapy because this is a concurrent disease.

At times, clinical patterns—especially with thick, tenacious secretions and polyps—resemble cystic fibrosis, suggesting a possible associative defect. In 1983, sweat chlorides were studied by iontophoresis in 12 patients with aspirin sensitivity selected at random in my office. All were within normal range. Ciliary function evaluated by Lewis et al.[32] because of similarities to ciliary dyskinesis were reported to be normal.

Pulmonary function studies are important, even in patients without overt asthma. Examination will reveal the presence or absence of wheezing. Spirometry values for forced vital capacity (FVC) and forced expiratory volume in one second (FEV_1) should be obtained as baseline values. Bronchodilator challenge provides a measure of pulmonary function responsiveness, and methacholine inhalation challenge will give predictive values of the bronchospastic response.

In 1982, Lumry and his group in Texas studied patients with perennial nasal symptoms including congestion and anosmia. Most had rhinorrhea, and 15 out of 19 had nasal polyps.[20] Often there was a history of multiple polypectomies and even of multiple surgery consisting of antrostomies, Caldwell-Luc procedures, and intranasal ethmoidectomies and sphenoidectomies. Importantly, they described distinct subgroups of patients with aspirin sensitive respiratory disease who have nonallergic eosinophilic hypertrophic rhinosinusitis with asthma. This might make one suspect that the category of nonallergic eosinophilic nasal and pulmonary diseases may be very early aspirin sensitivity syndromes, this being an unusual expression of it. Certainly more investigation is required.

PATHOPHYSIOLOGY

The pathogenesis of aspirin sensitivity is still unclear and controversial. It is known to be non–IgE-mediated and it does not appear to be any other immunologic phenomenon. The present theory is that of a metabolic defect.[33–37] In 1983, Drs. Vane, Samuelsson, and Bergstrom jointly won the Nobel Prize in Medicine and Physiology for their studies of the arachidonic acid metabolism. Dr. Vane studied the cyclo-oxygenase pathway with its generation of prostaglandins and thromboxanes and the relation to aspirin ingestion.[35, 36] A metabolic product of this pathway, PGE_2, is a bronchodilator. PGF_2 alpha and PGF_2 appear to be bronchoconstrictors. Bergstrom and Samuelsson described the lipo-oxygenase pathway and identified leukotrienes C_4, D_4, and E_4 as the chemical mediator we have known to be the slow reacting substance of anaphylaxis (SRS–A). These act as bronchoconstrictors. Aspirin and the nonsteroidal anti-inflammatory drugs block the cyclo-oxygenase pathway (Fig. 40–4). The first nonsteroidal anti-inflammatory drug (NSAID) that did not block this pathway but predominantly inhibited the lipo-oxygenase pathway, and therefore was recommended as a substitute for patients with arthritis, was benoxaprofen (Oraflex). However, it is now off the market because of toxic liver effects. Some of the more recently developed NSAIDs do not appear to cause problems in aspirin sensitive patients. Other inhibitors of the lipo-oxygenase pathway, specific leukotriene blockers, have been explored. They do not appear to inhibit the progression of the disease.

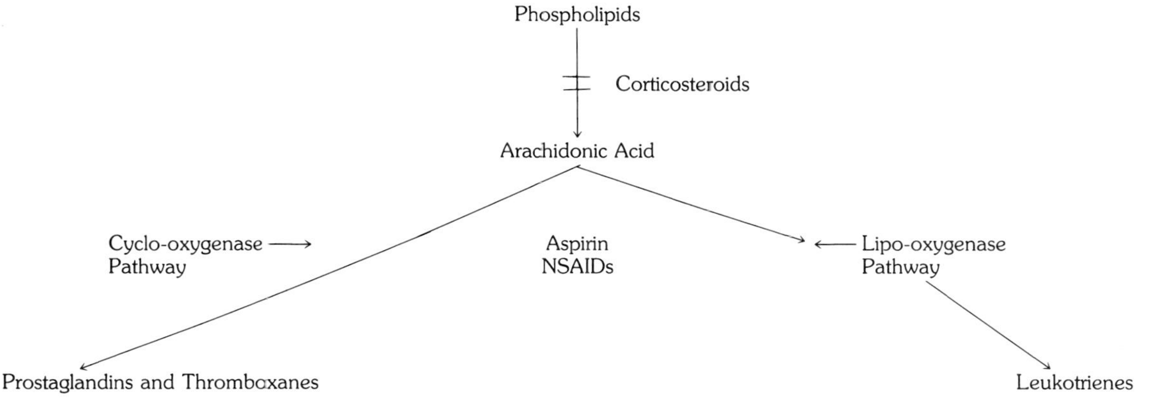

FIGURE 40–4. Arachidonic acid metabolism: blocking by corticosteroids and aspirin and nonsteroidal anti-inflammatory drugs (NSAIDs).

Tartrazine does not block the cyclo-oxygenase pathway. In the gastrointestinal tract it undergoes reduction cleavage, and in humans it appears to be completely excreted as sulfanilic acid within 48 hours. Tartrazine sensitivity has been found in some patients with aspirin sensitivity, but the mechanism is entirely unclear. Some studies have found no cross-reactivity of tartrazine with aspirin. Others indicate 8 to 15 per cent tartrazine sensitivity in proven aspirin sensitive patients.[9, 13–19, 21]

CHALLENGE AND DESENSITIZATION

The definitive diagnosis of aspirin sensitivity is by an oral challenge. All techniques are similar and require hospitalization with pulmonary function facilities and special monitoring with treatment of reactions as they occur. Stevenson, Mathison, and colleagues at the Scripps Institute in California have produced one of the most efficient tests, although others have been reported.[3, 12, 38] It may be done in about 10 hours on one day, but is safer done over 48 hours to prevent the accumulative effects of each dose. Placebo tests are done initially, and response to oral challenges are recorded. Zeiss and Lockey[39] reported in 1976 that the response to aspirin at the time of the challenge established only the presence or absence of aspirin sensitivity at that specific time. They felt it was dose-related and that patients do show a variability with repeated tests.

Four types of response to a challenge test are seen:[12] (1) a positive asthmatic response with a decline of the FEV_1 more than 25 per cent from baseline; (2) a positive naso-ocular response, especially of congestion and rhinorrhea; (3) a classic response of both asthmatic and naso-ocular symptoms; and (4) a negative response entirely. Pretreatment with antihistamines and sympathomimetic drugs and cromolyn may blunt the pulmonary challenge response, so they are withheld for 24 hours prior to the challenge. If the patient is on treatment for asthma with corticosteroids and theophylline, they are allowed to be continued. The asthma must be stabilized, under good control in a state of remission, before the challenge testing is started. Since corticosteroids inhibit both pathways of arachidonic acid metabolism and substantially improve the status of the asthma and rhinosinusitis, one wonders why the challenge test does not show interference in its presence.

Zeiss, Lockey, and others[39–43] have described a refractory period from two to seven days after challenge, during which time aspirin ingestion will not provoke symptoms. This led Stevenson and others to study the effects of continuing aspirin intake after achieving this tolerance state by such a challenge/desensitization program. They found initially that no asthma symptoms will occur in most patients who continue daily aspirin doses of 500 to 650 mg a day. Desensitization with NSAIDs has also been accomplished, and there is indeed a cross-reactivity of desensitization as well. A patient may be switched from aspirin to a comparable NSAID with no problem.

Stevenson et al.[44] studied the effect of desensitization on the rhinosinusitis. It appears that desensitization improves upper airway symptoms more than those of the lower airway. The improvement was subjective—by patient symptom scores and by the ability to reduce the prednisone and beclomethasone dosages. It indicated that congestion and sense of smell did improve, just as with steroid therapy. Eighty per cent (20 patients) had nasal polyps and 72 per cent (18 patients) had some previous nasal or sinus surgery. In the author's experience, the patient's symptoms in relation to the intranasal examination do not always correlate, and symptom scores would be less valid than a thorough otolaryngologic examination and computed tomography. Stevenson does state that "any explanations for benefit from ASA treatment in these ASA-desensitized patients are only speculative. . . . Perhaps a decrease in nasal congestion and a return of sense of smell are end-organ effects of ASA as an anti-inflammatory drug . . . or some additional effects on arachidonic acid metabolism." Purulent sinusitis may have been present in some of these patients. Five patients in Stevenson's study became worse in the treatment phase. Some patients undergoing daily aspirin treatment after desensitization have side effects of gastrointestinal symptoms or increase in asthma, necessitating cessation of the treatment. Nasal eosinophilia does not change during desensitization.

It appears that the interminably unrelenting disease that progresses in patients with rhinosinusitis might be slowed or halted by appropriate and extensive exenteration of the disease locally followed by desensitization and daily aspirin treatment. There are still many unanswered questions, such as how long it is necessary to stay on the aspirin after desensitization. It now appears that some patients gradually lose the benefits, and steroid doses must be increased.

MEDICAL MANAGEMENT

If infection is present, there must be extensive antibiotic treatment, possibly for months by sensitivity studies. If the intranasal polyps are massive, they may be reduced by an oral steroid burst, or with intranasal polyp injection. Occasionally, conservatively, an initial polypectomy is necessary just to allow the remaining polyps to be injected. Polyps are injected every six to eight weeks over a three- to four-month period utilizing 4 to 8 mg of Decadron-LA each time. Every patient reacts in a very individual manner. Some respond within days, others very slowly. Your author prefers Decadron-LA because it is long-acting, the size of the particles are the smallest, and the solution is thin compared with other injectable steroids available. No reactions to this preparation have been reported. A #23 1½-inch needle on a tuberculin or allergy syringe is very comfortable to use. A simple nasal polypectomy, as stated, is rarely of any long-term value in extensive rhinosinusitis.

In these cases, medically and surgically managed, aspirin and nonsteroidal anti-inflammatory drug avoidance is imperative. Probably tartrazine also should be avoided even though the rate of cross-reactivity appears to be low. Possibly, in severe cases, dietary management by a salicylate-free diet may be useful. Some patients respond well to such a diet. A few general allergists condemn the use of dietary restrictions; but patients who feel this helps, when nothing else has, refuse to change. A recent study in Switzerland indicated that a diet free of additives and nonsteroidal anti-inflammatory drugs resulted within five days in a marked improvement of symptoms that persisted eight to 14 months after the diet was started.[45] This may open an entirely new path of investigation.

Years ago, it was widely held that sinus surgery and even nasal polypectomy would precipitate asthma.[46] Now, understanding the natural course of this disease with the frequent late appearance of asthma and also with the improvement in anesthetics and antibiotics, this theory is no longer held. The clinical effect of surgery in known aspirin sensitivity patients has demonstrated that by removing the infection and clearing the upper airways surgically, all aspects of the disease improved, at least temporarily, and asthma was not precipitated.[47–49] If asthma was present, it often improved. This has very much been the author's experience. As a precaution, the pulmonary status should always be evaluated preoperatively and any active pulmonary disease treated before surgery.

If the infection cannot be controlled because of the obstruction, or conservative management is a failure, then comprehensive nasal and sinus surgery is indicated. Endoscopic surgery improves the control and extent of surgical management. The nasal polyps may return and must be anticipated. It is common in my practice to see a patient who has had three to 10 surgical procedures prior to being referred to me. One has had 32 operative procedures in seven years (Fig. 40–1).

Recently aspirin and other salicylate products have been implicated in pulmonary edema and even possibly in the adult respiratory distress syndrome (ARDS). These may be related to salicylate intoxication rather than an idiosyncrasy. The pathways, however, appear to be related also to arachidonic acid metabolism, with the blocking of the enzyme cyclo-oxygenase and prevention of the formation of thromboxanes and prostacyclin, and thereafter the prostaglandins. Heffner and Sahn[50] at the University of South Carolina suggest that prostacyclin may have membrane protective effects and that its absence leads to pathologic changes. In addition, if the metabolism stimulates the lipo-oxygenase pathway resulting in excess leukotriene production, these agents may increase membrane permeability leading to pulmonary edema and, I suggest, perhaps in the nose to mucosal edema and polyp formation.

In summary, it has been shown that the syndrome in the aspirin sensitivity patient

1. Is not IgE-mediated;
2. Is not related to complement activity; and
3. Cross-reacts with most NSAIDs.
4. The greater the drug inhibition of the prostaglandin synthetase, the greater its cross-reactivity with aspirin.

SUMMARY

Care of the aspirin sensitive patient is often a prolonged, frustrating experience for the clinician and the patient. With continuing basic and clinical research, the definitive etiology for aspirin sensitivity in all its ramifications may soon be proved. In the meantime, we must learn how to gain the best patient compliance and tolerance to the disease and continue our care.

REFERENCES

1. Samter M, Beers RF: Intolerance to aspirin. Ann Intern Med 68:975, 1968.
2. Speer F, Denison TR, Baptist JE: Aspirin allergy. Ann Allergy 46:123, 1981.
3. Mathison DA, Stevenson DD: Aspirin sensitivity in rhinosinusitis and asthma. Immunol Allergy Pract 5:340, 1983.
4. Taub SJ: Aspirin intolerance. EENT Monthly 49:53, 1970.
5. Lockey RF, Rucknagel DL, Vanselow NA: Familiar occurrence of asthma, nasal polyps and aspirin intolerance. Ann Intern Med 78:57, 1973.
6. Chafee FH, Settipane GA: Aspirin intolerance: I. Frequency in an allergic population. J Allergy Clin Immunol 53:193, 1974.
7. Settipane GA, Chafee FH, Klein DE: Aspirin intolerance: II. A prospective study in an atopic and normal population. J Allergy Clin Immunol 53:200, 1974.
8. Spector SL, Wangaard CH, Farr RS: Aspirin and concomitant idiosyncrasies in adult asthmatic patients. J Allergy Clin Immunol 64:500, 1979.
9. Spector SL, Farr RS: Aspirin idiosyncrasy: asthma and urticaria. *In* Middleton E, Reed LE, Ellis EF (eds): Allergy Principles and Practice. St Louis, CV Mosby, 1983, pp 1249–1273.
10. Szczeklik A, Gryglewski RJ, Czerniawska-Mysik G: Clinical patterns of hypersensitivity to nonsteroidal anti-inflammatory drugs and their pathogenesis. J Allergy Clin Immunol 60:276, 1977.
11. Szczeklik A, Gryglewski RJ, Czerniawska-Mysik G: Aspirin sensitivity: other drugs (letter to the editor). Ann Intern Med 82:286, 1975.
12. Mathison DA, Stevenson DD, Simon RA: Precipitating factors in asthma: aspirin, sulfites and other drugs and chemicals. Chest 87 [Suppl]:50S, 1985.
13. Chafee FH, Settipane GA: Asthma caused by FD&C approved drugs. J Allergy 40:65, 1967.
14. Settipane GA, Pudupakkam RK: Aspirin intolerance: III. Subtypes, familial occurrence and cross reactivity with tartrazine. J Allergy Clin Immunol 56:215, 1975.
15. Gerber JG, Payne NA, et al: Tartrazine and the prostaglandin system. J Allergy Clin Immunol 63:289, 1979.
16. Smith LJ, Slavin RG: Drugs containing tartrazine dye. J Allergy Clin Immunol 58:456, 1976.
17. Weber RW, Hoffman M, et al: Incidence of bronchoconstriction due to aspirin, azo dyes, nonazo dyes, and preservatives in a population of perennial asthmatics. J Allergy Clin Immunol 64:32, 1979.
18. Tse CST: Food products containing tartrazine (letter to the editor). N Engl J Med 306:681, 1982.
19. Hedman SE, Anderson RGG: Release of biological mediators by tartrazine from human leukocytes and polyps. Acta Pharmacol Toxicol 52:153, 1983.
20. Lumry WR, Curd JG, Zeiger RS: Aspirin sensitive rhinosinusitis: the clinical syndrome and effects of aspirin administration. J Allergy Clin Immunol 71:580, 1983.
21. Michel O, Naeige N, et al: Decreased sensitivity to tartrazine after aspirin desensitization in an asthmatic patient intolerant to both aspirin and tartrazine. Ann Allergy 52:368, 1984.
22. Jublin L, Michaëlsson G, Zetterström, O: Urticaria and asthma induced by food and drug additives in patients with aspirin sensitivity. J Allergy Clin Immunol 50:92, 1972.
23. Settipane GA: Aspirin and allergic diseases: a review. Am J Med 14:102, 1983.

24. English GM: Nasal polyposis. *In* Otolaryngology. Philadelphia, Harper & Row, 1983.
25. Rachelefsky GS, Coulson A, et al: Aspirin intolerance in chronic childhood asthma: detected by oral challenge. Pediatrics 56:443, 1975.
26. Tan Y, Collins-Williams C: Aspirin induced asthma in children. Ann Allergy 48:1, 1982.
27. Delaney JC: Asthma, nasal polyposis, and aspirin sensitivity (letter to the editor). Ann Intern Med 79:761, 1973.
28. Whiteside TL, Rabin BS, et al: The presence of IgE on the surface of lymphocytes in nasal polyps. J Allergy Clin Immunol 55:186, 1975.
29. Cunnette SL, Hall MM, et al: Microbiologic analysis of nasal polyp tissue. J Allergy Clin Immunol 78:102, 1986.
30. Pearon DJ, Stones NA, et al: Proctocolitis induced by salicylate and associated with asthma and recurrent nasal polyps. Br Med J 287:1675, 1983.
31. Hillerdal G, Lindholm H: Laryngeal edema as the only symptom of hypersensitivity to salicylic acid and other substances. J Laryngol Otol 98:547, 1984.
32. Lewis FH, Beals TF, et al: Ultrastructural and functional studies of cilia from patients with asthma, aspirin intolerance, and nasal polyps. Chest 63:487, 1983.
33. Szczeklik A, Gryglewski RJ, Czerniawska-Mysik G: Relationship of inhibition of prostaglandin biosynthesis by analgesics to asthma attacks in aspirin sensitive patients. Br Med J 11:67, 1975.
34. Casale TB, Kaliner M: Pathophysiology of asthma. ENT J 63:66, 1984.
35. Vane JR: Inhibition of prostaglandin synthesis as a mechanism of action for aspirin-like drugs. Nature New Biology 231:232, 1971.
36. Vane JR: The mode of action of aspirin and similar compounds. J Allergy Clin Immunol 58:691, 1976.
37. Samuelsson B: Oxygenation and further transformation of polyunsaturated fatty acids. Proceedings of the Fourth International Prostaglandin Conference. Washington, DC, 1979.
38. Stevenson DD, Simon RA, Mathison DA: Aspirin sensitive asthma: tolerance to aspirin after oral aspirin challenge. J Allergy Clin Immunol 66:82, 1980.
39. Zeiss CR, Lockey RF: Refractory period to aspirin in a patient with aspirin induced asthma. J Allergy Clin Immunol 57:440, 1976.
40. Szczeklik A: Aspirin and asthma. Eur J Resp Dis 63:376, 1982.
41. Pleskow WW, Stevenson DD: Aspirin desensitization in aspirin sensitive asthmatic patients: clinical manifestations and characterization of the refractory period. J Allergy Clin Immunol 69:11, 1982.
42. Chiu JT: Aspirin sensitive asthma. Immunol and Allergy Pract 5:389, 1983.
43. Sebastiano B, Mariella R, Guiseppe P: Treatment of aspirin idiosyncrasy (letter to the editor). J Allergy Clin Immunol 70:222, 1982.
44. Stevenson DD, Pleskow WW, et al: Aspirin sensitive rhinosinusitis asthma: a double blind crossover study of treatment with aspirin. J Allergy Clin Immunol 73:500, 1984.
45. Genton C, Frei PC, Pecound A: Value of oral provocation tests to aspirin and food additives in the routine investigation of asthma and chronic urticaria. J Allergy Clin Immunol 76:40, 1985.
46. Francis C: The prognosis of operation for removal of nasal polyps in cases of asthma. Practitioner 123:272, 1929.
47. Maloney JR: Nasal polyps, nasal polypectomy, asthma, and aspirin sensitivity. J Laryngol Otol 51:183, 1980.
48. Friedman WH, Katsantonis GP, et al: Sphenoethmoidectomy: the case for ethmoid marsupialization. Laryngoscope 96:473, 1986.
49. Lumry WR, Curd JG, Stevenson DD: Aspirin sensitive asthma and rhinosinusitis: current concepts and recent advances. ENT J 63:102, 1984.
50. Heffner JE, Sahn SA: Occult respiratory failure? Look for salicylate toxicity. J Resp Dis Jan:25, 1986.

Additional Suggested References

Research continues worldwide and published articles proliferate in an attempt to clarify the mechanism of and devise better clinical approaches for the aspirin sensitivity syndrome.

Asad SI, Kemeny DM, et al: Effect of aspirin in "aspirin sensitive" patients. Br Med J 288:745, 1984.

Bonne C, Moneret-Vautrim DA, et al: Arachidonic acid metabolism and inhibition of cyclooxygenase in platelets from asthmatic subjects with aspirin intolerance. Ann Allergy 54:158, 1985.

Cant AJ, Gibson P: Food hypersensitivity made life threatening by ingestion of aspirin. Br Med J 288:756, 1984.

Collins-Williams C: Clinical spectrum of adverse reactions to tartrazine. J Asthma 22:139, 1985.

Dor PJ, Vervloet D, et al: Aspirin intolerance and asthma induction of a tolerance and long term monitoring. Clin Allergy 15:37, 1985.

English GM: Nasal polypectomy and sinus surgery in patients with asthma and aspirin idiosyncrasies. Laryngoscope 96:374, 1986.

English GM, Spector S, et al: Histopathology and immunofluorescent immunoglobulins in asthmatics with aspirin idiosyncrasy. Arch Otolaryngol Head Neck Surg 113:377, 1987.

Kowalski ML, Grzelewsha-Pzymowska, et al: Fibrinolysis, blood coagulation and platelet function during aspirin induced bronchoconstriction in aspirin intolerant asthmatics. Ann Allergy 58:367, 1987.

McDonald TJ: Nasal disorders in children: allergic rhinitis, vasomotor rhinitis, and nasal polyps. Postgrad Med 81:65, 1987.

Morales MC, Basomba A, et al: Challenge tests with tartrazine in patients with asthma associated with intolerance to analgesics (ASA triad). Clin Allergy 15:55, 1985.

Nigam S, Kunke G, et al: Nasal polyps and their content of arachidonic acid metabolites. N Engl Regional Allergy Proc 7:109, 1986.

Settipane GA: Asthma, aspirin intolerance and nasal polyps. N Engl Regional Allergy Proc 7:32, 1986.

Settipane GA, Lapey A, Klein DE: Asthma, polyps and aspirin intolerance beginning in childhood. N Engl Regional Allergy Proc 7:2:122, 1986.

Slepian IK, Mathews KP, McLean JA: Aspirin sensitive asthma (review). Chest 87:386, 1985.

Stevenson DD: Diagnosis, prevention and treatment of adverse reactions to aspirin and non-steroidal anti-inflammatory drugs. J Allergy Clin Immunol 74:617, 1984.

Stevenson DD: Aspirin desensitization. N Engl Regional Allergy Proc 76:101, 1986.

Szmidt M, Grzelewska-Rzymowska, et al: Tolerance to acetylsalicylic acid (ASA) induced in ASA sensitive asthmatics does not depend on initial adverse reaction. Allergy 42:182, 1987.

Zeitz HJ, Garmoszuk I: Nasal polyps, bronchial asthma, and aspirin sensitivity: the Samter syndrome. Compr Ther 11:21, 1985.

CHAPTER 41

Management of Allergic Emergencies

Richard L. Mabry, M.D.

It is unfortunate that many physicians tend to treat a discussion of the management of allergic emergencies with the same cavalier attitude accorded to the emergency instructions recited by flight attendants before a plane trip—ignore it and hope the situation will not arise. However, although the likelihood of either set of instructions being needed is small, if they do come into play it will be at a time of maximum stress and confusion. Thus, if one is to practice allergy, the "reaction routine" must be so familiar as to be automatic. The discussion that follows is presented with the fervent hope that the reader will never need it, but that should the occasion arise, it will be effectively put into practice.

TYPES OF REACTIONS

Adverse reactions following an injection of allergenic extract may be immediate or delayed.

Delayed

Delayed reactions may be further divided into local and systemic types. A "significant" local reaction has been variously defined, ranging from induration or redness greater than about 30 mm in diameter (i.e., "the size of a half dollar") to pain and swelling sufficient to prevent the patient from raising his or her arm. Fortunately, most otolaryngic allergists espouse the former rather than the latter limits, and alter treatment accordingly.

Delayed systemic reactions are normally manifested as an increase in the patient's usual allergic symptoms, but may also include generalized urticaria, serum sickness–like manifestations, or constitutional symptoms involving virtually any organ system.

Delayed allergic reactions are most often of the Gel and Coombs type III, primarily mediated by IgG. The inhalant antigens most likely to produce delayed reactions are molds. Since these reactions occur from six to 36 or more hours after an injection, and thus outside the physician's office, patients must be educated as to the possibility of their occurrence, the forms they may take, and the proper measures for instituting treatment. The treatment of a delayed local reaction usually consists only of the administration of one or more doses of an antihistamine, plus reassurance. Severe symptoms of a systemic nature may necessitate corticosteroid therapy (to block further late-phase allergic reactions), although this is rare. In any case, patients should be advised to report any reactions promptly, both for confirmation of therapy by the physician and for appropriate adjustment of the dosage of extract given at the next injection.

Immediate

Immediate allergic reactions are of the Gel and Coombs type I (anaphylaxis), mediated by

IgE. They are important because they are potentially fatal and require prompt recognition and rapid, effective management. They are frightening to both patients and medical personnel, adding to the stress of the circumstances. However, to avoid withholding needed treatment or administering radical therapy unnecessarily, one must learn to quickly differentiate anaphylaxis from a vasovagal reaction.

The most common immediate adverse reaction to an injection of an allergen extract is a vasovagal one, ranging from minor apprehension to full-blown syncope. Patients experiencing such an event will typically appear pale and diaphoretic, with a slow pulse and normal or near-normal blood pressure. Loss of consciousness, if it does occur, lasts for no more than one or two minutes, and the patient awakens fully alert and lucid.

A true anaphylactic reaction implies the involvement of more than one organ system, but always including cardiovascular manifestations, typically tachycardia and hypotension. This may progress to arrhythmias, which can prove fatal. However, anaphylaxis most often also involves the respiratory system, and more deaths are due to upper and/or lower respiratory obstruction than to cardiovascular complications. The earliest sign of respiratory involvement is an itching of the mouth and throat, with increased nasal and bronchial secretions, progressing to hoarseness, nasal congestion, dysphagia, cough and wheezing, and stridor with labored respiration and intercostal retraction.

Cutaneous manifestations of anaphylaxis begin with a flushed, warm skin, with subsequent development of erythema, urticaria, and possible frank angioedema. Of course, if respiratory and cardiovascular distress are pronounced, cyanosis is noted.

Another hallmark of anaphylaxis is "angor animi," a feeling of impending doom (also seen in patients experiencing myocardial infarction). Gastrointestinal symptoms of anaphylaxis include nausea, vomiting, and diarrhea. Genitourinary involvement is signaled by a sense of urgency, and possible uterine cramps.

PREVENTION OF REACTIONS

Obviously it is more desirable to prevent an allergic reaction than to properly manage one. Several suggestions toward this end are worthy of consideration.

Some antigens are known to have the potential for causing severe systemic reactions. When possible, these should be tested for by the in vitro route. In vivo testing should be carried out with extreme caution if necessary. One must be especially cautious in dealing with some non-pollen antigens such as cottonseed, flaxseed, and castor bean.

Great care must be exercised in preparing antigen sets for testing and treatment. Mathematic miscalculations or physical errors in diluting, mixing, or injecting can have potentially disastrous results.

Allergists who base therapy on in vitro testing should always do a confirmatory skin test or vial test before therapy is begun. The first injection from any new treatment vial should ideally be given in the physician's office. If one has changed brands or suppliers for a stock antigen, it is wise to check the individual patient's sensitivity to the new antigen before preparing new individual treatment vials.

Finally, one should carefully and thoughtfully advance treatment doses to the optimal or maximally tolerated dose, realizing that local reactions (or systemic ones) necessitate alterations in dosage schedules. If continued reactions occur, it is often best and certainly safest to discard the patient's treatment vial and start again. Allergy must be understood and actively practiced, not performed by rote or formula. An ounce of prevention is worth ten minims of epinephrine!

PREPARING TO TREAT REACTIONS

Equipment

Cot or Table. After the patient is placed in a recumbent position and constricting clothing loosened, further measures may not be necessary.

Sphygmomanometer and Stethoscope. Pulse and blood pressure measurements are the best means of differentiating syncope from anaphylaxis and for following the cardiovascular status of patients with either condition. The blood pressure cuff should be placed on the arm opposite the injection site (where a tourniquet may be necessary).

Tourniquet. Apply above the injection site to slow absorption. Loosen every 15 to 20 minutes.

Oxygen and Airway Support. A small oxygen tank with mask should be readily at hand, and checked periodically to be sure it is properly charged.

An oral airway, Ambu bag, and some means of overcoming laryngeal obstruction (endotracheal tube and laryngoscope or cricothyrotomy set) should be available if further airway obstruction occurs.

Suction Apparatus. One of the hallmarks of anaphylaxis is an increase in upper and lower airway secretions, which often become thick and must be cleared, using a suction catheter.

IV Set-up. This becomes a "life line," with a large-bore needle connected to either 5 per cent dextrose in water or an electrolyte solution, for the administration of IV medications as necessary. Start the IV in the arm opposite the injection site, because of the tourniquet on that arm. The blood pressure cuff may be used to produce venous occlusion to start the IV. Alcohol sponges, tape, and an IV pole or hanger are also necessary.

Syringes and Needles. For subcutaneous and IM/IV injections, several 1 ml 25- or 27-gauge and 2½ ml 22-gauge needle-syringe units are necessary.

Drugs

Ammonia Ampules. Ammonia inhalation is highly effective in the treatment of vasovagal reactions and should be administered quickly at the first sign of such a reaction.

Epinephrine (1:1000, 1 mg/ml, for injection). This is the mainstay of treatment of anaphylactic reactions. It is available in 1 ml vials, in multiple dose vials, and as preloaded cartridge-syringe units that dispense a measured dose. The initial dose is usually 0.3 ml (range of 0.2 to 0.5 ml) intramuscularly or subcutaneously, repeated at intervals of 10 to 15 minutes as necessary, up to a maximum of 1 ml total.

In dire circumstances, epinephrine may be given intravenously by diluting 0.1 to 0.25 ml of epinephrine in a suitable intravenous solution for slow administration. If no intravenous line has been established, the direct injection of the same amount of undiluted epinephrine into the tongue will give virtually the same effect as intravenous administration.

Dopamine (40, 80, or 160 mg/ml vials, for injection). If using 500 ml of IV solution, add 5 ml of the 80 mg strength, and use this solution to maintain blood pressure if hypotension develops. Use corresponding amounts of the more or less concentrated forms for larger or smaller IV volumes.

Heparin (10,000 units/ml, for injection). This drug has a well-documented ability to neutralize histamine. The dosage of heparin should properly be described in units (the USP unit is 10 per cent greater than the International Unit), but 100 mg is roughly equivalent to 12,000 to 19,000 USP units. Although more conventional measures should precede its use in anaphylaxis, 10,000 USP units of heparin administered intravenously early in the treatment (and repeated later if necessary) has been said to have a marked salutary effect without compromising the clotting mechanism.

Diphenhydramine (50 mg/ml, for injection). Since antihistamines compete with histamine for H_1 receptor sites on effector cells, they do not reverse existing responses mediated by histamine, but may be useful in limiting further allergic reactions. The dose is 50 mg IM or IV. Antihistamines are not as effective against the actions of other vasoactive amines released during the anaphylactic reaction. Therefore, they are *not* the first drug to be given in treating such a reaction—that distinction goes to epinephrine!

Cimetidine (300 mg/2 ml, for injection). The efficacy of this H_2 antagonist in the treatment of anaphylaxis is supported by anecdotal reports and clinical experience; 300 mg may be given intramuscularly or intravenously. If the intravenous route is chosen, it must be diluted with an appropriate intravenous solution to a volume of

20 ml and given over a period of not less than two minutes. Episodes of hypotension and even shock following the rapid intravenous injection of cimetidine have been reported. Since the effect of a single dose continues for four to five hours, it is not usually necessary to administer a repeat parenteral dose.

Dexamethasone Sodium Phosphate (4 mg/ml, for injection). This rapidly acting corticosteroid is given to ameliorate late-phase reactions in anaphylaxis. It is available in ampules, in vials, or as a prefilled syringe containing 4 mg. The dose of 4 mg may be given intravenously or intramuscularly. As with the use of antihistamines, this preparation is not the initial drug of choice for treating anaphylaxis.

Albuterol Inhalation Aerosol. Although epinephrine is an alpha- and beta-adrenergic agonist, and normally reverses or diminishes bronchospasm, it may sometimes be necessary to supplement it with two inhalations from this inhaler. Beneficial effects are normally observed within five to 15 minutes, lasting up to four hours.

Neutralizing Dose of Allergen Extract. If known, this can dramatically reverse an allergic reaction, especially in the case of foods. However, conventional pharmacotherapy should also be administered.

TREATING A REACTION

The following "flow sheet" may be altered to suit the individual circumstances, but should give the physician treating a reaction following an injection of allergenic extract a plan of action, speeding proper treatment and guarding against omission of important steps.

1. Patient recumbent, loosen tight clothing.
2. Ammonia ampule, oxygen prn.
3. Apply BP cuff, check pulse and BP.
   a. Vasovagal reaction: observe, treat supportively.
   b. Suspected anaphylaxis: proceed as follows.
4. Call paramedics, get medical help!
5. Tourniquet above injection site (loosen q 20 min).
6. Epinephrine, 0.1 to 0.3 ml IM (this and all other injections in arm opposite injection site).*†
7. Start O_2 by mask; suction airway prn.
   a. Use oral airway, Ambu bag as needed.
   b. If glottic obstruction threatens, intubate or cricothyrotomy.
   c. Inhalation albuterol prn wheezing.
8. Start IV (large needle) in arm opposite injection site, run at keep-open rate.
9. Ready dopamine, add to IV prn hypotension.†
10. Heparin, 10,000 units subcutaneously or slow IV.
11. Repeat epinephrine, up to 0.3 ml IM prn (slow IV if necessary).*†
12. Diphenhydramine 50 mg IV.
13. Cimetidine 300 mg IM (or diluted and slow IV).
14. Dexamethasone 4 mg IV.
15. Repeat epinephrine, up to 0.3 ml IM prn (slow IV if necessary).*†
16. Administer neutralizing dose of provoking antigen (if known).
17. Transport as soon as possible to hospital—get help from emergency physician, internists. Observe at least 24 hours, with further pharmacotherapy as indicated.

SPECIAL CIRCUMSTANCES

Beta-Blockers

Anecdotal reports have implied that patients receiving beta-adrenergic blocking drugs may be prone to more severe allergic reactions than other patients. More important is the physiologic and pharmacologic evidence that such patients definitely are at risk for dire consequences from treatment of an anaphylactic reaction with epinephrine.

Adrenergic stimulation is mediated by three classes of receptors. Alpha-adrenergic stimulation causes smooth muscle constriction (vasoconstriction) in the arterial system, and $beta_1$ stimulation increases cardiac rate and contractility. $Beta_2$ stimulation causes bronchodilation by smooth muscle relaxation in the tracheobron-

*Omit or use with caution if on beta-blocker.
†Caution if on tricyclic antidepressant or MAO-inhibitor.

chial tree, while also relaxing smooth muscle in the vascular system and uterus.

Epinephrine has both alpha- and beta-adrenergic effects. The normal cardiovascular effects of epinephrine administration are a rise in systolic blood pressure and cardiac output (alpha- and $beta_1$-adrenergic stimulation) and a drop in diastolic blood pressure ($beta_2$ stimulation). Patients receiving beta-blockers, and especially noncardioselective preparations (propranolol, timolol, nadolol, pindolol, labetalol), when given epinephrine, sustain an unopposed alpha-adrenergic stimulation that may produce a hypertensive crisis. This will in turn activate vagal baroreceptors, causing cardiac slowing and possible asystole.

Additionally, beta-blockers will negate the $beta_2$ effect of bronchodilators administered during the treatment of anaphylaxis. The best bronchodilator for patients on beta-blocker therapy is a xanthine derivative such as aminophylline. This may be administered as aminophylline 400 mg (100 ml) in an IV drip over a 20-minute period. It should be noted that this solution is not compatible with epinephrine or some corticosteroids, and if these have been given intravenously, the tubing should be changed. Alternatively, an inhaled $beta_2$ agonist such as albuterol seems to be effective in these circumstances.

Thus, before instituting allergy immunotherapy in a patient receiving beta-blockers, one should contact the prescribing physician and discuss the feasibility of switching the patient to a different drug. Alternatively, it is preferable to change to a cardioselective beta-blocker (metaprolol, acebutolol, atenolol), which has greater $beta_1$ than $beta_2$ effects in normal doses.

The treatment of anaphylaxis in a patient who is on beta-blocking drugs should proceed as already outlined, except that epinephrine should be used with extreme caution, and repeat doses avoided. In the case of a patient on cardioselective beta-blockers, one is probably justified in using small amounts of epinephrine, in addition to heparin, antihistamines, and so forth, while carefully monitoring blood pressure and pulse. Should a hypertensive crisis occur in such a situation, the treatment is phentolamine, 5 to 20 mg IV, or, alternatively, sublingual nitroglycerin (which results in peripheral vasodilation to lower blood pressure, while also protecting from coronary vasospasm).

Tricyclic Antidepressants

These compounds interact with both direct-acting sympathomimetics (e.g., epinephrine) and indirect-acting or mixed action sympathomimetics (e.g., dopamine, phenylephrine) to potentiate their cardiovascular effects, resulting in tachycardia, hypertension, and possible arrhythmias. Thus, patients receiving tricyclic antidepressants (amitriptyline, imipramine, desipramine, nortriptyline, protriptyline, doxepin) should be treated for anaphylaxis with reduced doses of sympathomimetics, and using great caution.

Monoamine Oxidase (MAO) Inhibitors

These antidepressants (isocarboxazid, phenelzine, tranylcypromine, pargyline) also potentiate the effect of both direct- and indirect-acting adrenergic drugs, and this interaction can produce a hypertensive crisis. This effect may be seen up to 14 days after these compounds have been discontinued. If used to treat patients taking MAO-inhibitors, epinephrine and other sympathomimetics should be given in reduced doses and with caution.

In addition to the alteration of the treatment of allergic reactions, the interaction of tricyclic antidepressants or MAO-inhibitors with adrenergic drugs should be remembered when administering symptomatic therapy to patients taking these medications. The use of sympathomimetics in such instances may result in severe cardiovascular stimulation, with tachycardia and hypertension. Dosages should be reduced and therapeutic response closely monitored in such patients. Treatment of a hypertensive crisis resulting from such a drug interaction is with phentolamine, as noted previously.

REFERENCES

1. Guill MF: Allergy emergencies. Immunol Allergy Clin North Am 7:485, 1987.
2. Bellin JC (ed): AMA Drug Evaluations. 5th ed. Chicago, American Medical Association, 1983, pp 252–254; 581–582.
3. USP: Drug Information for the Health Care Provider. 7th ed. Rockville, MD, The United States Pharmacopeial Convention, 1987, pp 240–247; 398–401.
4. Warren CM: Treatment of allergic emergencies. Otolaryngol Clin North Am 4:599, 1971.

INDEX

Note: Page numbers in *italics* refer to figures; page numbers followed by t refer to tables.